# Prevention and Management of Postoperative Complications

*Editor*

JOHN D. MITCHELL

# THORACIC SURGERY CLINICS

www.thoracic.theclinics.com

*Consulting Editor*
M. BLAIR MARSHALL

November 2015 • Volume 25 • Number 4

**ELSEVIER**

1600 John F. Kennedy Boulevard ● Suite 1800 ● Philadelphia, Pennsylvania, 19103-2899

http://www.thoracic.theclinics.com

**THORACIC SURGERY CLINICS Volume 25, Number 4**
**November 2015 ISSN 1547-4127, ISBN-13: 978-0-323-41354-1**

**Editor:** John Vassallo (j.vassallo@elsevier.com)
**Developmental Editor:** Susan Showalter

*Thoracic Surgery Clinics* (ISSN 1547-4127) is published quarterly by Elsevier Inc., 360 Park Avenue South, New York, NY 10010-1710. Months of publication are February, May, August, and November. Business and editorial offices: 1600 John F. Kennedy Boulevard, Suite 1800, Philadelphia, PA 19103-2899. Periodicals postage paid at New York, NY, and additional mailing offices. Subscription prices are $350.00 per year (US individuals), $453.00 per year (US institutions), $165.00 per year (US Students), $435.00 per year (Canadian individuals), $585.00 per year (Canadian institutions), $225.00 per year (Canadian and international students), $465.00 per year (international individuals), and $585.00 per year (international institutions). Foreign air speed delivery is included in all Clinics' subscription prices. All prices are subject to change without notice. **POSTMASTER:** Send address changes to Thoracic Surgery Clinics, Elsevier Health Sciences Division, Subscription Customer Service, 3251 Riverport Lane, Maryland Heights, MO 63043. **Customer Service (orders, claims, online, change of address): Telephone: 1-800-654-2452 (U.S. and Canada); 314-447-8871 (outside U.S. and Canada). Fax: 314-447-8029. E-mail: journalscustomerservice-usa@elsevier.com (for print support); journalsonlinesupport-usa@elsevier.com (for online support).**

*Reprints.* For copies of 100 or more, of articles in this publication, please contact Commercial Rights Department, Elsevier Inc., 360 Park Avenue South, New York, NY 10010-1710. Tel: 212-633-3874; Fax: 212-633-3820; E-mail: reprints@elsevier.com.

*Thoracic Surgery Clinics* is covered in *MEDLINE/PubMed (Index Medicus), EMBASE/Excerpta Medica, Science Citation Index Expanded (SciSearch®), Journal Citation Reports/Science Edition,* and *Current Contents®/Clinical Medicine.*

# Contributors

## CONSULTING EDITOR

**M. BLAIR MARSHALL, MD, FACS**
Chief, Division of Thoracic Surgery; Associate
Professor of Surgery, Department of Surgery,
Georgetown University Medical Center,
Georgetown University School of Medicine,
Washington, DC

## EDITOR

**JOHN D. MITCHELL, MD, FACS**
Courtenay C. and Lucy Patten Davis Endowed
Chair in Thoracic Surgery, Professor and Chief,
Section of General Thoracic Surgery, Division
of Cardiothoracic Surgery, Consultant,
National Jewish Health, University of Colorado
School of Medicine, Aurora, Colorado

## AUTHORS

**RYAN V. ABBASZADEH, MD**
Department of General Surgery, University of
Washington, Seattle, Washington

**HUGH G. AUCHINCLOSS, MD, MPH**
Cardiothoracic Surgery Resident, Department
of Thoracic Surgery, Massachusetts General
Hospital, Boston, Massachusetts

**KATHLEEN S. BERFIELD, MD**
Division of Cardiothoracic Surgery, University
of Washington, Seattle, Washington

**SHANDA H. BLACKMON, MD, MPH**
Associate Professor, Department of Thoracic
Surgery, Mayo Clinic, Rochester, Minnesota

**RANDALL BLANK, MD**
Division of Thoracic & Cardiovascular Surgery,
Department of Anesthesia, University of
Virginia, Charlottesville, Virginia

**DANIEL J. BOFFA, MD**
Department of Thoracic Surgery, Yale
School of Medicine, New Haven,
Connecticut

**ROSS M. BREMNER, MD, PhD**
William Pilcher Chair, Department of Thoracic
Disease and Transplantation, Norton Thoracic
Institute, St. Joseph's Hospital and Medical
Center, Phoenix, Arizona

**BRYAN M. BURT, MD**
Assistant Professor, Division of Thoracic
Surgery, Baylor College of Medicine, Houston,
Texas

**KAREN J. DICKINSON, MBBS, BSc, MD,
FRCS**
Department of Thoracic Surgery, Mayo Clinic,
Rochester, Minnesota

**DEAN M. DONAHUE, MD**
Assistant Professor of Surgery, Harvard Medical
School; Associate Visiting Surgeon, Department
of Thoracic Surgery, Massachusetts General
Hospital, Boston, Massachusetts

**BRETT ELMORE, MD**
Division of Thoracic & Cardiovascular Surgery,
Department of Anesthesia, University of
Virginia, Charlottesville, Virginia

**SAMAD HASHIMI, MD**
Assistant Professor of Surgery, Department of Thoracic Disease and Transplantation, Norton Thoracic Institute, St. Joseph's Hospital and Medical Center, Phoenix, Arizona

**KWEKU HAZEL, MD**
Section of General Thoracic Surgery, Division of Cardiothoracic Surgery, University of Colorado Denver School of Medicine, Aurora, Colorado

**CAROLYN E. JONES, MD, FACS**
Associate Professor of Surgery, Division of Thoracic and Foregut Surgery, Department of Surgery, University of Rochester School of Medicine and Dentistry, Rochester, New York

**HARI B. KESHAVA, MD, MS**
Department of General Surgery, Cleveland Clinic Foundation, Cleveland, Ohio; Department of Thoracic Surgery, Yale School of Medicine, New Haven, Connecticut

**CHRISTINE LAU, MD, MBA**
Division of Thoracic & Cardiovascular Surgery, Department of Anesthesia, University of Virginia, Charlottesville, Virginia

**DONALD E. LOW, MD, FACS, FRCS(C), FRCSI (Hon), FRCS(Eng) (Hon)**
Head of Thoracic Surgery and Thoracic Oncology; Director, Digestive Disease Institute Esophageal Center of Excellence; Clinical Director, Ryan Hill Research Foundation, Virginia Mason Medical Center, Seattle, Washington

**NICOLA MARTUCCI, MD**
Staff Surgeon, Division of Thoracic Surgery, Department of Thoracic Surgery and Oncology, Istituto Nazionale Tumori, Fondazione Pascale, IRCCS, Naples, Italy

**DOUGLAS J. MATHISEN, MD**
Chief, Division of Thoracic Surgery, Department of Surgery, Massachusetts General Hospital, Harvard Medical School, Boston, Massachusetts

**JOHN D. MITCHELL, MD, FACS**
Courtenay C. and Lucy Patten Davis Endowed Chair in Thoracic Surgery, Professor and Chief, Section of General Thoracic Surgery, Division of Cardiothoracic Surgery, Consultant, National Jewish Health, University of Colorado School of Medicine, Aurora, Colorado

**KAMRAN MOHIUDDIN, MD**
Virginia Mason Medical Center, Seattle, Washington

**MICHAEL S. MULLIGAN, MD**
Division of Cardiothoracic Surgery, University of Washington, Seattle, Washington

**VAN NGUYEN, MD**
Division of Thoracic & Cardiovascular Surgery, Department of Anesthesia, University of Virginia, Charlottesville, Virginia

**HARALD C. OTT, MD**
Division of Thoracic Surgery, Department of Surgery, Massachusetts General Hospital, Harvard Medical School, Boston, Massachusetts

**GAETANO ROCCO, MD, FRCSEd**
Director of Department and Division Chief, Division of Thoracic Surgery, Department of Thoracic Surgery and Oncology, Istituto Nazionale Tumori, Fondazione Pascale, IRCCS, Naples, Italy

**JOSEPH B. SHRAGER, MD**
Professor of Cardiothoracic Surgery, Chief, Division of Thoracic Surgery, Stanford Hospitals and Clinics, Stanford University School of Medicine, Stanford, California; Division of Thoracic Surgery, VA Palo Alto Health Care System, Palo Alto, California

**SMITA SIHAG, MD**
Department of Thoracic Surgery, Harvard Medical School, Massachusetts General Hospital, Boston, Massachusetts

**LUIS F. TAPIAS, MD**
Division of Thoracic Surgery, Department of Surgery, Massachusetts General Hospital, Harvard Medical School, Boston, Massachusetts

**MAURA TRACEY, RN**
Division of Thoracic Surgery, Department of
Thoracic Surgery and Oncology, Istituto
Nazionale Tumori, Fondazione Pascale,
IRCCS, Naples, Italy

**THOMAS J. WATSON, MD, FACS**
Chief, Division of Thoracic and Foregut
Surgery; Professor, Department of Surgery,
University of Rochester School of Medicine
and Dentistry, Rochester, New York

**MICHAEL J. WEYANT, MD**
Associate Professor of Surgery, Section of
General Thoracic Surgery, Division of
Cardiothoracic Surgery, University of Colorado
Denver School of Medicine, Aurora, Colorado

**CAMERON D. WRIGHT, MD**
Professor of Surgery, Department of Thoracic
Surgery, Harvard Medical School,
Massachusetts General Hospital, Boston,
Massachusetts

**KENAN YOUNT, MD, MBA**
Division of Thoracic & Cardiovascular Surgery,
Department of Anesthesia, University of
Virginia, Charlottesville, Virginia

**GIORGIO ZANOTTI, MD**
Thoracic Surgical Resident, Division of
Cardiothoracic Surgery, University of
Colorado School of Medicine, Aurora,
Colorado

# Contents

respiratory failure, wound complications, and prosthetic complications. The main risk factors for complications are size of defect, age, and concomitant lung resection. Most complications related to either the wound or the prosthesis are late postoperative events. The identification of complications related to chest wall reconstruction requires clinical examination and the use of detailed imaging studies. The management of both prosthetic and wound complications often requires reoperation and removal of the prosthesis combined with soft tissue wound management.

Chylothorax is an unusual but serious complication of thoracic surgical procedures, and may carry considerable morbidity if not addressed in a timely fashion. Thoracic surgeons should be able to promptly diagnose this complication, and understand the implications of prolonged chyle loss to the patient. Conservative measures are often successful; direct intervention with percutaneous embolization of the cisterna chyli or thoracoscopic ligation is reserved for refractory cases. Some controversy exists regarding the timing of reintervention to limit the accumulated chyle loss. Prophylactic thoracic duct ligation has been examined but to date does not seem to reduce the incidence of chylothorax.

# THORACIC SURGERY CLINICS

---

**RELATED INTEREST**

*Radiologic Clinics,* Volume 52, Issue 1 (January 2014)
**Thoracic Imaging**
Jane P. Ko, *Editor*
Available at: www.radiologic.theclinics.com

---

**THE CLINICS ARE AVAILABLE ONLINE!**
Access your subscription at:
www.theclinics.com

# Preface
# Reducing the Footprint of Postoperative Complications

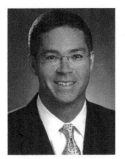

John D. Mitchell, MD, FACS
*Editor*

*No matter what measures are taken, doctors will sometimes falter, and it isn't reasonable to ask that we achieve perfection. What is reasonable is to ask that we never cease to aim for it.*
—*Atul Gawande, Complications: A Surgeon's Notes on an Imperfect Science*

If you operate, expect things to occasionally go wrong. This is a fact surgeons should learn early in their career—that no one is exempt from patient morbidity. It is possible, though, to minimize the *occurrence* of complications through thoughtful preventive measures in the perioperative time frame, and to reduce the *impact* of complications when they do occur through early recognition and decisive patient management. Surgeons adept at these strategies are often the most successful with the best patient outcomes.

This issue of *Thoracic Surgery Clinics* is dedicated to the prevention and management of complications that may occur following thoracic surgery. Some of the topics included, such as adverse cardiovascular events, respiratory failure, and chronic pain syndromes, are generic to any thoracic procedure. Other complications, such as prolonged air leak and anastomotic leak, are specific to particular operations. In each article, though, the contributing authors have tried to emphasize both prevention and management strategies to minimize patient morbidity. I believe they have been successful in achieving this goal.

I'd like to thank each of the contributing authors for their expertise and for their outstanding contributions to this issue. A special thanks goes to Blair Marshall, the Consulting Editor of *Thoracic Surgery Clinics*, for her gracious invitation to serve as guest editor and her gentle guidance after my acceptance of her offer. Finally, I'd like to express my appreciation to John Vassallo and Susan Showalter of Elsevier for their help and support throughout the preparation of this issue.

John D. Mitchell, MD, FACS
Section of General Thoracic Surgery
Division of Cardiothoracic Surgery
University of Colorado School of Medicine
Academic Office 1, C-310
12631 East 17th Avenue
Aurora, CO 80045, USA

E-mail address:
John.Mitchell@ucdenver.edu

Thorac Surg Clin 25 (2015) xiii
http://dx.doi.org/10.1016/j.thorsurg.2015.08.001
1547-4127/15/$ – see front matter © 2015 Published by Elsevier Inc.

# Cardiovascular Complications Following Thoracic Surgery

Hari B. Keshava, MD, MS[a,b], Daniel J. Boffa, MD[b,*]

## KEYWORDS

- Atrial fibrillation • Myocardial infarction • Pulmonary embolism

## KEY POINTS

- Cardiovascular complications occur in up to 30% of patients following noncardiac thoracic surgery.
- In patients with recent percutaneous coronary intervention, the risk of stent thrombosis must be weighed against the risk of bleeding if antiplatelet therapy is continued through surgery.
- Venous thromboembolism prophylaxis after thoracic surgery is optimized by the use of mechanical and pharmacologic prophylaxis.
- Several medications reduce the incidence of atrial fibrillation after thoracic surgery but may have significant side effects requiring surgeons to individualize the consideration for prophylaxis.
- When treating new-onset atrial fibrillation, it is critical to consider a potential process that is driving the rhythm change, such as pulmonary embolus or tension pneumothorax.

## INTRODUCTION

Cardiovascular complications occur in up to 30% of patients following noncardiac thoracic surgery, jeopardizing both the recovery and long-term function of this patient population.[1] As a result, considerable effort has been directed toward minimizing the incidence and consequences of cardiovascular complications after general thoracic surgical procedures. In the following article, several cardiovascular complications are discussed, including myocardial infarction (MI), deep vein thrombosis (DVT)/pulmonary embolism (PE), and atrial fibrillation. In addition, the impact of preoperative pulmonary hypertension on the postoperative course after lung surgery is briefly discussed.

Unfortunately, many of the clinical resources for complications (risk calculators, prophylaxis recommendations, and management guidelines) are not specific to the general thoracic patient population. The focus of this article is on major elective pulmonary and esophageal surgeries. The authors have attempted to identify relevant data-driven guidelines concerning the prevention and treatment of cardiovascular complications after these procedures (or list the population studied if general thoracic patients were not specified).

## MYOCARDIAL INFARCTION

MI has been reported to occur in less than 5% of nonpatients after lobectomy, pneumonectomy, or esophagectomy.[2,3] Although MI occurs less often than other cardiovascular complications, the mortality rate can be staggering (reported to be as high as 40% mortality rate after pneumonectomy[4]). Therefore, MI risk modulation and treatment are important considerations in the general thoracic surgery population.

---

Disclosures: The authors have no disclosures.
[a] Department of General Surgery, Cleveland Clinic Foundation, 9500 Euclid Avenue, A10, Cleveland, OH 44195, USA; [b] Department of Thoracic Surgery, Yale School of Medicine, 330 Cedar Street, BB205, New Haven, CT 06520-8062, USA
* Corresponding author.
*E-mail address:* Daniel.boffa@yale.edu

Thorac Surg Clin 25 (2015) 371–392
http://dx.doi.org/10.1016/j.thorsurg.2015.07.001
1547-4127/15/$ – see front matter © 2015 Elsevier Inc. All rights reserved.

## Risk Factors and Risk Stratification

The American College of Cardiology (ACC) and the American Heart Association (AHA) both consider noncardiac thoracic surgery to be an intermediate risk for postoperative cardiovascular death and nonfatal MI,[5] which is consistent with the reported range in the general thoracic surgical literature (1%–5%).[6,7] Preoperative risk assessment for MI in thoracic patients may be performed using the Revised Goldman Cardiac Risk Index (RCRI). The RCRI was derived using a broad noncardiac surgery patient population (12% general thoracic) and is one of the most validated and widely used risk models for postoperative events. This model uses 6 risk factors to predict the rate of cardiac death, nonfatal MI, and nonfatal cardiac arrest after noncardiac surgery as shown in **Table 1**.[8,9] In 2010 Brunelli and colleagues[10] proposed a modified version of the RCRI that was specific for patients undergoing lobectomy or pneumonectomy. In this scoring system, serum creatinine greater than 2 mg/dL, history of cardiac ischemia, cerebrovascular ischemia, and pneumonectomy as a surgical procedure were associated with an increased risk of major cardiac complications.

In addition to preoperative considerations, surgeons should attempt to minimize perioperative blood loss, as several studies have implicated transfusion as a risk factor for perioperative MI.[11,12] This point is particularly relevant as many patients may be at increased risk for bleeding because of the need for perioperative anticoagulation, as outlined in the following sections.

## Current Guidelines for Preoperative Cardiac Testing

Provocative cardiac testing (stress test) has the potential to identify coronary artery disease that places patients at a higher risk for perioperative MI. However, the desire to minimize MI risk must be tempered with the hazards of performing tests that are not indicated. Several specialty-specific societies have attempted to rectify the potential for risk modulation (chance the test will help the patients) with resource utilization (chance the test was not helpful). The 2013 American College of Cardiology Foundation (ACCF) consensus statement has addressed preoperative cardiac evaluation by risk of procedure (**Fig. 1**).[13,14] A brief synopsis is given next.

The following scenarios should proceed to surgery *without* further cardiac testing:

- All emergent procedures
- Elective low-risk procedures (ie, endoscopic, superficial procedures)
- Elective intermediate- to high-risk procedures (ie, lobectomy, pneumonectomy, esophagectomy) in patients without symptoms that can

**Table 1**
**RCRI and the risk of major cardiac events**

| | RCRI |
|---|---|
| Predictors/risk factors | High-risk surgery (vascular, thoracic, open intraperitoneal) History of ischemic heart disease[a] or history of coronary revascularization with current IHD symptoms History of heart failure[b] History of cerebrovascular disease[c] Insulin-dependent diabetes mellitus Preoperative serum Cr >2.0 mg/dL |
| Rate of major cardiac events | *No. of Risk Factors* 0: 0.5% 1: 1.3% 2: 4.0% ≥3: 9.0% |

*Abbreviations:* Cr, creatinine; IHD, ischemic heart disease.
  [a] Ischemic heart disease (defined by the presence of any of the following: history of MI, history of a positive exercise test, current complaint of chest pain considered to be secondary to myocardial ischemia, use of nitrate therapy, or electrocardiogram with pathologic Q waves).
  [b] Congestive heart failure (defined by the presence of any of the following: history of congestive heart failure, pulmonary edema, or paroxysmal nocturnal dyspnea; physical examination showing bilateral rales or S3 gallop; or chest radiograph showing pulmonary vascular redistribution).
  [c] History of cerebrovascular disease (transient ischemic attack or stroke).
  *Adapted from* Lee TH, Marcantonio ER, Mangione CM, et al. Derivation and prospective validation of a simple index for prediction of cardiac risk of major noncardiac surgery. Circulation 1999;100:1047.

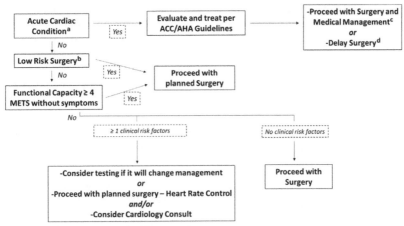

**Fig. 1.** Evaluation and care for thoracic surgery with cardiac risk factors. MET, metabolic equivalent. [a] Acute cardiac condition: MI/acute coronary syndrome. [b] Low-risk surgery: endoscopic, superficial, ambulatory surgery. [c] Proceed with surgery if work-up is negative, if patients are stabilized, and if there is an elevated risk of adverse outcomes with delaying surgery. [d] Delay surgery if patients have unstable coronary disease, decompensated heart failure, severe arrhythmia, or valvular heart disease or if patients undergo percutaneous coronary intervention. (*Adapted from* Report of the American College of Cardiology/American Heart Association Task Force on Practice Guidelines (Writing Committee to Revise the 2002 Guidelines on Perioperative Cardiovascular Evaluation for Noncardiac Surgery): developed in collaboration with the American Society of Echocardiography, American Society of Nuclear Cardiology, Heart Rhythm Society, Society of Cardiovascular Anesthesiologists, Society for Cardiovascular Angiography and Interventions, Society for Vascular Medicine and Biology, and Society for Vascular Surgery. Circulation 2007;116:e423.)

achieve 4 or greater metabolic equivalents (METS) (**Table 2**)

- Patients without cardiac risk factors

On the other hand, the following scenarios *should be evaluated* with further testing:

- Elective surgery (low, intermediate, or high risk) in patients with an *acute* cardiac condition
- Elective intermediate- to high-risk surgeries in patients with 1 or more cardiac risk factors that are unable to achieve 4 METS, but only

**Table 2**
**Metabolic equivalents and questions concerning activity**

| Energy Levels | Activity |
|---|---|
| 1 MET | Take care of yourself? <br> Eat, dress, and use the toilet? <br> Walk indoors around the house? <br> Walk a block or two on level ground at 2–3 mph? <br> Do light work around the house like dusting or washing dishes? |
| 4 METs | Climb a flight of stairs or walk up a hill? <br> Walk on level ground at 4 mph? <br> Run a short distance? <br> Do heavy work around the house like scrubbing floors or lifting or moving heavy furniture? <br> Participate in moderate recreational activities like golf, bowling, dancing, doubles tennis, or throwing a baseball or football? |
| >10 METs | Participate in strenuous sports like swimming, singles tennis, football, basketball or skiing? |

*Abbreviation:* MET, metabolic equivalent.

*Adapted from* Hlatky MA, Boineau RE, Higginbotham MB, et al. A brief self-administered questionnaire to determine functional capacity (the Duke Activity Status Index). Am J Cardiol 1989;64:651–4; and Fletcher GF, Balady G, Froelicher VF, et al. Exercise standards: statement for healthcare professionals from the American Heart Association. Circulation 1992;86:340–4.

if the results would change management (ie, if the team reacts to a positive stress test, with a coronary intervention, or direct patients to a lower-risk procedure)

With the increased use of computed tomography (CT) scanning, coronary calcifications are increasingly identified preoperatively in the thoracic surgery population. At this time, there is not a consensus with regard to the need for further testing for incidentally found coronary calcifications on thoracic imaging. The reported risk associated with incidentally found coronary calcifications is inconsistent but may be significant in the setting of type II diabetes.[15–17]

### Echocardiography

The 2014 ACC/AHA's guidelines recommend preoperative resting echocardiography only be performed if pursuing an established or suspected diagnosis (ie, to evaluate a murmur or worsening dyspnea). Clinically stable patients with previous left ventricular dysfunction may benefit from an echocardiogram if there has not been an assessment within a year before surgery.[1] Patients with known or suspected pulmonary hypertension (eg, marked pulmonary artery [PA] enlargement and impaired diffusion) may benefit from a preoperative echocardiogram to better assess PA pressure and right heart function for perioperative management.[18]

### Stress test considerations

The most appropriate stress test will depend on many factors, including the patients' ability to exercise, the resting electrocardiogram (EKG), the clinical indication for the test, the patients' body habitus, and any history of prior revascularization. Most patients in whom a stress test is indicated should undergo an exercise stress EKG (unless unable to exercise). Cardiopulmonary exercise testing may be considered for patients with unknown functional status. A low anaerobic threshold with a $Vo_2$ max less than 10 mL $O_2$/kg/min is associated with increased cardiovascular complications including MI.[1,19] If patients have an underlying EKG abnormality (eg, left bundle branch block), are paced, or have structural cardiac abnormalities, then stress test with imaging is recommended.

**Cautions with stress test and bronchospasm** Patients with significant bronchospasm may be at increased risk during pharmacologic stress testing. Intravenous dipyridamole and adenosine have been shown to cause bronchospasm in patients with asthma and chronic obstructive pulmonary disease (COPD).[20–22] Although the ACCF's 2013 guidelines discourage the use of adenosine as a pharmacologic agent in stress testing patients

with known COPD and asthma,[5] newer protocols with adenosine have been shown safe and effective for thoracic surgery patients.[22–24] It is also worth noting that theophylline (as well as caffeine) within 24 hours of a stress test can interfere with the effectiveness of pharmacologic stress test agents and, therefore, should be avoided.[14]

### Perioperative Management of Antiplatelet Medications for Coronary Stents

It is not uncommon for general thoracic surgery patients to be taking antiplatelet therapy for prior coronary stenting (given that smoking is a risk factor for both thoracic malignancies and coronary artery disease). Antiplatelet medications may increase the likelihood of perioperative bleeding (which is itself a risk for perioperative MI) creating a dilemma for thoracic surgeons. The risk of perioperative coronary events varies in accordance with the type of stent that was placed as well as the interval between stent placement and the thoracic surgery procedure. The ACC/AHA's 2014 guidelines recommend continued dual antiplatelet therapy (eg, aspirin and clopidogrel [Plavix]) for at least 12 months after drug-eluting stents (DES) placement and at least 4 to 6 weeks for bare-metal stents (BMS) to reduce the rate of major cardiac events.[1] The most common medications used as dual antiplatelet therapy are aspirin and clopidogrel, although several newer medications are increasingly being used (**Table 3**).[25]

There are currently no data-driven recommendations to guide the perioperative management of stent-related antiplatelet therapy that are specific for the general thoracic surgical population. The surgeon must balance the risk for bleeding with the likelihood and potential consequences of coronary stent thrombosis. There is a stent-specific (BMS or DES) correlation between the duration the stent has been in place and the likelihood of perioperative stent thrombosis. The American College of Chest Physicians (ACCP) has recommended that patients needing an operation within 6 weeks of a placement of a BMS or within 6 months to 1 year of DES placement should have antiplatelet therapy continued, especially for low- and intermediate-risk of bleeding.[26] Other factors the surgeon must consider include surgical challenges that could increase the bleeding risk (extensive prior surgery, prior pleurodesis, and so forth), coronary anatomy that could affect the consequences of stent thrombosis (stent location, collaterals, and so forth), and the options for nonsurgical treatment (eg, stereotactic radiosurgery for lung cancer). **Fig. 2** provides a flowchart regarding the management of dual antiplatelet therapy for patients who have received a DES.[25]

**Table 3**
**Antiplatelet medications and characteristics**

| Drug | Mechanism of Action | Half-life | Time to Recover Platelet Function After Drug Withdrawal | Platelet Inhibition | Administration Route |
|---|---|---|---|---|---|
| Aspirin | Cox-1 inhibition | 12–20 min | 4 d | Irreversible | Oral |
| Clopidogrel (Plavix) | $P2Y_{12}$ receptor inhibition | 7–9 h | 7–10 d | Irreversible | Oral |
| Prasugrel (Effient) | $P2Y_{12}$ receptor inhibition | 7 h | 2–3 d | Irreversible | Oral |
| Ticagrelor (Brilinta) | $P2Y_{12}$ and (partly) $P2Y_1$ receptor inhibition | 7–9 h | 3–4 d | Reversible | Oral |
| Cangrelor (Kengrexal) | ATP analogue with a high affinity for the $P2Y_{12}$ receptor | 3–6 min | Rapid (minutes to hours) | Reversible | IV |
| Abciximab (ReoPro) | Glycoprotein IIb/IIIa receptor inhibitor | 10–15 min | 12 h | Reversible | IV |
| Eptifibatide (Integrilin) | Glycoprotein IIb/IIIa receptor inhibitor | 2.5 h | 2–4 h | Reversible | IV |
| Tirofiban (Aggrastat) | Glycoprotein IIb/IIIa receptor inhibitor | 2 h | 2–4 h | Reversible | IV |

Abbreviations: COX, cyclooxygenase; IV, intravenous.
Adapted from Oprea AD, Popescu WM. Perioperative management of antiplatelet therapy. Br J Anaesth 2013;111(Suppl 1):i5; with permission.

### Holding antiplatelet therapy

If the surgeon elects to hold antiplatelet therapy, the duration of the preoperative time interval required for platelet function to normalize varies according to the half-life of the particular antiplatelet agent (see **Table 3**). At present, there is no indication to bridge antiplatelet therapy for coronary stents with shorter-acting agents (eg, low-molecular-weight heparin).[26] The antiplatelet therapy should be restarted after the surgery has taken place as soon as possible (once the surgeon is comfortable that the bleeding risk is no longer prohibitive).[27]

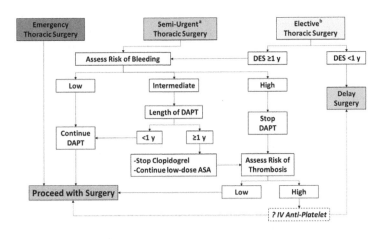

Fig. 2. Preoperative management of dual antiplatelet therapy after receiving a drug-eluting stent for patients undergoing thoracic surgery. ASA, aspirin; DAPT, dual antiplatelet therapy; IV, intravenous; ?, questionable. [a] Semiurgent thoracic surgery: surgery for nonemergent life-threatening condition (eg, cancer). [b] Elective thoracic surgery: surgery for nonemergent benign disease (eg, pectus excavatum surgery). (Adapted from Popescu WM. Perioperative management of the patient with a coronary stent. Curr Opin Anaesthesiol 2010;23:113; with permission.)

## Performing surgery with patients on antiplatelet therapy

There are numerous reports of performing thoracic procedures without discontinuing antiplatelet therapy (lobectomy,[28,29] esophagectomy[29,30]). It is also the authors' experience that with a bit more attention to hemostasis, it is typically possible to safely operate without discontinuing antiplatelet therapy (without increasing transfusion requirements or other bleeding complications). However, if the surgeon performs a thoracic procedure without discontinuing antiplatelet therapy, the surgeon must be aware of the potential reversibility of specific antiplatelet agents in the event of significant bleeding (see **Table 3**).

## Prophylaxis with Beta-Blockade

Several factors in the postoperative setting (pain, anemia, fluid volume shifts, and so forth) may increase cardiac work and perfusion demands. Beta-blockers may blunt some of the effects of postoperative cardiac stimulation,[31–33] which has motivated the empirical use of perioperative beta-blockers to reduce cardiac events. At this time, there is considerable debate over the role of beta-blockade in the perioperative setting to prevent MI.[34–36] In 2006, Lai and colleagues[32] illustrated the use of beta-blockers in elderly esophagectomy patients prevented postoperative cardiac events. Several subsequent meta-analyses illustrated a decrease in postoperative MI with beta-blockers started 1 day before surgery. However, they noted an increase in stroke, hypotension, bradycardia, and even death.[34] At the time of this article, it is the position of the ACC and AHA (per the 2014 guidelines) that there are insufficient data regarding the safety and efficacy of initiating (de novo) beta-blockers in the perioperative period and further research is needed. Patients chronically taking beta-blockers (before their surgical evaluation) should continue through surgery.

## Treatment of Postoperative Myocardial Infarction

The presentation of perioperative MI may be masked by chest pain from incisions and limitations in the patients' activity level. The diagnosis is typically made secondary to a change in clinical status that is accompanied by EKG changes. Within the differential diagnosis are acute hemorrhage and profound hypoxic respiratory failure both of which, if severe, could cause cardiac ischemia (which may or may not be distinguishable by EKG). It must be kept in mind that a negative stress test does not eliminate patients' chances of having coronary pathology (eg, coronary artery disease) and the risk of MI.

If an MI is highly suspected (and massive hemorrhage is not suspected), patients should be given aspirin 325 mg and morphine and should be evaluated by cardiology for possible catheterization and coronary intervention. The clinical impact of a perioperative MI may be highly variable, depending on patients' starting ventricular function and the territory involved in the event. The decision of whether or not to take patients for percutaneous intervention is an individual one recognizing any percutaneous coronary intervention is likely to require antiplatelet therapy (which has certainly been done successfully after thoracic surgical procedures[37]). Similar to the general acute coronary syndrome patient population (eg, not just patients recovering from surgery), the time to revascularization is crucial and must be weighed against the risk of perioperative bleeding.[5,13] For this reason, the use of fibrinolytics is not commonly used for postoperative MIs. The use of beta-blockers, angiotensin-converting enzyme inhibitors, and aspirin are recommended for all patients with an MI and low ejection fraction (per the ACC/AHA's guidelines for ST segment elevation MI and unstable angina[5]).

## Cardiac Herniation

Cardiac herniation through a defect in the pericardium is a very rare, potentially fatal complication of thoracic procedures that involves a resection of a portion of the pericardium. This complication has most commonly been described following a pneumonectomy that includes a pericardial resection. The average size of the defect associated with this complication is 4 cm.[38–47] The herniated ventricle can become constricted by the surrounding pericardium and become ischemic. The mortality for this complication reaches 50% for recognized cases and 100% for unrecognized cases.[48] For these reasons, surgeons should consider closing a pericardial defect created during a pneumonectomy. Fenestrated Gore-Tex (W.L. Gore and Associates, Inc, Newark, DE) has been frequently used for this purpose if the defect is too large to be closed primarily.[49] Patients presenting with suspected cardiac herniation require urgent evaluation with a low threshold to reoperate to prevent further cardiovascular collapse.

## DEEP VEIN THROMBOSIS/PULMONARY EMBOLISM
### Introduction

Venous thromboembolic events (VTEs) are important considerations after general thoracic surgery. Not only are many thoracic patients predisposed to develop VTEs (hypercoagulable from cancer, trauma, lack of mobility) but the patients' ability to tolerate a significant event after thoracic surgery may also be affected by reductions in pulmonary reserve. For example, in one study the 18-month survival after pneumonectomy complicated by VTE was only 13%.[50]

Similar to the previous section, the management of VTEs typically involves anticoagulation (and bleeding risk). This treatment can be particularly challenging when the cause of patients' status change (the underlying diagnosis) is unclear, as empirical treatment can lead to life-threatening hemorrhage. Therefore, great emphasis must be placed on preventing and diagnosing VTEs in patients recovering from general thoracic surgery.

### Incidence in Thoracic Surgery

The reported incidence of VTE after general thoracic surgical procedures is on the order of 5%. There is significant variability in VTE incidence (1%–26%) between different procedures, various surgical approaches, and the use of prophylaxis.[51–54] The Society of Thoracic Surgery (STS) databases report a 1.0% VTE incidence after lung cancer surgery[2] and 2.5% VTE incidence after esophagectomy.[3] In addition to the traditional risk factors for VTE (eg, Virchow triad of stasis, hypercoagulable state, and endothelial injury), the use of induction chemotherapy,[53,55,56] the use of a thoracotomy,[57–60] and smoking cessation[50,61,62] have all been suggested to increase the incidence of VTEs after general thoracic surgery. At one time video-assisted thoracic surgery (VATS) was thought to increase the risk for VTE by restricting venous return[63]; however, this observation has not been validated by the large database studies that have examined this question.[58]

### Prophylaxis

General thoracic surgery patients benefit from VTE prophylaxis. The ACCP's guidelines are specific to the thoracic surgical population[64] for VTE prophylaxis, which include early postoperative mobilization[65,66] and mechanical[66] and pharmacologic prophylaxis.[64,67]

#### Mechanical
Mechanical prophylaxis via pneumatic compression devices or stockings is an effective strategy to reduce VTEs (reducing the rate of DVT by up to 60%).[68] It is important to place compression devices or stocking at admission and in the operating room before surgery (with many studies advocating before anesthesia).[64,66,69] Once patients

reach the floor, compliance with pneumatic compression devices can vary significantly (53%–75%),[64] which can affect the effectiveness of this strategy. Using *both* mechanical and pharmacologic prophylaxis together seems to further decrease the incidence of DVT after thoracic surgery operations and is currently recommended by the ACCP.[64]

#### Pharmacologic
Pharmacologic prophylaxis by way of low-dose unfractionated heparin (LDUH) or low-molecular-weight heparin (LMWH) decreases the incidence of DVT and VTE in thoracic surgical patients.[51,64,70] The risk of surgical bleeding from pharmacologic prophylaxis seems to be outweighed by the far greater benefit of the VTE reduction.[64,70,71] There does not seem to be a significant difference in effectiveness of prophylactic low dose unfractionated heparin or LWMH.[64,72]

Several studies have attempted to optimize pharmacologic prophylaxis by varying the specific regimens. For example, several studies have examined the dose of pharmacologic prophylaxis given. There did not seem to be a difference between 10,000 units per day and 15,000 units per day of LDUH.[70,73] The dosage for LWMH used for VTE prophylaxis is 40 mg/d. Although weight-based LMWH prophylaxis (0.5 mg/kg/d) has been found to be efficacious in preventing VTE in obese bariatric patients,[74,75] the routine use of weight-based LMWH for thoracic surgery patients has not been fully studied.

The duration of pharmacologic prophylaxis has also been studied, and there does not seem to be a benefit to continuing prophylaxis after patients have been discharged. Extended VTE prophylaxis (longer than postoperative hospital stay) has only been shown beneficial for patients undergoing major abdominal or gynecologic surgery but has not been appreciated in thoracic surgery.[64]

The guidelines set forth by the ACCP are summarized later. In addition to these guidelines, early postoperative ambulation is imperative to help prevent DVT and VTE.[65]

Guidelines for VTE prophylaxis for thoracic surgery patients (adopted from the ACCP and the UK Royal College of Physicians)[62,64] are as follows:

- Start mechanical VTE prophylaxis at admission before surgery (intermittent pneumatic compression devices elastic stockings).
- Patients with low-risk for bleeding add pharmacologic prophylaxis: LDUH (10,000–15,000 units per day subcutaneous) or LMWH (40 mg subcutaneous daily).

- Patients with high-risk of bleeding (eg, pleural pneumonectomy) add mechanical prophylaxis only and add pharmacologic prophylaxis (LDUH or LMWH) when the risk of bleeding diminishes.
- Continue mechanical and pharmacologic prophylaxis until patients are ambulatory (~5–7 days).

### Inferior vena-cava filters

The primary role of inferior vena-cava (IVC) filters in the surgical population has been to prevent PEs (new or additional) in patients diagnosed with VTEs in whom anticoagulation was contraindicated.[50,55] IVC filters enable anticoagulation to be held perioperatively in thoracic surgery patients and are often placed in patients who are diagnosed with a VTE before surgery. Patients should have a retrievable IVC filter placed to allow the filter to be removed to prevent filter-related complications (~3–4 months in thoracic surgery patients).[64,76]

### Clinical Presentation

The diagnosis of VTE can be challenging in the thoracic surgical population. The classic signs and symptoms of a VTE (eg, asymmetric leg swelling, acute tachycardia, acute hypoxia) certainly should prompt a consideration for VTE evaluation. However, general thoracic surgery patients may experience events that mirror the classic presentation of a VTE. For example, thoracic patients often have tachycardia from pericarditis, pain, postoperative dysrhythmia, and so forth. Thoracic patients may be hypoxic from a mucous plug, splinting from incompletely controlled pain, a COPD flare, aspiration pneumonitis, or pneumonia. That being said, clinicians should have a relatively low threshold to pursue the VTE diagnosis (focused imaging evaluation) in light of these other potential diagnoses because

of the significant mortality associated with untreated VTEs.

### Diagnosis

The diagnostic evaluation for suspected PE should include a CT scan of the chest (specific PE protocol) if patients' renal function permits. A ventilation perfusion scan may be helpful in patients in which a PE is suspected but who cannot undergo CT scanning (because of impaired renal function or contrast allergy with insufficient time to premedicate patients). The downside of ventilation perfusion scanning is the significant variability between interpreting radiologists (resulting in variable sensitivity and specificity). There are high numbers of indeterminate scans and nondiagnostic studies (particularly in patients with COPD[77,78]). A transthoracic or transesophageal echocardiogram may also be used in patients who are either unable to have a CT scan or in patients with acute hemodynamic compromise in whom the diagnosis is unclear. Right heart strain is the main diagnostic parameter considered for these patients, but it is also possible at times to detect thrombus within the heart or the pulmonary artery. The main diagnostic imaging modality for a DVT is a duplex ultrasound, which can be used to assess for a source of subsequent PEs.

### Treatment

Prompt diagnosis and treatment is crucial for favorable outcomes for patients with VTE. PE requires the most urgent treatment (because of the risk of hemodynamic collapse). Treatment of any VTE must reconcile bleeding risk (with anticoagulation) and the risk of untreated VTE.

The patients' hemodynamic status is a critical determinant of the initial treatment of PE (**Fig. 3**). Unstable patients (those in shock or profoundly hypotensive) are unlikely to be transported for imaging studies; therefore, a suspected PE diagnosis

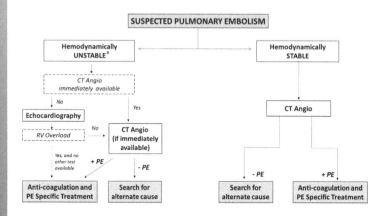

**Fig. 3.** Algorithm for PE after thoracic surgery if bleeding risk is low. CT Angio, CT angiography; RV, right ventricle. [a] If Echocardiography is unavailable and PE is highly suspected, consider empirical anticoagulation (as bleeding risk allows). (*Adapted from* Konstantinides SV, Torbicki A, Agnelli G, et al. ESC guidelines on the diagnosis and management of acute pulmonary embolism. Eur Heart J 2014;35:3046; with permission.)

is unlikely to be confirmed. A portable echocardiogram demonstrating right heart strain could support the diagnosis of PE, but treatment should not be held for this study if suspicion is high in hemodynamically compromised patients. The clinician must weigh the risks of bleeding from empirical anticoagulation (therapeutic intravenous heparin or subcutaneous LMWH) against the high mortality from an untreated PE in unstable patients. If patients' hemodynamics do not improve with resuscitation, then consideration may be given to thrombolysis (see later discussion) or (rarely) surgical embolectomy.

For hemodynamically stable patients, anticoagulation is the cornerstone of treatment. Anticoagulation after a PE effectively reduces mortality and recurrent embolic events. Acute treatment begins with unfractionated heparin or LMWH over the first 5 to 10 days. Subsequent treatment may include an oral vitamin K antagonist (eg, warfarin) or continuation of LMWH as an outpatient.[69] No difference has been appreciated with the treatment of PE with unfractionated heparin and LMWH. The advantage of intravenous (IV) unfractionated heparin drip is the ability to quickly interrupt and restore anticoagulation for necessary procedures or signs of hemorrhage. The absorption of subcutaneous (SQ) injections of LMWH may be variable in morbidly obese patients, which could also favor IV unfractionated heparin. For patients being treated managed with vitamin K antagonists, a heparin bridge is used to prevent any complications from the initial procoagulant phase of vitamin K antagonism.

Newer anticoagulants, such as factor Xa inhibitors (rivaroxaban, apixaban, edoxaban) and direct thrombin inhibitors (dabigatran), have been shown efficacious for the treatment of PE in nonsurgical patients.[79–81] **Table 4** describes common and newer anticoagulants used in the treatment of VTE, including risks, benefits, and reversing agents. There is a paucity of data regarding the safety and efficacy of using these agents to treat PE occurring after thoracic surgery. The lack of reversal agents may lead to greater blood loss should a bleeding complication arise.

### Thrombolysis

Thrombolysis restores pulmonary perfusion faster than anticoagulation with heparin alone. The maximum benefit occurs if patients undergo thrombolysis within 48 hours of presentation. Streptokinase, urokinase, and tissue plasminogen activator have been used with a reduction in mortality and recurrent PE.[82] The risk of bleeding is the major limitation to this form of treatment in the postoperative setting.

### Discharge and Follow-up

The ACCP recommends at least 3 months of anticoagulation for patients with an isolated single PE or DVT following surgery.[83] In patients with advanced cancer, there is some evidence to continue anticoagulation indefinitely.[83] Recent studies by Agnelli and colleagues[84,85] have shown a benefit in long-term anticoagulation for preventing further VTE in patients receiving chemotherapy or with stage 4 cancer particularly in lung and gastrointestinal malignancies. There are no data for empirical follow-up imaging for treated PE or DVT unless clinically indicated. (Although there is minimal risk associated with an extremity ultrasound for DVT, radiation exposure should be considered if clinicians are inclined to follow PE reabsorption in asymptomatic patients.)

### Pulmonary Artery Thrombosis After Vascular Sleeve Resection

A vascular sleeve resection of the PA carries a theoretic risk of artery thrombosis secondary to the period of clamping and trauma to the artery. Some investigators estimate this to be around 2%,[86,87] whereas others have not experienced an increase incidence of thrombosis after vascular sleeve resection.[88,89]

The use of prophylactic heparin in vascular sleeve resections has been debated, with some centers using routine anticoagulation,[86] whereas others not routinely using prophylactic anticoagulation.[87–89] At this point in time, there are no firm recommendations; but the authors currently administer 5000 units of IV heparin before clamping the PA for a vascular sleeve resection (as long as there are no contraindications).

The diagnosis of a PA thrombosis may be delayed, as the initial clinical indicators (eg, lobar opacity on chest radiograph, fever, increase in white blood cell count) are nonspecific and could represent mucus plugging or pneumonia. An IV contrast CT scan is the most common route to establish PA thrombosis.[86–88] The management depends on the patients' status and the suspicion of lobar infarct. If patients also underwent sleeve resection of the airway, the bronchial arterial supply to the lung has almost certainly been eliminated, resulting in a pulmonary infarct. Making a determination of pulmonary infarct is challenging, and bronchoscopy may not accurately reflect the status of the parenchyma. If the suspicion for infarct is high, then reoperation and inspection of the lung is indicated. If the remaining lobe is not

**Table 4**
Types of pharmacologic anticoagulation treatment of venous thromboembolism and atrial fibrillation

| Agent | Mechanism of Action | Route | Dosage | Laboratory Value | VTE Duration[c] | Afib Duration[c] | Half-life | Challenges/ Considerations | Reversal |
|---|---|---|---|---|---|---|---|---|---|
| UFH | Antithrombin III inhibitor | IV | Bolus: 80 units/kg Infusion: 18 units/kg Adjustment: aPTT range 60–80 | aPTT: every 6 h | Transition to oral therapy or LMWH | Transition to oral therapy or LMWH | 30–60 min | HIT IV route only | Protamine sulfate |
| LMWH (Lovenox) | Antithrombin III inhibitor | SQ | 1 mg/kg twice daily OR 1.5 mg/kg daily | Anti-Xa levels (only in select patients) | 3 mo OR Transition to oral | 4–6 wk after conversion to sinus OR transition to oral | 4.5 h | HIT Renal dysfunction Bleeding Cost | None |
| Warfarin (Coumadin) | Vitamin K antagonist | Oral | Variable, based on INR of 2–3 | INR | 3 mo Start with UFH or LMWH bridge | 4–6 wk after conversion to sinus Start with UFH or LMWH bridge | Up to 40 h | Bleeding Interactions with other medications Frequent blood testing | Vitamin K FFP |

| | | | | | | | | | Reversal |
|---|---|---|---|---|---|---|---|---|---|
| Rivaroxaban (Xarelto) Apixaban (Eliquis) Edoxaban (Savaysa) | Factor Xa inhibitors | Oral | Fixed[a] | n/a | 3–6 mo | 4–6 wk after conversion to sinus | 7–12 h | No testing needed. Increased chance of bleeding postop. Unknown if effective in surgical patients | None |
| Dabigatran | Direct thrombin inhibitor | Oral | 150 mg twice daily. If high CrCl[b]: 75 mg twice daily | n/a | 6 mo | 4–6 wk after conversion to sinus | 13 h | No testing needed. Increased chance of bleeding postop. Unknown if effective in surgical patients | None |

*Abbreviations:* Afib, atrial fibrillation; aPTT, activated partial thromboplastin time; CrCl, creatine clearance; FFP, fresh frozen plasma; HIT, heparin induced thrombocytopenia; INR, international normalized ratio; n/a, not applicable; postop, postoperatively; UFH, unfractionated heparin.

[a] Fixed = fixed dosing based on specific manufacturer guidelines and creatine clearance.

[b] High creatine clearance = 30–50 mL/min.

[c] May need longer duration of anticoagulation for patients with cancer.

*Adapted from* Frendl G, Sodickson AC, Chung MK, et al. 2014 AATS guidelines for the prevention and management of perioperative atrial fibrillation and flutter for thoracic surgical procedures. J Thorac Cardiovasc Surg 2014;148:e185; and Konstantinides SV, Torbicki A, Agnelli G, et al. 2014 ESC guidelines on the diagnosis and management of acute pulmonary embolism. Eur Heart J 2014;35:3054.

viable, then resection should take place to prevent further complications.

## ATRIAL ARRHYTHMIAS

Atrial arrhythmias are among the more common complications after thoracic surgery; although rarely life threatening, they may cause a significant derailment of an otherwise smooth recovery. The incidence varies significantly by the procedure performed (**Table 5**). Several investigators have evaluated the risk factors for postoperative atrial arrhythmias after thoracic surgery with mixed results. Some factors that have been identified to increase the risk of postoperative atrial fibrillation include preoperative atrial fibillration,[90] increased age,[91–95] male sex,[91,96] and coronary artery disease/congestive heart failure.[94,97–99]

### Causes of Atrial Fibrillation

Most atrial fibrillation after general thoracic surgery is presumed to be the result of surgical stress, anatomic manipulations, and other deviations from patients' normal physiologic state. However, there are important precipitating events in the general thoracic population that must be considered in patients with new-onset atrial fibrillation, such as pneumothorax, hemothorax, PE, aspiration, anastomotic leak, and MI. Although atrial fibrillation carries risk to patients' recovery, failure to recognize a precipitating complication could be devastating.

### Prophylaxis for Postoperative Atrial Fibrillation

Several randomized trials and multiple meta-analyses have evaluated the efficacy of atrial fibrillation prophylaxis after thoracic surgery, with mixed results. The STS' 2012 and the American Association of Thoracic Surgeons' (AATS) 2014 guidelines for the prevention and management of atrial fibrillation and flutter for thoracic surgery procedures were based on these data and give recommendations for prophylaxis outlined next.[90,98–103]

### Beta-blockers

Class 1 evidence is recognized by both the STS' and AATS' guidelines for continuing patients on preoperative beta-blocker before thoracic surgery to prevent potential beta-blocker withdrawal syndrome and increased risk of postoperative atrial fibrillation. The administration of prophylactic beta-blockers for patients who are beta-blocker naïve is unclear. There is some evidence pointing to prophylactic beta-blocker use and the prevention of postoperative atrial fibrillation; however, the incidence of postoperative hypotension, bradycardia, and stroke-related mortality is high.[1,100,102] For this reason, prophylactic beta-blockers for beta-blocker–naïve patients is not currently recommended by the STS or the AATS.[98,99] The STS' guidelines state that postoperative administration of a new beta-blocker *can* be used to prevent postoperative atrial

---

**Table 5**
**Risk of postoperative atrial fibrillation after thoracic surgery**

| Low Risk (<5% Incidence) | Intermediate Risk (5%–15% Incidence) | High Risk (>15% Incidence) |
|---|---|---|
| • Bronchoscopy ± biopsy<br>• Tracheal stenting<br>• Thoracostomy tube/ Tunneled tube thoracostomy<br>• Pleurodesis<br>• Mediastinoscopy<br>• VATS wedge resection<br>• PEG tube/esophagoscopy<br>• Esophageal diltation/ stenting | • Thoracoscopic sympathectomy<br>• Segmentectomy<br>• Laparoscopic Nissen fundoplication/myotomy<br>• Zenker diverticulectomy | • Resection of anterior mediastinal mass<br>• Thoracoscopic lobectomy<br>• Open thoracotomy/open lobectomy<br>• Pneumonectomy<br>• Pleurectomy<br>• Lung volume reduction surgery/bullectomy<br>• Bronchopleural fistula repair<br>• Clagett window<br>• Esophagectomy<br>• Lung transplantation<br>• Pericardial window |

*Abbreviation:* PEG, percutaneous endoscopic gastrostomy.
*Adapted from* Frendl G, Sodickson AC, Chung MK, et al. 2014 AATS guidelines for the prevention and management of perioperative atrial fibrillation and flutter for thoracic surgical procedures. J Thorac Cardiovasc Surg 2014;148:e156.

fibrillation; however, the side effects (bradycardia, hypotension) should be monitored closely.[98]

### Calcium channel blockers
The STS' guidelines recognize 5 different randomized controlled trials for patients not taking beta-blockers preoperatively that show the initiation of diltiazem is beneficial for the prevention of postoperative atrial fibrillation in the thoracic surgical population with a reduction of atrial fibrillation by half (10.6% incidence of atrial arrhythmias compared with a control group of 21.5%).[98,104] Both the AATS' and STS' guidelines state calcium channel blockers can be used preoperatively to prevent atrial fibrillation, especially in patients undergoing a PA resection not already taking a beta-blocker.[98,99] The concomitant use of beta-blockers and calcium channel blockers is not advised as prophylaxis because of the risk of profound hypotension.

### Amiodarone
Both the STS' and AATS' guidelines state that postoperative administration of IV amiodarone may help reduce the risk of atrial fibrillation after lobectomy and esophagectomy.[98,99] The STS' guidelines do not recommend prophylactic amiodarone in the setting of pneumonectomy because of the paucity of data and the potential risks of pulmonary toxicity and acute respiratory distress syndrome.[98] QTc prolongation with amiodarone can be severe, especially with administration with other medications predisposing patients to torsades de pointes. Other side effects include thyroid dysfunction and pancreatitis.

### Other
Several other pharmacologic interventions have been studied for the prevention of postoperative atrial arrhythmias. Magnesium supplementation is recommended for patients with preoperative hypomagnesaemia by both the STS and AATS before thoracic surgery.[98,99] Digoxin has no role in prophylaxis against the development of atrial fibrillation, as it seems to *increase* the incidence of postoperative atrial fibrillation in thoracic surgical patients.[98,99] Statin use before surgery in statin-naïve patients has been shown to reduce postoperative atrial fibrillation in cardiac and noncardiac surgery.[105,106] At the time of writing this article, only one study has shown a decrease in postoperative atrial fibrillation with prophylactic statin use in thoracic surgery patients with a 3-fold decrease.[107] The AATS' guidelines state atorvastatin may be considered for intermediate- and high-risk thoracic surgery patients for the prevention of postoperative atrial fibrillation; however, this is not a class 1 recommendation at this time.[99]

### Treatment
The treatment of postoperative atrial fibrillation must take into account the patients' hemodynamic status and the duration of time the patients have been in atrial fibrillation. There is an urgency to treat unstable patients, but the surgeon must also consider a driving event that precipitated the atrial fibrillation (and is also contributing the hemodynamic instability, such as a PE). An intravenous fluid bolus is typically helpful in patients with hypotension and atrial fibrillation. Many patients with a decrease in blood pressure will respond to fluid and tolerate negative chronotropes without much additional decline in pressure.

New-onset atrial fibrillation that is associated with profound hemodynamic collapse (hypotension, malperfusion) should be treated with direct current (DC) cardioversion while the surgeon rapidly evaluates for a potentially catastrophic precipitating event (PE, tension pneumothorax, and so forth).[98,99] If patients are stable, there is the flexibility to attempt pharmacologic rate- and rhythm-control maneuvers. With rate- and rhythm-control strategies, 85% revert to sinus during the hospitalization.[99] The AATS devised an algorithm for the management of atrial fibrillation after thoracic surgery (**Fig. 4**).[99]

### Medical treatment
The initial goal of the medical treatment of atrial fibrillation is rate control for a goal heart rate of less than 110 beats per minute before rhythm control. Many patients convert to sinus rhythm with rate-control strategies alone. Both beta-blockers and calcium channel blockers have class 1 evidence supporting their use for postoperative atrial fibrillation in normotensive patients. If patients have moderate or severe COPD, then calcium channel blockers should be trialed first (as opposed to beta-blockers because of the incidence of bronchospasm). Use of a beta-blocker and a calcium channel blocker together can cause profound hypotension, bradycardia, and heart block; thus, use should be individualized.[99] Digoxin should not be used as a single agent; however, its use together with a beta-blocker or calcium channel blocker may be effective.

Amiodarone is used frequently for thoracic surgery patients with atrial fibrillation. A benefit of amiodarone is the potential for pharmacologic cardioversion, thereby avoiding the need for anticoagulation (if converted within 48 hours of onset). Guidelines from the STS warn against the use of amiodarone with ventilated patients, patients who have undergone pneumonectomy, or in

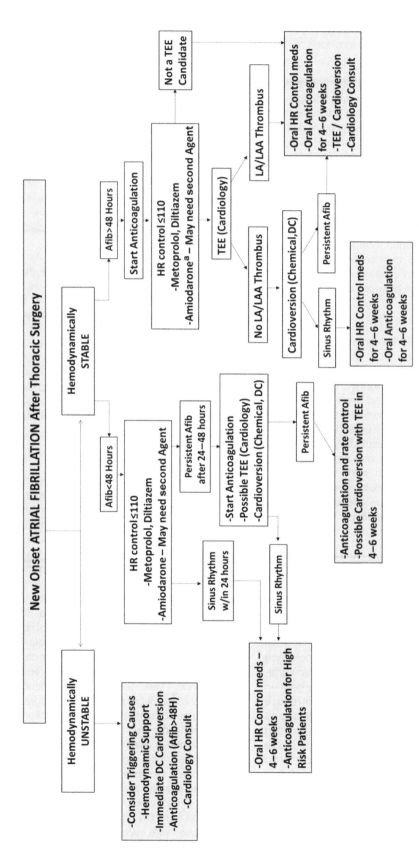

**Fig. 4.** Algorithm for postoperative atrial fibrillation after thoracic surgery. Afib, atrial fibrillation; HR, heart rate; LA/LAA, left atrium/left atrial appendage; meds, medications; sTEE, transesophageal echocardiogram. [a] Caution should be exercised and a transesophageal echocardiogram considered if amiodarone is used after 48 hours after the onset of atrial fibrillation as there is a possibility that the rhythm could convert with the risk of thromboembolism. (*Adapted from* Frendl G, Sodickson AC, Chung MK, et al. AATS guidelines for the prevention and management of perioperative atrial fibrillation and flutter for thoracic surgical procedures. J Thorac Cardiovasc Surg 2014;148:e170; with permission.)

patients with substantial preexisting lung disease, primarily because of the risk of pulmonary toxicity with amiodarone that may occur in up to 10% of patients.[98]

Rate-control agents should be continued for 4 to 8 weeks after discharge if the heart rate is in sinus rhythm. If patients are still in rate-controlled atrial fibrillation, cardiology consultation is warranted for further assessment and possible cardioversion for rhythm control.[98,99]

### Cardioversion

Within the first 48 hours of onset, hemodynamically unstable patients should be cardioverted without the need for anticoagulation.

For patients in atrial fibrillation for more than 48 hours, cardioversion, chemical cardioversion with flecainide or amiodarone, or DC cardioversion is reasonable in hemodynamically stable patients. However, the STS and AATS recommend obtaining a transesophageal echocardiogram (TEE) to rule out left atrial thrombus. If a thrombus is identified, patients should be rate controlled and anticoagulated for 4 to 6 weeks before attempting cardioversion.[98,99] For esophagectomy patients

and other patients who cannot undergo a TEE, 4 to 6 weeks of anticoagulation before cardioversion is recommended.[99]

### Anticoagulation

Anticoagulation for postoperative atrial fibrillation is indicated to prevent thrombus formation in the left atrium and subsequent thromboembolism (eg, cerebrovascular accident). One predictive model commonly used to assess the risk for thromboembolic events from patients in atrial fibrillation is called the $CHA_2DS_2$-VASc score (congestive heart failure, hypertension, age $\geq 75$ years, diabetes mellitus, prior stroke, vascular disease, age 65–74 years, female sex category). The $CHA_2DS_2$-VASc score is a clinical prediction tool estimating the annual risk of stroke in patients with nonrheumatic atrial fibrillation using points allocated to known risk factors. A higher $CHA_2DS_2$-VASc score indicates an increasing risk of stroke (**Tables 6** and **7**). The AATS' 2014 recommendations for anticoagulation depend on the timing of postoperative atrial fibrillation, the patients' $CHA_2DS_2$-VASc score, the duration of postoperative atrial fibrillation, and the risk of

**Table 6**
**Stroke risk stratification using the $CHA_2DS_2$-VASc score**

|  | Risk Factor | Points |
|---|---|---|
| C | Congestive Heart Failure (LV Dysfunction) | 1 |
| H | Hypertension | 1 |
| $A_2$ | Age $\geq 75$ | 2 |
| D | Diabetes Mellitus | 1 |
| $S_2$ | Prior Stroke or TIA or Thromboembolism | 2 |
| V | Vascular Disease (eg, MI, PVD) | 1 |
| A | Age 65-74 | 1 |
| Sc | Sex Category (Female) | 1 |

| $CHA_2DS_2$VASc Score | Adjusted Annual Stroke Risk (%)[a] |
|---|---|
| 0 | 0 |
| 1 | 0.7 |
| 2 | 1.9 |
| 3 | 4.7 |
| 4 | 2.3 |
| 5 | 3.9 |
| 6 | 4.5 |
| 7 | 10.1 |
| 8 | 14.2 |
| 9 | 100 |

Abbreviations: LV, left ventricular; PVD, peripheral vascular disease; TIA, transient ischemic attack.

[a] Adjusted for patients receiving aspirin to give annual risk of stroke without therapy.

Adapted from Lip GYH. Implications of the CHA2DS2-VASc and HAS-BLED scores for thromboprophylaxis in atrial fibrillation. Am J Med 2011;124:112; with permission.

**Table 7**
**Commonly used rate/rhythm control agents for postoperative atrial fibrillation**

| Agent | Mechanism of Action | Dosage | Rate/Rhythm Control | Duration | Side Effects |
|---|---|---|---|---|---|
| Metoprolol | Beta-blocker | • 2.5–5.0 mg IV × 3 doses<br>• Followed by 12.5–100 mg oral every 6–12 h | Rate | 4–8 wk | Bradycardia, hypotension, bronchospasm, heart failure exacerbation |
| Diltiazem | Calcium channel blocker | • 0.25 mg/kg IV loading dose over 2 min, then 5–15 mg/h IV continuous infusion<br>• Followed by 30–60 mg every 6–8 h | Rate | 4–8 wk | Hypotension, bradycardia, heart failure exacerbation |
| Amiodarone | Class III antiarrhythmic | • 150 mg/10 min IV; then 1 mg/min for 6 h; then 0.5 mg/min IV for 18 h<br>• Followed by 400 mg twice oral daily | Rate/Rhythm | 4–8 wk | Bradycardia, QTc prolongation, pulmonary toxicity, thyroid toxicity, pancreatitis |
| Digoxin | Na+/K + ATPase in myocardium | • Total IV dose of 1.25–1.5 mg in the first 24 h<br>• Followed by 0.125–0.5 mg oral daily | Rate | 4–8 wk | Nausea, vomiting, anorexia, confusion, AV block |
| Flecainide | Class IC antiarrhythmic | • 200–300 mg single oral dose<br>• Followed by 50–150 mg oral every 12 h | Rhythm | 4–8 wk | Dizziness, blurred vision, sinus bradycardia, AV block, contraindicated with low left ventricular function or coronary artery disease |
| Procainamide | Class IA antiarrhythmic | • 20–50 mg/min IV continuous, until Afib terminated<br>• OR 100 mg IV every 5 min until Afib terminated | Rhythm | Until Afib terminated | Hypotension, QTc prolongation, torsades de pointes, contraindicated with low left ventricular function |

*Abbreviations:* Afib, atrial fibrillation; AV, atrioventricular.
  *Data from* Frendl G, Sodickson AC, Chung MK, et al. 2014 AATS guidelines for the prevention and management of perioperative atrial fibrillation and flutter for thoracic surgical procedures. J Thorac Cardiovasc Surg 2014;148:e153–93.

postoperative bleeding.[99] For patients with atrial fibrillation of less than 48 hours duration, anticoagulation is typically not recommended (see **Fig. 4**).

For patients with atrial fibrillation extending beyond 48 hours, anticoagulation should be considered (particularly if there is consideration for cardioversion). Unfractionated heparin, LMWH, and warfarin result in equivalent risk reduction of thrombosis.[99] Warfarin and LMWH are the mainstay for long-term anticoagulation, with LMWH having restrictions on patients with renal insufficiency and its high cost.

**Table 4** describes both common and some of the newer anticoagulants used for atrial fibrillation along with risks, benefits, and reversing agents. Recent guidelines from the AATS consider the data in support of these newer agents to warrant a class II recommendation as an alternative to warfarin.[99] These agents should be used with caution in the perioperative setting as their anticoagulation effects are not immediately reversible.

Anticoagulation should be continued for 4 to 6 weeks once patients have returned to sinus rhythm. Longer anticoagulation may be needed for patients with a higher $CHA_2DS_2$-VASc score. For patients that remain in atrial fibrillation, a TEE may be performed after 4 to 6 weeks of anticoagulation to rule out atrial thrombus. If no thrombus is identified, patients may be DC cardioverted to sinus rhythm. Patients who fail electrical and pharmacologic cardioversion and remain in atrial fibrillation should remain anticoagulated to reduce the risk of a cerebral vascular accident.

## OTHER CONSIDERATIONS
### Pulmonary Hypertension and Lung Surgery

Preoperative pulmonary hypertension is associated with an increase in morbidity and mortality after noncardiac thoracic surgery.[108,109] Hemodynamic compromise has been suggested to be the result of changes in intrathoracic pressures, lung volumes, and oxygenation that can acutely increase pulmonary vascular resistance and lead to right ventricular failure.[109,110] Currently, specific guidelines do not exist for general thoracic surgery in patients with pulmonary hypertension because of the paucity of data.

Symptoms for pulmonary hypertension are nonspecific (eg, dyspnea). Echocardiography is an important screening tool if pulmonary hypertension is suspected, yet right heart catheterization is the gold standard for diagnosis and assessment of vasodilator response in pulmonary hypertension. Specific risk factors for surgical complications associated with pulmonary hypertension include an echocardiogram demonstrating a right ventricular systolic pressure greater than 70 mm Hg or a mean PA pressure of greater than or equal to 50 mm Hg or right heart catheterization showing PA hypertension.[109,111]

For patients with severe pulmonary hypertension, even procedures ordinarily considered to be low risk may be dangerous. For example, numerous patients with pulmonary hypertension have been described to have severe bleeding from wedge resections.[18] This postoperative bleeding potentially reflects the hemostatic capability of the staples, which are not designed for elevated pressures. Although no specific guidelines exist for performing thoracic surgery on patients with pulmonary hypertension, a multidisciplinary approach with cardiology, anesthesiology, and thoracic surgery is crucial for optimum diagnosis, treatment, and management.

## SUMMARY

Cardiovascular events after thoracic surgery can result in increased morbidity, mortality, length of stay, and increased overall cost. The prevention of postoperative cardiovascular complications is an area of intense study, and the body of evidence guiding clinicians continues to grow. Early diagnosis and management of cardiovascular events can minimize the consequences of these complications.

## REFERENCES

1. Fleisher LA, Fleischmann KE, Auerbach AD, et al. 2014 ACC/AHA guideline on perioperative cardiovascular evaluation and management of patients undergoing noncardiac surgery: a report of the American College of Cardiology/American Heart Association Task Force on Practice Guidelines. J Am Coll Cardiol 2014;64:e77–137.
2. Boffa DJ, Allen MS, Grab JD, et al. Data from the Society of Thoracic Surgeons general thoracic surgery database: the surgical management of primary lung tumors. J Thorac Cardiovasc Surg 2008;135:247–54.
3. Wright CD, Kucharczuk JC, O'Brien SM, et al. Predictors of major morbidity and mortality after esophagectomy for esophageal cancer: a Society of Thoracic Surgeons general thoracic surgery database risk adjustment model. J Thorac Cardiovasc Surg 2009;137:587–96 [discussion: 596].
4. Marret E, Miled F, Bazelly B, et al. Risk and protective factors for major complications after pneumonectomy for lung cancer. Interactive Cardiovasc Thorac Surg 2010;10:936–9.
5. Fleisher LA, Beckman JA, Brown KA, et al. ACC/AHA 2007 guidelines on perioperative cardiovascular

evaluation and care for noncardiac surgery: a report of the American College of Cardiology/American Heart Association Task Force on Practice Guidelines (Writing Committee to Revise the 2002 Guidelines on Perioperative Cardiovascular Evaluation for Noncardiac Surgery): developed in collaboration with the American Society of Echocardiography, American Society of Nuclear Cardiology, Heart Rhythm Society, Society of Cardiovascular Anesthesiologists, Society for Cardiovascular Angiography and Interventions, Society for Vascular Medicine and Biology, and Society for Vascular Surgery. Circulation 2007; 116:e418–99.

6. Rentz J, Bull D, Harpole D, et al. Transthoracic versus transhiatal esophagectomy: a prospective study of 945 patients. J Thorac Cardiovasc Surg 2003;125:1114–20.

7. Bailey SH, Bull DA, Harpole DH, et al. Outcomes after esophagectomy: a ten-year prospective cohort. Ann Thorac Surg 2003;75:217–22 [discussion: 222].

8. Lee TH, Marcantonio ER, Mangione CM, et al. Derivation and prospective validation of a simple index for prediction of cardiac risk of major noncardiac surgery. Circulation 1999;100:1043–9.

9. Devereaux PJ, Goldman L, Cook DJ, et al. Perioperative cardiac events in patients undergoing noncardiac surgery: a review of the magnitude of the problem, the pathophysiology of the events and methods to estimate and communicate risk. CMAJ 2005;173:627–34.

10. Brunelli A, Varela G, Salati M, et al. Recalibration of the revised cardiac risk index in lung resection candidates. Ann Thorac Surg 2010;90:199–203.

11. Devereaux PJ, Xavier D, Pogue J, et al. Characteristics and short-term prognosis of perioperative myocardial infarction in patients undergoing noncardiac surgery: a cohort study. Ann Intern Med 2011;154:523–8.

12. Kamel H, Johnston SC, Kirkham JC, et al. Association between major perioperative hemorrhage and stroke or Q-wave myocardial infarction. Circulation 2012;126:207–12.

13. Fihn SD, Blankenship JC, Alexander KP, et al. 2014 ACC/AHA/AATS/PCNA/SCAI/STS focused update of the guideline for the diagnosis and management of patients with stable ischemic heart disease: a report of the American College of Cardiology/American Heart Association Task Force on Practice Guidelines, and the American Association for Thoracic Surgery, Preventive Cardiovascular Nurses Association, Society for Cardiovascular Angiography and Interventions, and Society of Thoracic Surgeons. J Am Coll Cardiol 2014;64: 1929–49.

14. Ronan G, Wolk MJ, Bailey SR, et al. ACCF/AHA/ASE/ASNC/HFSA/HRS/SCAI/SCCT/SCMR/STS 2013 multimodality appropriate use criteria for the detection and risk assessment of stable ischemic heart disease: a report of the American College of Cardiology Foundation Appropriate Use Criteria Task Force, American Heart Association, American Society of Echocardiography, American Society of Nuclear Cardiology, Heart Failure Society of America, Heart Rhythm Society, Society for Cardiovascular Angiography and Interventions, Society of Cardiovascular Computed Tomography, Society for Cardiovascular Magnetic Resonance, and Society of Thoracic Surgeons. J Nucl Cardiol 2014;21:192–220.

15. Ovrehus KA, Jasinskiene J, Sand NP, et al. Coronary calcification among 3477 asymptomatic and symptomatic individuals. Eur J Prev Cardiol 2015. [Epub ahead of print].

16. Loffroy R, Bernard S, Serusclat A, et al. Noninvasive assessment of the prevalence and characteristics of coronary atherosclerotic plaques by multidetector computed tomography in asymptomatic type 2 diabetic patients at high risk of significant coronary artery disease: a preliminary study. Arch Cardiovasc Dis 2009;102:607–15.

17. Becker A, Leber AW, Becker C, et al. Predictive value of coronary calcifications for future cardiac events in asymptomatic patients with diabetes mellitus: a prospective study in 716 patients over 8 years. BMC Cardiovasc Disord 2008;8:27.

18. Ross AF, Ueda K. Pulmonary hypertension in thoracic surgical patients. Curr Opin Anaesthesiol 2010;23:25–33.

19. Hall A, Older P. Cardiopulmonary exercise testing accurately predicts risk of major surgery including esophageal resection: letter 1. Ann Thorac Surg 2009;87:670–1.

20. Husain Z, Palani G, Cabrera R, et al. Hemodynamic response, arrhythmic risk, and overall safety of regadenoson as a pharmacologic stress agent for myocardial perfusion imaging in chronic obstructive pulmonary disease and bronchial asthma patients. Int J Cardiovasc Imaging 2012;28:1841–9.

21. Leitha T, Gwechenberger M, Falger-Banyai S. Does dyspnoea during dipyridamole cardiac stress testing indicate bronchospasm and is the pretest clinical history predictive of this side-effect? Eur J Nucl Med 1995;22:1408–10.

22. Balan KK, Critchley M. Is the dyspnea during adenosine cardiac stress test caused by bronchospasm? Am Heart J 2001;142:142–5.

23. Fricke E, Esdorn E, Kammeier A, et al. Respiratory resistance of patients during cardiac stress testing with adenosine: is dyspnea a sign of bronchospasm? J Nucl Cardiol 2008;15:94–9.

24. Reyes E, Loong CY, Wechalekar K, et al. Side effect profile and tolerability of adenosine myocardial perfusion scintigraphy in patients with mild asthma

or chronic obstructive pulmonary disease. J Nucl Cardiol 2007;14:827–34.

25. Popescu WM. Perioperative management of the patient with a coronary stent. Curr Opin Anaesthesiol 2010;23:109–15.

26. Douketis JD, Spyropoulos AC, Spencer FA, et al. Perioperative management of antithrombotic therapy: antithrombotic therapy and prevention of thrombosis, 9th ed: American College of Chest Physicians evidence-based clinical practice guidelines. Chest 2012;141:e326S–50S.

27. Grines CL, Bonow RO, Casey DE Jr, et al. Prevention of premature discontinuation of dual antiplatelet therapy in patients with coronary artery stents: a science advisory from the American Heart Association, American College of Cardiology, Society for Cardiovascular Angiography and Interventions, American College of Surgeons, and American Dental Association, with representation from the American College of Physicians. J Am Coll Cardiol 2007;49:734–9.

28. Ceppa DP, Welsby IJ, Wang TY, et al. Perioperative management of patients on clopidogrel (Plavix) undergoing major lung resection. Ann Thorac Surg 2011;92:1971–6.

29. Cerfolio RJ, Minnich DJ, Bryant AS. General thoracic surgery is safe in patients taking clopidogrel (Plavix). J Thorac Cardiovasc Surg 2010;140:970–6.

30. Namasivayam V, Prasad GA, Lutzke LS, et al. The risk of endoscopic mucosal resection in the setting of clopidogrel use. ISRN Gastroenterol 2014;2014:494157.

31. Jakobsen CJ, Bille S, Ahlburg P, et al. Preoperative metoprolol improves cardiovascular stability and reduces oxygen consumption after thoracotomy. Acta Anaesthesiol Scand 1997;41:1324–30.

32. Lai RC, Xu MX, Huang WQ, et al. Beneficial effects of metoprolol on perioperative cardiac function of elderly esophageal cancer patients. Ai Zheng 2006;25:609–13 [in Chinese].

33. Mangano DT, Layug EL, Wallace A, et al. Effect of atenolol on mortality and cardiovascular morbidity after noncardiac surgery. Multicenter study of perioperative ischemia research group. N Engl J Med 1996;335:1713–20.

34. Wijeysundera DN, Duncan D, Nkonde-Price C, et al. Perioperative beta blockade in noncardiac surgery: a systematic review for the 2014 ACC/AHA guideline on perioperative cardiovascular evaluation and management of patients undergoing noncardiac surgery: a report of the American College of Cardiology/American Heart Association Task Force on Practice Guidelines. J Am Coll Cardiol 2014;64:2406–25.

35. Dai N, Xu D, Zhang J, et al. Different beta-blockers and initiation time in patients undergoing noncardiac surgery: a meta-analysis. Am J Med Sci 2014;347:235–44.

36. Talati R, Reinhart KM, White CM, et al. Outcomes of perioperative beta-blockade in patients undergoing noncardiac surgery: a meta-analysis. Ann Pharmacother 2009;43:1181–8.

37. Anwaruddin S, Askari AT, Saudye H, et al. Characterization of post-operative risk associated with prior drug-eluting stent use. JACC Cardiovasc Interv 2009;2:542–9.

38. Fenstad ER, Anavekar NS, Williamson E, et al. Twist and shout: acute right ventricular failure secondary to cardiac herniation and pulmonary artery compression. Circulation 2014;129:e409–12.

39. Shimizu J, Ishida Y, Hirano Y, et al. Cardiac herniation following intrapericardial pneumonectomy with partial pericardiectomy for advanced lung cancer. Ann Thorac Cardiovasc Surg 2003;9:68–72.

40. Ponten JE, Elenbaas TW, ter Woorst JF, et al. Cardiac herniation after operative management of lung cancer: a rare and dangerous complication. Gen Thorac Cardiovasc Surg 2012;60:668–72.

41. Terauchi Y, Kitaoka H, Tanioka K, et al. Inferior acute myocardial infarction due to acute cardiac herniation after right pneumonectomy. Cardiovasc Interv Ther 2012;27:110–3.

42. Kamiyoshihara M, Nagashima T, Baba S, et al. Serial chest films are needed after a diagnosis of pneumopericardium because of risk of cardiac herniation. Ann Thorac Surg 2010;90:1705–7.

43. Kawamukai K, Antonacci F, Di Saverio S, et al. Acute postoperative cardiac herniation. Interactive Cardiovasc Thorac Surg 2011;12:73–4.

44. Steinmann D, Rohr E, Kirschbaum A. Acute tension pneumothorax following cardiac herniation after pneumonectomy. Case Rep Med 2010;2010:213818.

45. Holloway B, Mukadam M, Thompson R, et al. Cardiac herniation and lung torsion following heart and lung transplantation. Interactive Cardiovasc Thorac Surg 2010;10:1044–6.

46. Karalapillai D, Larobina M, Stevenson K, et al. A change of heart: acute cardiac dextroversion with cardiogenic shock after partial lung resection. Crit Care Resuscitation 2008;10:140–3.

47. Kiev J, Parker M, Zhao X, et al. Cardiac herniation after intrapericardial pneumonectomy and subsequent cardiac tamponade. Am Surg 2007;73:906–8.

48. Mehanna MJ, Israel GM, Katigbak M, et al. Cardiac herniation after right pneumonectomy: case report and review of the literature. J Thorac Imaging 2007;22:280–2.

49. Zandberg FT, Verbeke SJ, Snijder RJ, et al. Sudden cardiac herniation 6 months after right pneumonectomy. Ann Thorac Surg 2004;78:1095–7.

50. Mason DP, Quader MA, Blackstone EH, et al. Thromboembolism after pneumonectomy for

malignancy: an independent marker of poor outcome. J Thorac Cardiovasc Surg 2006;131: 711–8.

51. Ziomek S, Read RC, Tobler HG, et al. Thromboembolism in patients undergoing thoracotomy. Ann Thorac Surg 1993;56:223–6 [discussion: 227].

52. Dentali F, Malato A, Ageno W, et al. Incidence of venous thromboembolism in patients undergoing thoracotomy for lung cancer. J Thorac Cardiovasc Surg 2008;135:705–6.

53. Bosch DJ, Van Dalfsen QA, Mul VE, et al. Increased risk of thromboembolism in esophageal cancer patients treated with neoadjuvant chemoradiotherapy. Am J Surg 2014;208:215–21.

54. Connolly GC, Dalal M, Lin J, et al. Incidence and predictors of venous thromboembolism (VTE) among ambulatory patients with lung cancer. Lung Cancer 2012;78:253–8.

55. Patel A, Anraku M, Darling GE, et al. Venous thromboembolism in patients receiving multimodality therapy for thoracic malignancies. J Thorac Cardiovasc Surg 2009;138:843–8.

56. Verhage RJ, van der Horst S, van der Sluis PC, et al. Risk of thromboembolic events after perioperative chemotherapy versus surgery alone for esophageal adenocarcinoma. Ann Surg Oncol 2012;19:684–92.

57. Scott WJ, Allen MS, Darling G, et al. Video-assisted thoracic surgery versus open lobectomy for lung cancer: a secondary analysis of data from the American College of Surgeons Oncology Group Z0030 randomized clinical trial. J Thorac Cardiovasc Surg 2010;139:976–81 [discussion: 981–3].

58. Boffa DJ, Dhamija A, Kosinski AS, et al. Fewer complications result from a video-assisted approach to anatomic resection of clinical stage I lung cancer. J Thorac Cardiovasc Surg 2014;148: 637–43.

59. Cao C, Manganas C, Ang SC, et al. A meta-analysis of unmatched and matched patients comparing video-assisted thoracoscopic lobectomy and conventional open lobectomy. Ann Cardiothorac Surg 2012;1:16–23.

60. Flores RM, Park BJ, Dycoco J, et al. Lobectomy by video-assisted thoracic surgery (VATS) versus thoracotomy for lung cancer. J Thorac Cardiovasc Surg 2009;138:11–8.

61. Daddi G, Milillo G, Lupattelli L, et al. Postoperative pulmonary embolism detected with multislice computed tomography in lung surgery for cancer. J Thorac Cardiovasc Surg 2006;132:197–8.

62. National Clinical Guideline Centre A, Chronic C, National Institute for Health and Clinical Excellence: Guidance. Venous thromboembolism: reducing the risk of venous thromboembolism (deep vein thrombosis and pulmonary embolism) in patients admitted to hospital. London: Royal College of Physicians (UK) National Clinical Guideline Centre - Acute and Chronic Conditions; 2010.

63. Brock H, Rieger R, Gabriel C, et al. Haemodynamic changes during thoracoscopic surgery the effects of one-lung ventilation compared with carbon dioxide insufflation. Anaesthesia 2000;55:10–6.

64. Gould MK, Garcia DA, Wren SM, et al. Prevention of VTE in nonorthopedic surgical patients: antithrombotic therapy and prevention of thrombosis, 9th ed: American College of Chest Physicians evidence-based clinical practice guidelines. Chest 2012;141:e227S–77S.

65. Agnelli G, Bolis G, Capussotti L, et al. A clinical outcome-based prospective study on venous thromboembolism after cancer surgery: the @RISTOS project. Ann Surg 2006;243:89–95.

66. Giannoukas AD, Labropoulos N, Michaels JA. Compression with or without early ambulation in the prevention of post-thrombotic syndrome: a systematic review. Eur J Vasc Endovasc Surg 2006;32: 217–21.

67. Collins R, Scrimgeour A, Yusuf S, et al. Reduction in fatal pulmonary embolism and venous thrombosis by perioperative administration of subcutaneous heparin. Overview of results of randomized trials in general, orthopedic, and urologic surgery. N Engl J Med 1988;318:1162–73.

68. Vanek VW. Meta-analysis of effectiveness of intermittent pneumatic compression devices with a comparison of thigh-high to knee-high sleeves. Am Surg 1998;64:1050–8.

69. Konstantinides SV, Torbicki A, Agnelli G, et al. 2014 ESC guidelines on the diagnosis and management of acute pulmonary embolism. Eur Heart J 2014;35: 3033–69, 3069a–k.

70. Prevention of fatal postoperative pulmonary embolism by low doses of heparin. An international multicentre trial. Lancet 1975;2:45–51.

71. Mismetti P, Laporte S, Darmon JY, et al. Meta-analysis of low molecular weight heparin in the prevention of venous thromboembolism in general surgery. Br J Surg 2001;88:913–30.

72. Arnold JD, Dart BW, Barker DE, et al. Gold Medal Forum winner. Unfractionated heparin three times a day versus enoxaparin in the prevention of deep vein thrombosis in trauma patients. Am Surg 2010;76:563–70.

73. Phung OJ, Kahn SR, Cook DJ, et al. Dosing frequency of unfractionated heparin thromboprophylaxis: a meta-analysis. Chest 2011;140:374–81.

74. Ikesaka R, Delluc A, Le Gal G, et al. Efficacy and safety of weight-adjusted heparin prophylaxis for the prevention of acute venous thromboembolism among obese patients undergoing bariatric surgery: a systematic review and meta-analysis. Thromb Res 2014;133:682–7.

75. Jamal MH, Corcelles R, Shimizu H, et al. Thromboembolic events in bariatric surgery: a large multi-institutional referral center experience. Surg Endosc 2015;29:376–80.

76. Sarosiek S, Crowther M, Sloan JM. Indications, complications, and management of inferior vena cava filters: the experience in 952 patients at an academic hospital with a level I trauma center. JAMA Intern Med 2013;173:513–7.

77. Srivastava SD, Eagleton MJ, Greenfield LJ. Diagnosis of pulmonary embolism with various imaging modalities. Semin Vasc Surg 2004;17:173–80.

78. Hartmann IJ, Hagen PJ, Melissant CF, et al. Diagnosing acute pulmonary embolism: effect of chronic obstructive pulmonary disease on the performance of D-dimer testing, ventilation/perfusion scintigraphy, spiral computed tomographic angiography, and conventional angiography. ANTELOPE Study Group. Advances in New Technologies Evaluating the Localization of Pulmonary Embolism. Am J Respir Crit Care Med 2000;162:2232–7.

79. Schulman S, Kearon C, Kakkar AK, et al. Dabigatran versus warfarin in the treatment of acute venous thromboembolism. N Engl J Med 2009; 361:2342–52.

80. Lee AY, Bauersachs R, Janas MS, et al. CATCH: a randomised clinical trial comparing long-term tinzaparin versus warfarin for treatment of acute venous thromboembolism in cancer patients. BMC Cancer 2013;13:284.

81. Loffredo L, Perri L, Del Ben M, et al. New oral anticoagulants for the treatment of acute venous thromboembolism: are they safer than vitamin K antagonists? A meta-analysis of the interventional trials. Intern Emerg Med 2015;10(4):499–506.

82. Kameyama K, Huang CL, Liu D, et al. Pulmonary embolism after lung resection: diagnosis and treatment. Ann Thorac Surg 2003;76:599–601.

83. Guyatt GH, Akl EA, Crowther M, et al. Introduction to the ninth edition: antithrombotic therapy and prevention of thrombosis, 9th ed: American College of Chest Physicians evidence-based clinical practice guidelines. Chest 2012;141:48s–52s.

84. Agnelli G, George DJ, Kakkar AK, et al. Semuloparin for thromboprophylaxis in patients receiving chemotherapy for cancer. N Engl J Med 2012; 366:601–9.

85. Agnelli G, Verso M. Thromboprophylaxis during chemotherapy in patients with advanced cancer. Thromb Res 2010;125(Suppl 2):S17–20.

86. Ma Q, Liu D, Guo Y, et al. Surgical techniques and results of the pulmonary artery reconstruction for patients with central non-small cell lung cancer. J Card Surg 2013;8:219.

87. Rendina E, Venuta F. Sleeve resection and prosthetic reconstruction of the pulmonary artery for lung cancer. Ann Thorac Surg 1999;68:995–1001.

88. Alifano M, Cusumano G, Strano S, et al. Lobectomy with pulmonary artery resection: morbidity, mortality, and long-term survival. J Thorac Cardiovasc Surg 2009;137:1400–5.

89. Shrager J, Lambright E, McGrath C, et al. Lobectomy with tangential pulmonary artery resection without regard to pulmonary function. Ann Thorac Surg 2000;70:234–9.

90. Amar D. Prevention and management of perioperative arrhythmias in the thoracic surgical population. Anesthesiol Clin 2008;26:325–35, vii.

91. Roselli EE, Murthy SC, Rice TW, et al. Atrial fibrillation complicating lung cancer resection. J Thorac Cardiovasc Surg 2005;130:438–44.

92. Amar D. Postthoracotomy atrial fibrillation. Curr Opin Anaesthesiol 2007;20:43–7.

93. Mason DP, Marsh DH, Alster JM, et al. Atrial fibrillation after lung transplantation: timing, risk factors, and treatment. Ann Thorac Surg 2007;84:1878–84.

94. Ivanovic J, Maziak DE, Ramzan S, et al. Incidence, severity and perioperative risk factors for atrial fibrillation following pulmonary resection. Interactive Cardiovasc Thorac Surg 2014;18:340–6.

95. Neragi-Miandoab S, Weiner S, Sugarbaker DJ. Incidence of atrial fibrillation after extrapleural pneumonectomy vs. pleurectomy in patients with malignant pleural mesothelioma. Interactive Cardiovasc Thorac Surg 2008;7:1039–42.

96. Vaporciyan AA, Correa AM, Rice DC, et al. Risk factors associated with atrial fibrillation after noncardiac thoracic surgery: analysis of 2588 patients. J Thorac Cardiovasc Surg 2004;127:779–86.

97. Stougard J. Cardiac arrhythmias following pneumonectomy. Thorax 1969;24:568–72.

98. Fernando HC, Jaklitsch MT, Walsh GL, et al. The Society of Thoracic Surgeons practice guideline on the prophylaxis and management of atrial fibrillation associated with general thoracic surgery: executive summary. Ann Thorac Surg 2011;92: 1144–52.

99. Frendl G, Sodickson AC, Chung MK, et al. 2014 AATS guidelines for the prevention and management of perioperative atrial fibrillation and flutter for thoracic surgical procedures. J Thorac Cardiovasc Surg 2014;148:e153–93.

100. Flynn BC, Vernick WJ, Ellis JE. β-Blockade in the perioperative management of the patient with cardiac disease undergoing non-cardiac surgery. Br J Anaesth 2011;107(Suppl 1):i3–15.

101. Bagshaw SM, Galbraith PD, Mitchell LB, et al. Prophylactic amiodarone for prevention of atrial fibrillation after cardiac surgery: a meta-analysis. Ann Thorac Surg 2006;82:1927–37.

102. Bouri S, Shun-Shin MJ, Cole GD, et al. Meta-analysis of secure randomised controlled trials of beta-blockade to prevent perioperative death in non-cardiac surgery. Heart 2014;100:456–64.

103. Cook RC, Yamashita MH, Kearns M, et al. Prophylactic magnesium does not prevent atrial fibrillation after cardiac surgery: a meta-analysis. Ann Thorac Surg 2013;95:533–41.

104. Amar D, Roistacher N, Rusch VW, et al. Effects of diltiazem prophylaxis on the incidence and clinical outcome of atrial arrhythmias after thoracic surgery. J Thorac Cardiovasc Surg 2000;120:790–8.

105. Dehghani MR, Kasianzadeh M, Rezaei Y, et al. Atorvastatin reduces the incidence of postoperative atrial fibrillation in statin-naive patients undergoing isolated heart valve surgery: a double-blind, placebo-controlled randomized trial. J Cardiovasc Pharmacol Ther 2015;20(5): 465–72.

106. Zheng H, Xue S, Hu ZL, et al. The use of statins to prevent postoperative atrial fibrillation after coronary artery bypass grafting: a meta-analysis of 12 studies. J Cardiovasc Pharmacol 2014;64:285–92.

107. Amar D, Zhang H, Heerdt PM, et al. Statin use is associated with a reduction in atrial fibrillation after noncardiac thoracic surgery independent of C-reactive protein. Chest 2005;128:3421–7.

108. Lai HC, Lai HC, Wang KY, et al. Severe pulmonary hypertension complicates postoperative outcome of non-cardiac surgery. Br J Anaesth 2007;99: 184–90.

109. Ramakrishna G, Sprung J, Ravi BS, et al. Impact of pulmonary hypertension on the outcomes of noncardiac surgery: predictors of perioperative morbidity and mortality. J Am Coll Cardiol 2005; 45:1691–9.

110. Pritts CD, Pearl RG. Anesthesia for patients with pulmonary hypertension. Curr Opin Anaesthesiol 2010;23:411–6.

111. Minai OA, Yared JP, Kaw R, et al. Perioperative risk and management in patients with pulmonary hypertension. Chest 2013;144:329–40.

# Pain Management Following Thoracic Surgery

Brett Elmore, MD, Van Nguyen, MD, Randall Blank, MD,
Kenan Yount, MD, Christine Lau, MD*

## KEYWORDS

- Postoperative pain • Thoracic surgery • Pain management • Chronic pain

## KEY POINTS

- Managing postoperative pain is critical in reducing postoperative respiratory.
- Postoperative pain results from multiple etiologic factors. There is no one modality that addresses each contributing factor.
- Optimizing pain control while minimizing sedation and respiratory depression are challenging and competing goals, and neuraxial or regional techniques are strongly preferred over primary parenteral analgesia in the immediate postoperative period.
- Epidural anesthesia is the gold standard for treatment; paravertebral nerve blocks are gaining popularity, but can be technically difficult to perform for an inexperienced anesthesiologist.
- Chronic pain complicates all types of thoracic procedures; once established, chronic postthoracotomy pain is difficult to treat. Preventive approaches include regional and neuraxial analgesia and careful surgical technique.

## INTRODUCTION

Postoperative pain following thoracic surgery presents a significant challenge, and multiple factors complicate recovery and pain management for this population. Although opioids are often sufficient for managing pain after other surgical procedures, patients who are candidates for thoracic surgery often suffer from serious pulmonary pathology and are consequently less likely to tolerate adverse effects of opioids on the respiratory system. Considerable comorbidities often exist in thoracic surgical patients, thus further limiting therapeutic options. Thoracic surgical incisions, even those used for video-assisted thoracic surgery (VATS), can result in significant, long-lasting, and intense discomfort, which may lead to so-called postthoracotomy pain syndrome (PTPS) that may persist for years.[1] In addition, postoperative cardiovascular complications from thoracic operations may also complicate pain management. Tailoring a treatment regimen that adequately addresses these issues can be overwhelming.

Postoperative pain in thoracic patients is multifactorial and incompletely understood. Elements of nociceptive and neuropathic pain may contribute greatly to patient discomfort. The multilayer intercostal incisions, thoracostomy tube insertion, and pleural irritation are intensely painful. Iatrogenic factors, such as inadvertent rib fractures, intentional rib resection, chest tube positioning, and injuries from unrecognized suboptimal intraoperative positioning, can further exacerbate postoperative pain. This diversity of insults can lead to a variety of pain symptoms including stabbing chest pain and pleurisy, throbbing shoulder pain, and burning rib pain. In the chronically opioid-dependent patient, these symptoms may be far more challenging to treat effectively. There is no single pharmaceutical agent

Division of Thoracic & Cardiovascular Surgery, Department of Anesthesia, University of Virginia, Charlottesville, VA 22908, USA
* Corresponding author.
E-mail address: cll2y@virginia.edu

Thorac Surg Clin 25 (2015) 393–409
http://dx.doi.org/10.1016/j.thorsurg.2015.07.005
1547-4127/15/$ – see front matter © 2015 Elsevier Inc. All rights reserved.

or route of administration that addresses every individual contributor to pain, and thus treatment regimens should be multimodal and tailored to the patient and procedure. Treating these individual contributors to achieve patient satisfaction is an important primary perioperative goal, and failure to address acute postoperative pain may lead to the development of chronic pain syndromes.

It is now well-established that effective pain prophylaxis and treatment regimens begin with regional and neuraxial anesthesia techniques. Thoracic epidural anesthesia (TEA) is still considered the gold standard for treating postoperative pain. However, the complications of TEA are many and, in rare cases, can be devastating. Although paravertebral nerve block (PVB) has gained popularity as a treatment modality, too few anesthesiologists are comfortable with PVBs. If performed by inexperienced personnel, the patient can suffer from complications including epidural and intrathecal spread of local anesthetic, pneumothorax, nerve injury, and inadequate pain relief. Furthermore, the advent of diverse and numerous oral anticoagulant and antiplatelet agents have increased the potential for neuraxial hematoma and, hence, the contraindications for epidural and paravertebral techniques. Although systemic opioids are repeatedly vilified in this population, they may become the cornerstone of the treatment regimen when the risk of catastrophic bleeding prohibits the use of regional techniques. This article outlines systemic agents, regional techniques (and attendant complications), etiologies of pain following thoracic procedures, and the development and treatment of chronic pain.

## ETIOLOGIES OF PAIN

The major component of acute postthoracotomy pain is attributed to the intercostal incision that spans the skin, subcutaneous tissue, muscle layers (including intercostal muscles, latissimus dorsi, serratus anterior, and the pectoralis major), and parietal pleura.[2] These layers are innervated by nerves with unique origins. Skin, subcutaneous tissues, and intercostal muscles are innervated by the intercostal nerves. The latissimus dorsi and serratus anterior are supplied by the brachial plexus (thoracodorsal and long thoracic nerves, respectively). The parietal pleura has contributions from the intercostal nerves and the phrenic nerve. Intraoperatively, the incision is forcibly retracted, which can lead to crushing of cutaneous or intercostal nerves and further muscle trauma.[3] Although VATS operations decrease the extent of the incision, identical tissue layers are traversed. During inspiration, the chest wall expands causing

stretching of the incision. Without adequate analgesia, the resulting intense pain frequently leads patients to breathe shallowly.

Rib fractures can exacerbate an already painful incision. Patients in this population are often aging and have poor bone mineral density, which can place them at increased risk for fractures. A careful surgeon takes measures to avoid unintended fractures, but vigorous rib spreader insertion and retraction can lead to such injuries. The extensive exposure sometimes required to operate in the thoracic cavity may necessitate sectioning or excising segments of rib (ie, "shingling"). This can certainly reduce postoperative pain, but the periosteal compromise itself is painful nonetheless.

Thoracostomy tubes, frequently placed away from the primary incision, are used to drain blood and reduce iatrogenic pneumothorax. The additional incision is an obvious contributor to pain, but the tube also makes contact with the highly innervated visceral and parietal pleura. During inspiration, the tube can mechanically irritate parietal and more sensitive visceral pleura, resulting in intense discomfort. If the tube is inserted too deeply or malpositioned, the resultant friction can be excruciating. In severe cases, lung injury can occur.

Ipsilateral shoulder pain is a nearly ubiquitous complaint after all types of thoracic operations involving thoracotomy or thoracoscopy incisions and may be the result of phrenic nerve injury or diaphragmatic trauma. Although these two etiologies are especially sinister given their impact on respiratory function and complications postoperatively, it is unlikely that they are solely responsible for all cases of shoulder pain. The elderly frequently have shoulder pathologies that are easily worsened by lateral decubitus positioning. Chest tube irritation can also be referred to the shoulder area. Brachial plexopathies are common in supine procedures, but even more common in the lateral position if pressure points and exaggerated shoulder extension are not closely monitored intraoperatively. It is prudent to perform a focused neurologic examination before and after thoracic surgery.

### Thoracotomy Versus Video-Assisted Thoracic Surgery

Minimally invasive thoracic surgical techniques have improved considerably in the past two decades. In general, patients recovering from VATS operations have fewer respiratory complications and have lower pain scores postoperatively. Generally, length of stay following lobectomy via thoracotomy for lung cancer averages 4 to 5 days, but only 3 to 4 days following VATS lobectomy.[4] Many advocate thoracic epidural use for VATS lobectomies, although its utility when compared with systemic analgesia remains controversial. Development of PTPS is somewhat similar in the two groups.[5] Muscle-sparing thoracotomy approaches have also gained popularity, but data are conflicting regarding the development of PTPS for this approach when compared with posterolateral approach.[6]

## Systemic Versus Regional Analgesia

Although TEA is recognized to be the gold standard for pain prevention and treatment among thoracic surgery patients, this modality fails to address all the components of acute pain following thoracic surgery. For example, pain contributions from thoracic dermatomes can be reliably muted with thoracic epidural or multilevel paravertebral analgesia, but shoulder discomfort and pleural discomfort often persist. Other therapeutic agents may also be useful in treating pain following thoracic surgery. Whether systemically or regionally administered, these therapies possess beneficial and potentially detrimental qualities that must be weighed when tailoring a treatment regimen (**Tables 1** and **2**).

## SYSTEMIC AND PARENTERAL THERAPIES
## Opioids

Whether administered intravenously, orally, or neuraxially, opioids are an important component of most treatment regimens following thoracic operations. Both systemic and neuraxial routes provide reliable analgesia, although systemic opioids are more likely to increase the risk of pulmonary complications, such as atelectasis, pneumonia, and hypoxic or hypercarbic respiratory failure. Opioid overdose can be devastating in this population. Serious morbidity can result even with minimal opioid-induced respiratory depression. The adverse effects of opioids are not well tolerated in patients with obstructive pulmonary disease, particularly following lung resection. Unless contraindicated, the benefits of regional and neuraxial techniques using a combination of local anesthetic and opioid outweigh the risks and should be considered superior to a parenteral opioid technique.

Intravenous (IV) patient-controlled analgesia (PCA) systems have become a mainstay of treatment of postsurgical pain in the modern era. Although this therapy does allow the patient to titrate relief to perceived pain level and reduce the risk of overdose, PCAs are not dynamic

enough to address pain while the patient sleeps, participates in physical therapy, or practices necessary pulmonary toilet measures (eg, incentive spirometry, deep-breathing, coughing, and so forth) However, recent work[7] suggests that PCAs, when paired with nonopioid adjuvant medications, can be effective in providing adequate analgesia without increasing the risk of PTPS. Nonetheless, if systemic opioids are to be used in place of regional anesthesia, the patient should be monitored at even more frequent intervals in a critical care setting with tight titration and liberal use of nonopioid adjuvants.

## Nonsteroidal Anti-inflammatory Drugs

Adjunctive analgesic medications that do not suppress ventilatory drive are of particular interest in this population. Nonsteroidal anti-inflammatory drugs (NSAIDs) provide analgesia by reversibly inhibiting cyclooxygenase (COX), which reduces prostaglandin synthesis. NSAIDs have varying degrees of specificity for inhibiting the subtypes of COX inhibitors: COX-1 and COX-2. COX-1, present in several tissues at baseline, is central in the synthesis of various prostaglandins from arachidonic acid, including those responsible for regulating inflammation, platelet aggregation, renal vascular vasodilation, and gastric acid secretion. COX-2 is upregulated in states of inflammation and was of considerable interest as a pharmaceutical target in hopes of reducing inflammation with fewer side effects than traditional nonselective COX-inhibitors. Unfortunately, COX-2 inhibitors (eg, celecoxib and rofecoxib) were found to significantly increase risk for adverse cardiac and cerebrovascular events, thus limiting their therapeutic role in postthoracotomy pain. At least one study[8] suggests an increase in patient satisfaction with analgesia when celecoxib was combined with TEA, but the study was not sufficiently powered to evaluate cardiac morbidity.

Nonselective NSAIDs are more routinely used in supplementing opioids perioperatively. When administered concurrently with acetaminophen, NSAIDs were noted to reduce opioid requirements by roughly 30% to 35%.[9] Indomethacin administration was shown[10] to significantly reduce opioid consumption and reduce pain scores after thoracotomy. IV ketorolac, if given preoperatively, was noted to reduce morphine consumption by 36% when compared with placebo, although it had no effect on pulmonary function postoperatively.[11] If used, significant attention must be given to their potential side effects including not only increased risk of cardiovascular events, but also bleeding, renal    impairment,    dyspepsia,    and    gastric

**Table 1**
**Nonopioid analgesics**

| Systemic Analgesics | Benefits | Risks | Recommendations |
|---|---|---|---|
| Acetaminophen | Safe, effective analgesic and antipyretic<br>Reduces pain scores and opioid requirements<br>No increased incidence in hemorrhage, gastric ulceration, cardiovascular, and renal adverse effects<br>Has "ceiling effect" | Liver toxicity | Recommended in combination with other analgesics |
| NSAIDs | Improves pain relief<br>Reduces opioid consumption by 30% and decreases opioid-related adverse effects | Impaired coagulation, gastric irritation, renal dysfunction, and cardiovascular adverse effects | Recommended in combination with other analgesics |
| COX-2 inhibitors | Improves pain scores, decreases opioid consumption, and reduces opioid-related adverse effects<br>Similar efficacy as NSAIDs<br>No effects on platelet function and perioperative bleeding | Potential gastric irritation, renal dysfunction, and cardiovascular adverse effects | Recommended in combination with other analgesics |
| Glucocorticoids (dexamethasone) | Reduces inflammation, improves pain relief, prolongs time to first analgesic, and modest reduction in opioid requirements | Increase blood glucose levels up to 24 h, but may not be clinically relevant | Recommended as an adjunct |
| Ketamine | Analgesic properties without respiratory depressive effects, reduces pain scores, and opioid consumption, and prolongs time to first analgesic<br>Optimal dose and duration of administration remain controversial | Sympathomimetic and neurocognitive side effects | Not recommended for routine use |
| Gabapentinoids (gabapentin and pregabalin) | Reduced pain scores and opioid requirements<br>Optimal dose and duration of administration remain controversial | Sedation, dizziness, and visual disturbances | Not recommended for routine use |

Abbreviations: COX, cyclooxygenase; NSAIDs, nonsteroidal anti-inflammatory drugs.

From Romero A, Garcia JE, Joshi GP. The state of the art in preventing postthoracotomy pain. Semin Thorac Cardiovasc Surg 2013;25(2):119; with permission.

**Table 2**
**Regional analgesia techniques for thoracic surgery**

| Regional Anesthesia Techniques | Benefits | Risks | Recommendations |
|---|---|---|---|
| Thoracic paravertebral analgesia | Superior dynamic analgesia during coughing and physical therapy<br>Improved postoperative outcome<br>Equally effective as TEA<br>Trend toward lower incidence of major complications compared with TEA and lower block failure rate<br>Limited value with single-shot injection | Epidural spread of local anesthetic with associated risks, vascular injury, and pleural injury<br>Potential for catastrophic neurologic complications is remote | Recommended |
| TEA | Superior analgesia during coughing and physical therapy, and improved postoperative outcome | High (15%) failure rate, complicates postoperative anticoagulation, hypotension, nausea, urinary retention, pruritus, accidental intrathecal spread, epidural hematoma, and epidural abscess | Recommended |
| Intrathecal opioid analgesia | Better static and dynamic pain scores compared with systemic opioid analgesia specifically in first 24 h postoperatively | Risk of respiratory depression, pruritus, urinary retention, nausea, and vomiting | Recommended, if paravertebral block or TEA is contraindicated or not possible |
| Intercostal analgesia | Simple and easy to perform, superior pain scores, reduced opioid requirements, and improved postoperative outcome | Systemic local toxicity, better pain scores with continuous catheter, or multiple injections | Recommended in combination with nonopioid analgesics, such as acetaminophen and NSAIDs or COX-2-specific inhibitors, if paravertebral block or TEA is contraindicated or not possible |
| Interpleural analgesia | Easy to perform but not efficacious | Potential of local anesthetic toxicity | Not recommended |
| Intercostal nerve cryoanalgesia | Effective in perioperative period in improving pain scores compared with placebo | Implicated in increasing incidence of chronic pain | Not recommended |

*Abbreviations:* COX, cyclooxygenase; NSAIDs, nonsteroidal anti-inflammatory drugs.
   *From* Romero A, Garcia JE, Joshi GP. The state of the art in preventing postthoracotomy pain. Semin Thorac Cardiovasc Surg 2013;25(2):188; with permission.

ulceration. Restrictive fluid management for lung resection surgeries may increase the susceptibility to NSAID-induced acute renal injury and other hypoperfusion-related side effects. When used, our typical IV regimen is 15 to 30 mg scheduled every 6 hours for six doses.

### Acetaminophen

Acetaminophen has long been used to reduce opioid requirements in the postoperative period for various painful procedures.[12–14] Like NSAIDs, it provides analgesia without increasing the incidence of pulmonary complications. It also avoids the adverse side effects of NSAIDs, such as renal function, gastric ulceration, or platelet aggregation. Its use is only limited by its potential for liver toxicity and, accordingly, patients with hepatic impairment should receive it only sparingly. Recently, an IV formulation of acetaminophen has generated considerable interest in the perioperative use of acetaminophen. Administration in critically ill patients has shown to decrease time to extubation, reduce opioid-related side effects (nausea and sedation), and decrease meperidine consumption.[15] In a recent, double-blind, randomized, placebo-controlled study, Mac and colleagues[16] demonstrated that 48 hours of perioperative acetaminophen significantly reduced ipsilateral shoulder pain compared with placebo. Given its relatively safe profile and proved benefit when used in multimodal analgesia, acetaminophen should be incorporated into most multimodal pain regimens. When used, our typical IV regimen is 1000 mg every 6 hours (maximum, 4000 mg in 24 hours).

### Benzodiazepines

Not surprisingly, patients can have debilitating anxiety if suffering from severe pain that is exacerbated simply with inhalation and coughing. Although benzodiazepines can be used for severe cases of anxiety (especially in patients previously on daily regimens), this category of drugs has fallen out of favor because of its strong association with postoperative delirium. The elderly are particularly sensitive to the effects, which can be long-lasting and exaggerated in this subgroup.[17] Furthermore, benzodiazepines are known to cause respiratory depression, especially when used in combination with systemic opioids. Although benzodiazepines may be useful in attenuating the dysphoric effects of ketamine, the use of true analgesics and multimodal adjuncts should be considered preferable to the routine use of benzodiazepines in this context.

### Ketamine

Ketamine is an N-methyl-D-aspartate receptor antagonist that has long been used to reduce opioid requirements. Ketamine is particularly useful as an adjunct in this population because it is known to stimulate respiratory drive even with low-dose administration. A systematic review by Laskowski and colleagues[18] suggests that ketamine, when used intraoperatively, shows improved quality of pain control independent of timing, dose, and route of opioid administration in major operations. Its role in reducing PTPS is still unclear. Suzuki and colleagues[19] evaluated ketamine-potentiation of epidural analgesia with

ropivacaine and morphine. Forty-nine patients were randomized to low-dose ketamine infusion versus saline placebo. Patients receiving low-dose ketamine demonstrated lower pain scores at 24 hours, 48 hours, 1 month, and 3 months. If regional anesthesia is contraindicated, providers should strongly consider ketamine as an adjunct because of its favorable side effect profile and demonstrated analgesic efficacy in this context.[20] Although ketamine is known to sometimes lead to intense dysphoria, this is less likely at doses traditionally used as an adjunct for pain treatment (0.5–1 mg/kg dose or <10 mg/h infusion).[21–23] Still, this adverse effect should be respected in an aging population that is already at increased risk for postoperative delirium.

### Dexmedetomidine

Dexmedetomidine is a selective $\alpha_2$-agonist that has a sedative effect without affecting respiratory drive. Wahlander and colleagues[24] assessed whether an IV infusion of dexmedetomidine reduced epidural use in postthoracotomy patients. Although there was no difference in pain scores or epidural use compared with placebo, the placebo group required more supplemental epidural fentanyl. A study by Ramsay and colleagues[25] had similar results: pain scores were similar in the dexmedetomidine infusion group and place group, but the dexmedetomidine group used 41% less opioids, comparatively. Limiting its usefulness is the association of dexmedetomidine with hypotension and bradycardia. This population is already at risk for severe hypotension secondary to epidural-induced sympathectomy, almost universal $\beta$-blocker administration for tachyarrhythmia prophylaxis, and fluid restriction. Administration should be limited to continuous low-dose infusions to avoid hypotension.

### Gabapentinoids

Gabapentin and pregabalin are the two clinically available gabapentinoids used in the management of neuropathic pain. In a recent review, Humble and colleagues[26] found that gabapentinoids reduced postoperative pain in cases without concomitant epidural anesthesia. Kinney and colleagues[27] in a double-blind, randomized, controlled trial showed that a single dose of gabapentin (600 mg) preoperatively had no effect on pain scores or opioid consumption. Studies by Omran and Mohamed[28] and Solak and coworkers[29] noted that longer preoperative and postoperative gabapentinoid regimens did result in reductions in opioid requirements. The role of gabapentinoids on PTPS is discussed later.

## Intravenous Lidocaine Infusion

Lidocaine infusions have been used to reduce opioid requirements in many surgical procedures with consistent benefit per a meta-analysis by Vigneault and coworkers.[30] Cui and colleagues[31] demonstrate a reduction in PCA morphine use for the first 6 hours following thoracic surgery, but no benefit for the remainder of the initial 48-hour postoperative period. A study evaluating its usefulness in VATS, where epidural use is less likely, is ongoing.

## REGIONAL ANESTHESIA TECHNIQUES

Regional anesthesia techniques can offer excellent pain management for patients undergoing thoracic operations. Both thoracic epidural analgesia and paravertebral analgesia are often regarded as optimal modalities for postthoracotomy analgesia given their superior track record of pain control and improved outcomes. Other regional techniques, including but not limited to intrathecal opioid analgesia, intercostal nerve block (ICNB), intercostal cryoanalgesia, and intrapleural analgesia, can aid in improving pain scores and reducing opioid consumption.

## Thoracic Epidural Analgesia

TEA has long been considered the gold standard regimen for patients undergoing thoracic operations given its proved record of excellent dynamic pain relief and prevention of postoperative pulmonary complications. Depending on the size of the surgical incisions (VATS vs thoracotomy) and the tolerance of the patient (opioid-dependent vs naive), epidurals can be placed either preoperatively or postoperatively. Although the timing of initiation of TEA remains controversial, its continuous use for at least 48 hours postthoracotomy has been shown to provide the benefits of optimal pain control and improved outcomes.[32] Our typical practice is to leave epidurals in place until removal of chest tube drains.

In a randomized controlled trial, Bauer and colleagues[33] followed patients undergoing lobectomy or bilobectomy via thoracotomy with pain control regimens of either TEA with ropivacaine and sufentanil or IV morphine PCA. Patients with epidurals showed greater postoperative forced vital capacity and forced expiratory volume in 1 second than patients with PCA. The epidural group also had better pain control as expressed by lower visual analog scores (VAS) at rest and with deep inspiration or coughing. In another randomized control trial, Ali and colleagues[34] confirmed that patients undergoing thoracic or upper abdominal operations (>50% of surgeries were thoracic) with TEA versus IV morphine PCA had significant lower pain scores at all measured time points. The epidural group also had a higher sense of physical and mental well-being at 24 hours and 1 week postoperatively, as measured by the SF-8 and SF-36 short-form health surveys. The author hypothesized that the superior pain control offered by TEA, in combination with its opioid-sparing effects, served to maximize physical mobility and minimize undesirable side effects often associated with IV opioids (ie, drowsiness, nausea, vomiting, sleep disturbances).

TEA can be used in combination with other modes of analgesia to provide superior pain control. Senard and colleagues[8] in a recent study demonstrated that TEA, when paired with celecoxib, can result in lower resting and dynamic pain scores, and higher patient satisfaction, during first 48 hours postoperatively without an increased incidence of bleeding. The use of local anesthetic in TEA may also decrease the incidence of postoperative arrhythmia, as suggested in a study by Oka and colleagues.[35] In this study, patients undergoing thoracic surgeries were randomized to receiving TEA with bupivacaine versus morphine. The group receiving TEA with bupivacaine had significant lower incidence of tachyarrhythmia (taking into consideration episodes lasting >60 minutes) compared with the group receiving TEA with morphine.

The use of TEA is not without drawbacks. Among the most common side effects is the increased incidence of hypotension. Hypotension is driven primarily by the sympathectomy caused by local anesthetic in the epidural space, and it may be exacerbated by hypovolemia. This side effect further limits its use in patients who depend on higher coronary or cerebral perfusion pressures. Furthermore, hypotension in patients after thoracic operations frequently leads to temporary or permanent discontinuation of epidural local anesthetic infusions, which ultimately compromises pain control.

Other common side effects of TEA include nausea, vomiting, pruritus, and urinary retention, all of which are likely attributable to the opioid component of most epidural infusions.[32] Knowledge of the cause of TEA common side effects is therefore necessary in the trouble-shooting process, which may involve the modification of the epidural infusion drugs, infusion rate, or administration of adjunct medications. Additionally, TEA can have a failure rate ranging from roughly 10% to 15% in a review by Hermanides and coworkers[36] to as high as 32% from all causes (predominantly caused by dislodged catheter,

catheter not in the epidural space, or incomplete block per Ready[37]). Epidurals also can complicate the postoperative plan for anticoagulation. Our typical practice is to schedule prophylactic enoxaparin at 18:00 daily (single-dose) for all patients with epidurals in place to facilitate their timely removal and optimal management of anticoagulation.

Catastrophic complications of TEA, such as epidural hematoma and abscess, are rare. However, studies suggest that the incidence of epidural hematoma has increased over the past two decades. A multicenter, retrospective study in North America academic hospitals by Bateman and colleagues[38] indicates that incidence of epidural hematoma requiring emergent laminectomy is between 1 in 4330 and 1 in 22,189 placements. In four of the seven documented epidural hematomas (out of 62,450 patients), current American Society of Regional Anesthesia (ASRA) anticoagulation guidelines were not followed. Time to development of symptoms in this study varied widely from 11 to 71 hours after epidural placement. Horlocker and Kopp[39] note that prior studies from 1993 early show a much lower incidence (in one case, <1 in 150,000). This is at least in part caused by current medical practice of aggressive venous thromboembolic prophylaxis with modern potent anticoagulants. This warrants serious concern in patients receiving TEA (or even PVB) after thoracic operations, because they often require concurrent anticoagulation therapy for other conditions, such as atrial fibrillation, coronary stents, and history of deep vein thrombosis. The ASRA has developed consensus guidelines to assist physicians in managing regional anesthesia techniques concurrently with anticoagulation therapy.[40] These guidelines should be adhered to whenever possible in this population to minimize the likelihood of epidural hematoma. **Table 3** summarizes some of these recommendations when using common modern anticoagulants. Development of new or exaggerated neurologic symptoms any time after placement should warrant further neurologic examination, neuraxial imaging, or consultation of neurosurgery, especially when anticoagulants are administered in high-risk patients or patients with coagulopathy.

Epidural abscess is extraordinarily uncommon, but it can be more sinister because symptoms are often nonspecific.[43] Incidence of epidural abscess complicating epidural placement is difficult to estimate, with studies ranging from 1 in 1000 to 1 in 100,000.[44–46] Grewal and colleagues[44] assert that certain risk factors may predispose to epidural abscess: compromised immunity (ie, diabetes mellitus, immunosuppression therapy, cancer),

disruption of the spinal column by previous surgery or instrumentation, duration of catheterization, and coexisting sources of infection. Patients undergoing thoracic operations frequently possess one or more of these risk factors. Presenting symptoms of epidural abscess show remarkable inconsistency, despite traditional teaching that a patient will classically present with new neurologic symptoms, fever, and back pain.[47] The importance of vigilance and a high index of suspicion for these complications in patients with a recent neuraxial intervention cannot be overstated. Many reported cases presented well after the patient was discharged from inpatient care, so patients should be instructed to self-monitor for concerning signs and symptoms.[47]

The benefits of TEA in reducing postsurgical pulmonary complications over the past few decades have been eroded by a combination of improved surgical technique, prophylactic antibiotics, early mobilization, and more aggressive pulmonary physiotherapy.[48] TEA is still the most preferred thoracic pain management technique, but its routine use has been increasingly questioned.[49–51]

### Paravertebral Analgesia

Although TEA has long been considered the gold standard for thoracic operations, PVB has been increasing steadily in popularity. Reasons for the increasing popularity of paravertebral analgesia include the emergence of ultrasound guidance to facilitate easier and more accurate paravertebral catheter placement (PVB has been traditionally been placed using landmark/loss of resistance technique, and, intraoperatively, under direct visualization), and a more favorable side effect profile as compared with TEA. Multiple reviews and meta-analysis have shown no difference in pain scores, postoperative pulmonary function, and postoperative pulmonary complications in patients undergoing thoracic procedures between PVB and TEA.[32,52]

Joshi and colleagues[32] concluded in their systemic reviews of randomized controlled trials that continuous PVB provides comparable pain relief to continuous TEA when local anesthetic alone was used in both infusions. The evidence for superiority between the two modalities was inconclusive when it came to continuous infusions containing both local anesthetic and opioid. A more recent randomized controlled trial by Grider and colleagues[53] studied patients undergoing thoracotomy receiving either continuous PVB with bupivacaine alone, TEA with bupivacaine alone, or TEA with bupivacaine and hydromorphone. Although the groups receiving PVB with bupivacaine and TEA with bupivacaine alone had similar VAS scores, the group with TEA with bupivacaine and hydromorphone had statistically significant lower VAS scores than the other two groups. This suggests that although PVB and TEA modalities may offer similar pain control, bupivacaine and hydromorphone can work synergistically in the epidural space to provide better analgesia.

Multiple studies have demonstrated that PVB results in better postoperative pulmonary function and less adverse effects on hemodynamics compared with TEA. The prospective, multicenter, observational trial by Powell and colleagues[54] comparing the effect of PVB versus TEA on major postoperative complications in patients undergoing pneumonectomy concluded that the PVB group experienced lower incidence of hypotension requiring inotropes, arrhythmia requiring antiarrhythmics, respiratory complications requiring ventilator support, and need for surgical re-exploration. From a technical standpoint, placement of a paravertebral catheter is unlikely to result in accidental dural puncture that can lead to postdural puncture headache, a complication infrequently associated with the placement of thoracic epidural catheters. Position of the paravertebral catheter outside the rigid epidural space also means that the possibility of catastrophic neurologic injuries associated with TEA, such as epidural hematoma or epidural abscess, is less likely. Still, the most recent ASRA guidelines[39,40] recommend that the same anticoagulation guidelines for neuraxial procedures also be applied to "deep peripheral" blocks (such as PVB). Strict application of these guidelines limits the use of PVB when TEA is also contraindicated because of existing coagulopathy. **Table 3** shows current recommendations for the discontinuation of common anticoagulant and antiplatelet therapies before neuraxial and paravertebral procedures.[55] However, in the setting of thrombocytopenia, PVB has been used safely.[56] It should be noted that many anesthesiologists are more comfortable placing epidural catheters than PVBs. However, the reported failure rate of PVB (~6% per[57]) is lower than that of TEA (10%–15% per[36]).

Injection of medication within the paravertebral space may spread less reliably when compared with that in the epidural space. Up to 70% of patients with PVB have some degree of epidural spread. Spread of infusion from the paravertebral space into the epidural space through the vertebral foramen has limited side effects, such as transient hypotension and/or contralateral numbness, which may mimic the effects of TEA. The incidence of epidural spread of PVB seems to be higher with larger volume of injectate (single large-volume

bolus in the paravertebral space is more susceptible to epidural spread compared with small, repeated boluses or continuous infusions through a catheter) and with the use of ultrasound guidance.[58] Another potential risk of PVB is pleural injury resulting in pneumothorax, which can be minimized under intraoperative, direct visualization. The use of ultrasound does not guarantee safe, extrapleural PVB catheter placement,[59] but likely reduces the incidence of pneumothorax in the hands of an experienced anesthesiologist. Vascular injury is also a concern given the highly vascular nature of the paravertebral space. However, because of the large volume of the paravertebral space, the likelihood of a hematoma causing significant adverse effects is remote.

It should be noted that a continuous infusion through a paravertebral catheter should be preferred over a single injection for patients undergoing thoracic operations given its ability extend the duration of pain management. If only a single paravertebral injection is possible, longer-acting local anesthetics, such as bupivacaine or ropivacaine, should be considered to give the patient longer duration of pain control. The commonly used local anesthetics lidocaine, bupivacaine, and ropivacaine seem equally efficacious when infused continuously in the paravertebral space. Unlike TEA, the addition of opioids to local anesthetics has not been shown to improve pain control in PVB, and therefore is not recommended.[60]

Several studies have demonstrated that PVB is superior to TEA in reducing the incidence of hypotension without compromising quality of analgesia.[61–63] PVB was also shown to lead to less nausea/vomiting and urinary retention than TEA.[61]

Although it can be argued that TEA and PVB are both viable options for many unilateral thoracic procedures, certain operations favor TEA because of its bilateral and arguably more complete analgesia. Examples include bilateral lung transplant or heart-lung transplant (bilateral thoracotomy with sternal transection), Ivor-Lewis esophagectomy (right thoracotomy with midline laparotomy), and thoracoabdominal aneurysm repair (left thoracotomy with variable midline incision). Although more labor intensive, bilateral PVB still remains an option for these procedures. Richardson and colleagues[64] reviewed 12 studies that used bilateral PVB and concluded that this method was a reasonable alternative to epidural anesthesia with complications, such as hypotension and pneumothorax (3.6% and 1%, respectively; N = 196), deemed low-risk. Ostensibly, level of comfort with performing PVB considerably limits use of bilateral PVB and likely raises the risk of complications.

**Table 3**
Anticoagulation guidelines for regional anesthesia and analgesia: Wake Forest University RAAPM recommendations to avoid increasing the risk of neuraxial hematoma following neuraxial analgesic/anesthetic procedures

| Anticoagulant (Half-Life) | Anticoagulant Type | Minimum Delay Between Last Dose of Anticoagulant and Performance of Neuraxial Technique | Minimum Delay Between Neuraxial Technique or Catheter Removal and Next Anticoagulant Dose | Other Precautions |
|---|---|---|---|---|
| Heparin (unfractionated)[b] Intravenous (1.5 h) | Pro–antithrombin III (anti-II,X) | 2–4 h and aPTT WNL[a] | ≥1 h[40] | c |
| Heparin (unfractionated)[b] (1.5 h) SQ BID ≤10,000 U/day | Pro–antithrombin III (anti-II,X) | No restriction,[40] caution during peak 1–4 h postdose[a] | No restriction[40] | c |
| Heparin (unfractionated)[b] (1.5 h) SQ TID ≥10,000 U/d | Pro–antithrombin III (anti-II,X) | Insufficient data and caution advised[40] >6 h[a] | ≥1 h[40] (unless first dose then no restriction)[a] | c |
| Enoxaparin (Lovenox) (3–6 h) prophylaxis 40 mg QD or 30 mg BID | LMWH anti-Xa | 12 h[40] | Initiate ≥4 h postremoval[40] (BID use not recommended with indwelling catheter)[40,41] | c |
| Enoxaparin (Lovenox) (3–6 h) therapeutic 1 mg/kg BID or 1.5 mg/kg QD | LMWH anti-Xa | 24 h[40] | Not recommended with catheter[40] Initiate ≥4 h postremoval[a,41] | c |
| Fondaparinux (Arixtra) (17–21 h) | Pentasaccharide anti-Xa | 4.5 d and/or heparin assay[a] | Contraindicated with catheter[40] Initiate ≥2 h postremoval[a] | c |
| Rivaroxaban (Xarelto) (5–13 h) | Anti-Xa | 48–72[a] For catheter removal 22–26 h[42] | 6 h, or 24 h if traumatic insertion (package insert)[42] | c,d |
| Warfarin (Coumadin) (60 h) | Vitamin K–dependent factor inhibition | 4–5 d and INR WNL (≤1.2)[40] for removal INR ≤1.5[40] | Guided by INR[40] | c |
| Aspirin/NSAIDS (>72 h) | Antiplatelet | No restrictions[40] | No restrictions[40] | — |
| Clopidogrel (Plavix) (6–8 h) | Irreversible platelet aggregation inhibitor | 7 d[40] | Not recommended with catheter[40] Initiate ≥2 h postremoval[a] | — |
| Ticlopicline (Ticlid) (4–5 d with repeated doses) | Irreversible platelet aggregation inhibitor | 14 d[40] | Not recommended with catheter[40] Initiate ≥2 h postremoval[a] | — |

| | | | | |
|---|---|---|---|---|
| Prasugrel (Effient) (7 h) | Irreversible platelet aggregation inhibitor | 7–10 d[42] | Not recommended with catheter[42] Initiate $\geq$2 h postremoval[a] | — |
| Ticagrelor (Brilinta) (7–12 h) | ADP reversible receptor blocker | 5 d[42] | Not recommended with catheter[42] Initiate $\geq$2 h postremoval[a] | d |
| Abciximab (Reopro) (30 min) | Glycoprotein IIb/IIIa inhibitor | 48 h[40] | Not recommended with catheter[40] Initiate $\geq$2 h postremoval[a] | — |
| Eptifibatide (Integrilin) (2.5 h) | Glycoprotein IIb/IIIa inhibitor | 8 h[40] | Not recommended with catheter[40] Initiate $\geq$2 h postremoval[a] | — |
| Tirofiban (Aggrastat) (2 h) | Glycoprotein IIb/IIIa inhibitor | 8 h[40] | Not recommended with catheter[40] Initiate $\geq$2 h postremoval[a] | — |
| Bivalrudin (Augiomax) Desirudi (Iprivask) Argatroban (Acova) | Thrombin (II) Inhibitor (IV) | Insufficient data[40] Neuraxial techniques not recommended[a] | Insufficient data[40] | — |
| Dabigatran (Pradaxa) (17 h) (prolonged with CRI) | Thrombin (II) Inhibitor (oral) | 5 d[a] | Not recommended with catheter[40] Initiate $\geq$6 h postremoval[42] | c |
| Apixaban (Eliquis) (12–15 h) | Oral factor Xa inhibitor | 4 d[a] | $\geq$6 h[42] | d |

*Note:* Recommendations are based on single drug use, combinations increase risk. Caution if traumatic neuraxial technique. Recommendation compliance does not eliminate the risk for neuraxial hematoma.

*Abbreviations:* ADP, adenosine diphosphate; aPTT, activated partial thromboplastin time; BID, twice daily; CRI, continuous rate infusion; INR, international normalized ratio; LMWH, low-molecular-weight heparin; QD, every day; SQ, subcutaneous; TID, three times a day; WNL, within normal limits.

[a] Our current practice, no current published guidelines.
[b] Patients receiving unfractionated heparin should have platelet count checked after 4 days to monitor for possible heparin-induced thrombocytopenia.
[c] Caution with CRI, low weight, elderly.
[d] T 1/2 doubled with strong CYP3A4 inhibitors (antifungals, antiretrovirals).

*From* Henshaw DS, Jaffe JD, Weller RS. Quick Reference Guide for Regional Anesthesia in the Anticoagulated Patient. Available at: http://www.nysora.com/newsletterz/2014/4313-july-2014-newsletter.html. Accessed July 27, 2015; with permission.

## Intrathecal Opioid Analgesia

Intrathecal opioids can also be used to control postoperative pain. This technique typically involves the administration of a small amount of morphine, often as a single injection, into the intrathecal space. Because of its hydrophilic characteristic, morphine spreads rostrally in the cerebrospinal fluid. Therefore an injection at the lumbar level can produce analgesia for thoracic and upper abdominal operations. Pain relief from intrathecal morphine typically lasts up to 24 hours after injection.

Meylan and colleagues,[65] in a recent meta-analysis of 27 studies on intrathecal morphine analgesia in major thoracic and abdominal operations, concluded that intrathecal morphine can effectively reduce pain at rest and on movement postoperatively, with pain reduction most significant during the first 4 hours, extending up to 24 hours. The authors found that the total opioid requirement was decreased intraoperatively and up to 48 hours postsurgery after intrathecal morphine. However, this decrease in opioid use was more statistically significant for major abdominal surgeries compared with thoracic surgeries, and there was an increased risk of respiratory depression and pruritus.

Dango and colleagues,[66] in a more recent randomized controlled trial, compared intrathecal morphine in combination with paravertebral analgesia against TEA for thoracotomy. The author showed that postthoracotomy pain relief in both groups was similar. The need to combine paravertebral analgesia with intrathecal morphine in this particular study, however, makes it more difficult to assess the effectiveness of intrathecal morphine alone.

Suksompong and colleagues,[67] most recently, studied the effectiveness of two different dosages of intrathecal morphine, 0.2 mg versus 0.3 mg, for postthoracotomy analgesia in a group of 40 patients. The authors found no significant difference between the two groups in pain-free time, time to first drinking, eating, sitting, or walking. Total opioid consumption was also equivalent between the two groups at 24 and 48 hours postsurgery. Of note, one patient in the 0.3-mg intrathecal morphine group developed respiratory depression but did not require intubation, prompting the authors to conclude that higher intrathecal morphine may lead to increased risk of respiratory depression without concomitant benefits of opioid reduction. Other common side effects of intrathecal morphine include pruritus, nausea, vomiting, and urinary retention.

## Intercostal Analgesia

ICNB analgesia is a well-established technique for controlling postthoracotomy pain. ICNB is easy to perform, and can be done quickly with the patient in a variety of positions. This stands in stark contrast to the neuraxial techniques described previously (TEA, PVB, and intrathecal opioid analgesia), where optional patient positioning is necessary to safely access the neuraxis. Placement of an intercostal nerve block or catheter (eg, On-Q pump) therefore can be done either preoperatively, postoperatively, or intraoperatively at the end of the operation under direct visualization by the surgeon.

Joshi and colleagues,[32] in their systematic review of regional techniques for postthoracotomy analgesia, concluded that intercostal analgesia was superior to systemic analgesia. Postoperative pain scores with ICNB were superior to placebo, particularly when administered as repeated boluses or infusions. The disadvantages of ICNB include an insufficient duration of action because a large percentage of the local anesthetic injected is absorbed into the bloodstream, leading to high risk of local anesthetic systemic toxicity. Although ICNB catheters may extend the duration of analgesia, multiple catheters (one per each rib) would be needed to provide coverage equivalent to a single catheter placed in the neuraxis, and would theoretically lead to an even higher risk of local anesthetic toxicity.

Studies comparing ICNB with TEA have generally been conflicting with respect to analgesic effectiveness, total opioid consumption, and postoperative pulmonary function.[68] Taken as a whole, ICNB is an attractive alternate to TEA and PVB, especially when neuraxial techniques are not possible or contraindicated. Our typical practice is to use ICNB in all thoracic operations, including open and VATS approaches, when technically feasible.

## Intrapleural Analgesia

Intrapleural analgesia involves the injection of local anesthetic into the pleural space between the parietal and visceral pleura, with the goal of having the local anesthetic diffuse across the parietal pleura to block thoracic nerves. Intrapleural nerve block, even when performed correctly, has a much lower level of effectiveness in controlling postthoracotomy pain when compared with TEA or PVB techniques.[32] As such, this method of regional anesthesia is not recommended because of its analgesic inferiority combined with its potential for local anesthetic systemic toxicity.

## Cryoanalgesia

Cryoanalgesia involves the freezing of intercostal nerves, resulting in axonal disintegration and neurolysis, to provide postthoracotomy pain relief. The most recent review by Khanbhai and colleagues[69] examined 12 separate studies on cryoanalgesia. The author concluded that half of the studies fail to show cryoanalgesia to be better than other methods when it comes to pain control. Furthermore, there was an increased incidence of postoperative neuropathic pain in patients receiving cryoanalgesia. Because of its tendency to potentiate PTPS, cryoanalgesia is not a recommended regional technique for controlling pain post thoracic surgeries.

## CHRONIC POSTTHORACOTOMY PAIN

The incidence of PTPS after thoracotomy is approximately 30% to 50%. The International Association for the Study of Pain defines PTPS as pain that recurs or persists along a thoracotomy scar greater than 2 months after surgery. PTPS is believed to be the result of intercostal nerve injury, resulting in the transmission of pain signals from chest wall and pleura. Injury to these intercostal nerves can occur during the course of surgical incision, rib retraction, trocar placement, or suturing. Like most neuropathic pain syndromes, PTPS is a challenging diagnosis. Predicting which patients will develop PTPS is difficult and prevention of PTPS is confounded by lack of understanding of the pathophysiologic mechanism underlying the development of neuropathic pain. Modalities used in the treatment of PTPS have yielded mostly disappointing results.

## Prevention

Many patients with inadequately treated pain during the perioperative period go on to develop PTPS. Therefore, optimal pain management in the acute setting is paramount. The concept of preventive analgesia (the prevention of central pain sensitization by blockade of all pain signals from reaching the central nervous system from the onset of surgical incision until final wound healing) is generally accepted as the best way to prevent PTPS. Systematic reviews of published literature have suggested that the best method for thoracotomy pain control involves the use of a regional anesthesia technique, such as TEA or PVB analgesia. If these techniques are contraindicated or impossible, intrathecal opioid analgesia or intercostal analgesia can be considered, typically in conjunction with a multimodal analgesic regimen that uses other analgesic therapies,

such as systemic opioid, acetaminophen, NSAIDs, COX-2 selective inhibitors, and other analgesic adjuncts.[70] Overall, there is evidence that TEA can be helpful in the prevention of PTPS, although the timing of initiation of TEA has not been shown to be clinically significant. PVB, although clearly effective in the acute treatment of postthoracotomy pain, has not been adequately investigated in the prevention of PTPS. Similarly, intercostal analgesia and intrathecal analgesia lack adequate evidence in their ability to affect long-term outcome. Cryoanalgesia, meanwhile, has been found to increase the incidence of PTPS in several studies.

Definitive studies regarding the effectiveness of adjunct medications in preventing PTPS are likewise lacking. Low-dose ketamine has been shown to be quite effective in reducing postoperative pain in the immediate term (up to 1 week postoperatively), but fails to prevent development of chronic pain at long-term follow-up (at 3 months and 6 months postoperatively).[20] Besides anecdotal evidence, there is little literature supporting the effectiveness of acetaminophen, COX-2 inhibitors, or NSAIDs in preventing PTPS.[70] Future studies on the subject are therefore warranted.

Refinements in surgical technique have been thought to potentially reduce postthoracotomy pain and subsequent development of PTPS. It is still unclear, however, whether any thoracotomy approaches can actually decrease the incidence of PTPS. Two retrospective studies by Nomori and colleagues[71,72] suggested that the anterior approach may result less in PTPS, whereas separate studies by Landreneau and colleagues[73] and Khan and colleagues[74] each concluded no difference between muscle-sparing thoracotomy and standard posterolateral thoracotomies. The lack of prospective randomized controlled trials means that this area may be an interesting topic for future research. Meanwhile, data regarding VATS and PTPS are conflicting, with two prospective trials suggesting no difference in the incidence of PTPS when compared with the classic or muscle-sparing posterolateral approach, and one retrospective trial finding a lower incidence of PTPS for VATS when compared with muscle-sparing thoracotomy.[6]

Wildgaard and colleagues,[75] in their critical review, concluded that specific surgical techniques that may reduce the incidence of PTPS include harvesting an intercostal muscle flap (eg, "dangle" the intercostal nerve bundle away from the rib spreader to prevent it from being crushed), free dissection of intercostal nerves, and the use of intracostal sutures for closing the incision. The use of intracostal sutures and the harvesting of intercostal muscle flap to reduce PTPS are supported by Cerfolio and colleagues,[76,77] who arrive at the same conclusion in separate studies.

## Treatment

The treatment of PTPS, like other neuropathic pain syndromes, can be challenging. There are few studies designed to specifically investigate the treatment of PTPS, and most suffer from a variety of methodologic flaws. Broadly speaking, the management of PTPS is divided into pharmacologic and interventional modalities.

### Pharmacologic

Because chronic persistent surgical pain, such as PTPS, is thought to be neuropathic in nature, systemic opioid therapy may not be effective. Gabapentinoids, however, theoretically have benefits. Solak and colleagues[29] showed in their prospective, randomized, controlled study of 40 patients with PTPS that those receiving gabapentin showed significantly lower pain scores after 60 days with treatment when compared with those receiving naproxen. The authors concluded that gabapentin is safe and effective in treatment of PTPS, with high patient compliance and tolerability. Pregabalin, like gabapentin, is a structural analog of $\gamma$-aminobutyric acid and is commonly used to treat neuropathic pain. Studies have demonstrated that pregabalin can reduce opioid consumption perioperatively; however, it has high incidence of visual disturbances. It should be noted that both gabapentin and pregabalin can cause drowsiness and dizziness.

Other medications typically used in the treatment of PTPS include tricyclic antidepressant, serotonin-norepinephrine reuptake inhibitors, tramadol, and lidocaine. Unfortunately, their effectiveness is mostly anecdotal and further research is necessary.

### Interventional

Beyond pharmacologic treatment, case reports and retrospective studies have suggested that interventions, such as ICNB, pulsed radiofrequency of the dorsal root ganglion, and spinal cord and peripheral nerve stimulation, can provide some benefits in the treatment of PTPS. In a randomized controlled trial, the use of acupuncture for the treatment of PTPS was found to be ineffective.[78] Epidural steroid injection, a technique common in the management of neuropathic pain, does not have any formal literature supporting its use in the treatment of PTPS.

## REFERENCES

1. Gerner P. Postthoracotomy pain management problems. Anesthesiol Clin 2008;26:355–67.

2. Ochroch EA, Gottschalk A. Impact of acute pain and its management for thoracic surgical patients. Thorac Surg Clin 2005;15(1):105–21.

3. Sapkota R, Shrestha UK, Sayami P. Intercostal muscle flap and intracostal suture to reduce post-thoracotomy pain. Asian Cardiovasc Thorac Ann 2013;22(6):706–11.

4. Flores RM, Park BJ, Dycoco J, et al. Lobectomy by video-assisted thoracic surgery (VATS) versus thoracotomy for lung cancer. J Thorac Cardiovasc Surg 2009;138(1):11–8.

5. Landreneau RJ, Mack MJ, Hazelrigg SR, et al. Prevalence of chronic pain after pulmonary resection by thoracotomy or video-assisted thoracic surgery. J Thorac Cardiovasc Surg 1994;107(4):1079–85.

6. Rogers ML, Duff JP. Surgical aspects of chronic post-thoracotomy pain. Eur J Cardiothorac Surg 2000;18:711–6.

7. Tiippana E, Nelskylä K, Nilsson E, et al. Managing post-thoracotomy pain: epidural or systemic analgesia and extended care: a randomized study with an "as usual" control group. Scand J Pain 2015;5(4):240–7.

8. Senard M, Deflandre EP, Ledoux D, et al. Effect of celecoxib combined with thoracic epidural analgesia on pain after thoracotomy. Br J Anaesth 2010;105(2):196–200.

9. Ong CK, Seymour RA, Lirk P, et al. Combining paracetamol (acetaminophen) with nonsteroidal antiinflammatory drugs: a qualitative systematic review of analgesic efficacy for acute postoperative pain. Anesth Analg 2010;110(4):1170–9.

10. Pavy T, Medley C, Murphy DF. Effect of indomethacin on pain relief after thoracotomy. Br J Anaesth 1990;65(5):624–7.

11. Boussofara M, Mtaallah MH, Bracco D, et al. Co-analgesic effect of ketorolac after thoracic surgery. Tunis Med 2006;84(7):427–31.

12. Peduto VA, Ballabio M, Stefanini S. Efficacy of propacetamol in the treatment of postoperative pain: morphine-sparing effect in orthopedic surgery. Acta Anaesthesiol Scand 1998;42(3):293–8.

13. Hernández-Palazón J, Tortosa JA, Martínez-Lage JF, et al. Intravenous administration of propacetamol reduces morphine consumption after spinal fusion surgery. Anesth Analg 2001;92:1473–6.

14. Khalili G, Janghorbani M, Saryazdi H, et al. Effect of preemptive and preventive acetaminophen on postoperative pain score: a randomized, double-blind trial of patients undergoing lower extremity surgery. J Clin Anesth 2013;25(3):188–92.

15. Memis D, Inal MT, Kavalci G, et al. Intravenous paracetamol reduced the use of opioids, extubation time, and opioid-related adverse effects after major surgery in intensive care unit. J Crit Care 2010;25(3):458–62.

16. Mac TB, Girard F, Chouinard P, et al. Acetaminophen decreases early post-thoracotomy ipsilateral

shoulder pain in patients with thoracic epidural analgesia: a double-blind placebo-controlled study. J Cardiothorac Vasc Anesth 2005;19(4):475–8.

17. Pisani MA, Murphy TE, Araujo KL, et al. Benzodiazepine and opioid use and the duration of intensive care unit delirium in an older population. Crit Care Med 2009;37(1):177–83.

18. Laskowski K, Murphy TE, Araujo KL, et al. A systematic review of intravenous ketamine for postoperative analgesia. Can J Anaesth 2011; 58(10):911–23.

19. Suzuki M, Haraguti S, Sugimoto K, et al. Low-dose intravenous ketamine potentiates epidural analgesia after thoracotomy. Anesthesiology 2006;105(1):111–9.

20. Mendola C, Cammarota G, Netto R, et al. S (+) ketamine for control of perioperative pain and prevention of post-thoracotomy pain syndrome: a randomized, double-blind study. Minerva Anestesiol 2012;78:757–66.

21. Himmelseher S, Durieux ME. Ketamine for perioperative pain management. Anesthesiology 2005; 102(1):211–20.

22. Guillou N, Tanguy M, Seguin P, et al. The effects of small-dose ketamine on morphine consumption in surgical intensive care unit patients after major abdominal surgery. Anesth Analg 2003;97:843–7.

23. Chia YY, Liu K, Liu YC, et al. Adding ketamine in a multimodal patient-controlled epidural regimen reduces postoperative pain and analgesic consumption. Anesth Analg 1998;86:1245–9.

24. Wahlander S, Frumento RJ, Wagener G, et al. A prospective, double-blind, randomized, placebo-controlled study of dexmedetomidine as an adjunct to epidural analgesia after thoracic surgery. J Cardiothorac Vasc Anesth 2005;19(5):630–5.

25. Ramsay MA, Newman KB, Leeper B, et al. Dexmedetomidine infusion for analgesia up to 48 hours after lung surgery performed by lateral thoracotomy. Proc (Bayl Univ Med Cent) 2014;27(1):3–10.

26. Humble SR, Dalton AJ, Li L. A systematic review of therapeutic interventions to reduce acute and chronic post-surgical pain after amputation, thoracotomy or mastectomy. Eur J Pain 2015;19(4):451–65.

27. Available at: http://www.ncbi.nlm.nih.gov/pubmed/21676165.

28. Omran AF, Mohamed AE. A randomized study of the effects of gabapentin versus placebo on post-thoracotomy pain and pulmonary function. Eg J Anaesth 2005;21:277–81.

29. Solak O, Metin M, Esme H, et al. Effectiveness of gabapentin in the treatment of chronic post-thoracotomy pain. Eur J Cardiothorac Surg 2007; 32:9–12.

30. Vigneault L, Turgeon AF, Côté D, et al. Perioperative intravenous lidocaine infusion for postoperative pain control: a meta-analysis of randomized controlled trials. Can J Anaesth 2011;58(1):22–37.

31. Cui W, Turgeon AF, Côté D, et al. Systemic administration of lidocaine reduces morphine requirements and postoperative pain of patients undergoing thoracic surgery after propofol-remifentanil-based anaesthesia. Eur J Anaesthesiol 2010;27(1):41–6.

32. Joshi GP, Bonnet F, Shah R, et al. A systematic review of randomized trials evaluating regional techniques for postthoracotomy analgesia. Anesth Analg 2008;107:1026–40.

33. Bauer C, Hentz JG, Ducrocq X, et al. Lung function after lobectomy: a randomized, double-blinded trial comparing thoracic epidural ropivacaine/sufentanil and intravenous morphine for patient-controlled analgesia. Anesth Analg 2007;105:238–44.

34. Ali M, Winter DC, Hanly AM, et al. Prospective randomized, controlled trial of thoracic epidural or patient-controlled opiate analgesia on perioperative quality of life. Br J Anaesth 2010;104:292–7.

35. Oka T, Ozawa Y, Ohkubo Y. Thoracic epidural bupivacaine attenuates supraventricular tachyarrhythmias after pulmonary resection. Anesth Analg 2001;93:153–9.

36. Hermanides J, Hollmann MW, Stevens MF, et al. Failed epidural: causes and management. Br J Anaesth 2012;109(2):144–54.

37. Ready LB. Acute pain: lessons learned from 25,000 patients. Reg Anesth Pain Med 1999;24:499–505.

38. Bateman BT, Mhyre JM, Ehrenfeld J, et al. The risk and outcomes of epidural hematomas after perioperative and obstetric epidural catheterization: a report from the Multicenter Perioperative Outcomes Group Research Consortium. Anesth Analg 2013; 116(6):1380–5.

39. Horlocker T, Kopp S. Epidural hematoma after epidural blockade in the United States: it's not just low molecular heparin following orthopedic surgery anymore. Anesth Analg 2013;116(6):1195–7.

40. Horlocker T, Wedel DJ, Rowlingson JC, et al. Regional anesthesia in the patient receiving antithrombotic or thrombolytic therapy: American Society of Regional Anesthesia and Pain Medicine evidence-based guidelines (third edition). Reg Anesth Pain Med 2010;35(1):64–101.

41. ASRA Safety Announcement: Updated recommendations to decrease risk of spinal column bleeding and paralysis in patients on low molecular weight heparins, 11/6/13.

42. Regional anesthesia and Antithrombotic agents: recommendations of the European Society of Anesthesiology.

43. Chan YC, Dasey N. Iatrogenic spinal epidural abscess. Acta Chir Belg 2007;107(2):109–18.

44. Grewal S, Hocking G, Wildsmith JAW. Epidural abscesses. Br J Anaesth 2006;96(3):292–302.

45. Grieve JP, Ashwood N, O'Neill KS, et al. A retrospective study of surgical and conservative treatment for spinal extradural abscess. Eur Spine J 2000;9:67–71.

46. Phillips JM, Stedeford JC, Hartsilver E, et al. Epidural abscess complicating insertion of epidural catheters. Br J Anaesth 2002;89:778–82.

47. Darouiche RO. Spinal epidural abscess. N Engl J Med 2006;355(19):2012–20.

48. Popping DM, Elia N, Marret E, et al. Protective effects of epidural analgesia on pulmonary complications after abdominal and thoracic surgery: a meta-analysis. Arch Surg 2008;143:990–9.

49. Low J, Johnston N, Morris C. Epidural analgesia: First do no harm. Anaesthesia 2008;63:1–3.

50. Freise H, Van Aken HK. Risks and benefits of thoracic epidural anaesthesia. Br J Anaesth 2011;107:859–68.

51. Rawal N. Epidural technique for postoperative pain gold standard no more? Reg Anesth Pain Med 2012;37:310–7.

52. Kotze A, Scally A, Howell S. Efficacy and safety of different techniques of paravertebral block for analgesia after thoracotomy: a systematic review and metaregression. Br J Anaesth 2009;103:626–36.

53. Grider JS, Mullet TW, Saha SP, et al. A randomized double-blind trial comparing continuous thoracic epidural bupivacaine with and without opioid in contrast to a continuous paravertebral infusion of bupivacaine for post-thoracotomy pain. J Cardiothorac Vasc Anesth 2012;26:83–9.

54. Powell ES, Cook D, Pearce AC, et al. A prospective, multicentre, observational cohort study of analgesia and outcome after pneumonectomy. Br J Anaesth 2011;106:364–70.

55. Henshaw D, Jaffe J, Weller R. Quick reference guide for regional anesthesia in the anticoagulated patient. New York School of Regional Anesthesia; 2014. Available at: http://www.nysora.com/newsletterz/2014/4313-july-2014-newsletter.html. Accessed July 27, 2015.

56. Nguyen VH, de Souza DG, Blank RS, et al. Ultrasound-guided thoracic paravertebral catheter placement in a patient undergoing thoracotomy who had the relative contraindication of thrombocytopenia to epidural placement. J Cardiothorac Vasc Anesth 2012;26:666–8.

57. Naja Z, Lönnqvist PA. Somatic paravertebral nerve blockade. Incidence of failed block and complications. Anaesthesia 2001;56(12):1184–8.

58. Chelly JE. Paravertebral blocks. Anesthesiol Clin 2012;30:75–90.

59. Kus A, Gurkan Y, Gul Akgul A, et al. Pleural puncture and intrathoracic catheter placement during ultrasound guided paravertebral block. J Cardiothorac Vasc Anesth 2013;27(2):11–2.

60. Romero A, Garcia JE, Joshi GP. The state of the art in preventing postthoracotomy pain. Semin Thorac Cardiovasc Surg 2013;25:116–24.

61. Ding X, Jin S, Niu X, et al. A comparison of the analgesia efficacy and side effects of paravertebral compared with epidural blockade for thoracotomy: an updated meta-analysis. PLoS One 2014;9(5): e96233.

62. Baidya DK, Khanna P, Maitra S. Analgesic efficacy and safety of thoracic paravertebral and epidural analgesia for thoracic surgery: a systematic review and meta-analysis. Interact Cardiovasc Thorac Surg 2014;18(5):626–35.

63. Okajima H, Tanaka O, Ushio M, et al. Ultrasound-guided continuous thoracic paravertebral block provides comparable analgesia and fewer episodes of hypotension than continuous epidural block after lung surgery. J Anesth 2015;29(3):373–8.

64. Richardson J, Lönnqvist PA, Naja Z. Bilateral thoracic paravertebral block: potential and practice. Br J Anaesth 2011;106(2):164–71.

65. Meylan N, Elia N, Lysakowski C, et al. Benefits and risks of intrathetcal morphine without local anaesthetic in patients undergoing major surgery: meta-analysis of randomized trials. Br J Anaesth 2009; 102:156–67.

66. Dango S, Harris S, Offner K, et al. Combined paravertebral and intrathecal vs thoracic epidural analgesia for post-thoracotomy pain relief. Br J Anaesth 2013;110:443–9.

67. Suksompong S, Pongpayuha P, Lertpaitoonpan W, et al. Low-dose spinal morphine for post-thoracotomy pain: a prospective randomized study. J Cardiothorac Vasc Anesth 2013;27:417–22.

68. Meierhenrich R, Hock D, Kuhn S, et al. Analgesia and pulmonary function after lung surgery: Is a single intercostal nerve block plus patient-controlled intravenous morphine as effective as patient-controlled epidural anesthesia? A randomized non-inferiority clinical trial. Br J Anaesth 2011;106:580–9.

69. Khanbhai M, Yap KH, Mohamed S, et al. Is cryoanalgesia effective for post-thoracotomy pain? Interact Cardiovasc Thorac Surg 2014;18:202–9.

70. Doan LV, Augustus J, Androphy R, et al. Mitigating the impact of acute and chronic post-thoracotomy pain. J Cardiothorac Vasc Anesth 2014;28:1060–8.

71. Nomori H, Horio H, Suemasu K. Anterior limited thoracotomy with intrathoracic illumination for lung cancer: its advantages over anteroaxillary and posterolateral thoracotomy. Chest 1999;115:874–80.

72. Nomori H, Horio H, Suemasu K. Intrathoracic light-assisted anterior limited thoracotomy in lung cancer surgery. Surg Today 1999;29:606–9.

73. Landreneau RJ, Pigula F, Luketich JD, et al. Acute and chronic morbidity differences between muscle-sparing and standard lateral thoracotomies. J Thorac Cardiovasc Surg 1996;112:1346–50.

74. Khan IH, McManus KG, McCraith A, et al. Muscle sparing thoracotomy: a biomechanical analysis confirms preservation of muscle strength but no improvement in wound discomfort. Eur J Cardiothorac Surg 2000;18:656–61.

75. Wildgaard K, Ravn J, Kehlet H. Chronic post-thoracotomy pain: a critical review of pathogenic mechanisms and strategies for prevention. Eur J Cardiothorac Surg 2009;36:170–80.

76. Cerfolio RJ, Bryant AS, Patel B, et al. Intercostal muscle flap reduces the pain of thoracotomy: a prospective randomized trial. J Thorac Cardiovasc Surg 2005;130:987–93.

77. Cerfolio RJ, Bryant AS, Maniscalco LM. A nondivided intercostal muscle flap further reduces pain of thoracotomy: a prospective randomized trial. Ann Thorac Surg 2008;85:1901–6.

78. Deng G, Rusch V, Vickers A, et al. Randomized controlled trial of a special acupuncture technique for pain after thoracotomy. J Thorac Cardiovasc Surg 2008;136:1464–9.

# The Prevention and Management of Air Leaks Following Pulmonary Resection

Bryan M. Burt, MD[a], Joseph B. Shrager, MD[b,c],*

## KEYWORDS

- Pulmonary resection • Postoperative • Air leak • Alveolar pleural fistula

## KEY POINTS

- Based on preoperative risk factors, selected patients should be considered for intraoperative techniques to minimize air leaks and the residual spaces that predispose to prolonged air leaks, including pleural tenting and pneumoperitoneum.
- There is insufficient evidence for the routine use of surgical sealants following pulmonary resection; we recommend buttressing staple lines in nonanatomic pulmonary resections for patients with moderate to severe emphysema (forced expiratory volume in 1 second <60% of predicted) to prevent prolonged air leaks.
- In postoperative patients with less than a large air leak and no more than a small pneumothorax, algorithms incorporating no applied external suction or alternating suction likely reduce the duration of air leak.
- Initial evaluation of digital drainage systems suggest that their use may result in shorter duration of air leak, duration of chest tube, and length of stay.
- Most prolonged alveolar air leaks resolve with time and tube drainage alone, and a trial of a few weeks of watchful waiting incorporating a Heimlich valve is reasonable in the outpatient setting.

## INTRODUCTION

Alveolar air leaks after pulmonary resection are a common problem in thoracic surgery. A variety of reports have shown that an air leak is present immediately on completion of a routine pulmonary resection in 28% to 60% of patients, after both lobectomies and lesser resections. On the morning of postoperative day 1, an air leak is present in 26% to 48% of patients; on the morning of postoperative day 2, an air leak is present in 22% to 24% of patients; and on the morning of postoperative day 4, an air leak is present in 8% of patients.[1]

A contemporary, practical definition of prolonged air leak (PAL) is an air leak that persists beyond postoperative day 5. This definition is used by the Society of Thoracic Surgeons database and represents a leak whose duration exceeds the average length of stay (LOS) for lobectomy. Several studies have found that PAL is associated with an increased rate of postoperative complications following routine pulmonary resection. Brunelli and colleagues[2] reported an 8.2% to 10.4% rate of empyema in patients who had an air leak lasting more than 7 days, compared with a 0% to 1.1% in patients with lesser air leaks. Similarly,

Disclosures: Dr J.B. Shrager is a consultant for Maquet, Inc.
[a] Division of Thoracic Surgery, Baylor College of Medicine, One Baylor Plaza, BCM 390, Houston, TX 77030, USA; [b] Division of Thoracic Surgery, Stanford Hospitals and Clinics, Stanford University School of Medicine, 300 Pasteur Drive, Falk Building CV-207, Stanford, CA 94305, USA; [c] Division of Thoracic Surgery, VA Palo Alto Health Care System, Palo Alto, CA, USA
* Corresponding author. Division of Thoracic Surgery, Stanford Hospitals and Clinics, Stanford University School of Medicine, 300 Pasteur Drive, Falk Building CV-207, Stanford, CA 94305.
E-mail address: shrager@stanford.edu

Thorac Surg Clin 25 (2015) 411–419
http://dx.doi.org/10.1016/j.thorsurg.2015.07.002
1547-4127/15/$ – see front matter Published by Elsevier Inc.

Varela and colleagues[3] found that air leaks lasting at least 5 days postoperatively were associated with increased pulmonary morbidity, including atelectasis, pneumonia, or empyema. In the lung volume reduction surgery (LVRS) population, postoperative complications occur more often in patients experiencing air leak (57%) than in those who do not (30%).[4]

Several risk factors for PAL following pulmonary resection have been identified. The most consistently identified risk factor for PAL is chronic obstructive pulmonary disease (COPD). Preoperative tests reflecting the severity of COPD and that are associated with PAL include reduced postoperative predicted forced expiratory volume in 1 second ($FEV_1$), $FEV_1$ less than 79% of predicted, $FEV_1$ less than 1.5 L, $FEV_1$ less than 70%, and both $FEV_1$ and forced vital capacity less than 70%.[1] Other risk factors with proven associations with PAL include carbon monoxide diffusion in the lung less than 80%, presence of adhesions, upper lobectomy and bilobectomy, presence of a pneumothorax coinciding with an air leak, and steroid use.[1]

## THERAPEUTIC OPTIONS AND CLINICAL OUTCOMES
### Intraoperative Prevention of Air Leaks

Because PALs are common, clearly increase LOS, and likely cause associated complications, several surgical strategies have been developed to prevent them. The general principles underlying these surgical techniques involve an elimination of residual space and achieving apposition of the visceral pleura, either to the parietal pleura or to transposed tissue (**Table 1**). Other techniques include addressing pulmonary resection beds and staple lines with adhesives and/or buttressing material.

Routine performance/use of these techniques is not advisable; not all patients are expected to benefit from these intraoperative adjuncts, which can be time consuming and/or costly. A careful selection of patients for such techniques should be based on underlying risk factors and probability of PAL and pleural space problems. For example, small or moderate residual spaces after pulmonary resection in many patients are physiologic and inconsequential; they resolve over time without ill effect. However, a large residual space in the context of a patient at high risk for air leak, which may result in infection of that space, can lead to a cascade of untoward events and morbidity. There are several intraoperative measures for preventing residual air spaces with which a thoracic surgeon should be familiar and many of

| Table 1 | |
|---|---|
| **Intraoperative procedures to manage residual thoracic air spaces** | |
| **Anatomic Structure** | **Intraoperative Procedure** |
| Parietal pleura | Pleural tent Pleurectomy or pleurodesis |
| Visceral pleura | Adhesiolysis Decortication |
| Diaphragm | Pneumoperitoneum Phrenic nerve paralysis |
| Muscular chest wall | Intrathoracic transposition of muscle |
| Osteotendinous chest wall | Rib resection at thoracotomy level Tailored thoracoplasty |
| Omentum | Omental transposition |

these have randomized studies establishing their effectiveness.

### Lung mobilization

Although less often a problem after sublobar resection compared with lobectomy, attaining pleural apposition without having to resort to high levels of suction seems to be an effective strategy for preventing PALs. There are several techniques that are commonly used to minimize residual space. Mobilization of all intrapleural adhesions and division of the inferior pulmonary ligament are the simplest of these, and should be routinely practiced because they are helpful. Similarly, decortication of the remaining lung, in rare instances and when required, may facilitate pleural apposition.

### Pleural tent

Creation of an apical pleural tent at the time of upper lobectomy or upper bilobectomy (resection of upper and middle lobes) is a proven technique for decreasing PAL. A pleural tent is created by detachment of the parietal pleura from the endothoracic fascia, usually beginning at the level of the thoracotomy or one of the upper thoracoscopic port sites. The pleura is elevated circumferentially along the chest wall, being careful not to tear it. The resulting pleural tent falls directly onto the staple lines along the interlobar fissures. It compartmentalizes the chest cavity by separating the caudally located, fully drained space, which contains the residual lung, from the cranially located undrained space, which is allowed to fill with serum. Three randomized trials in patients undergoing lung resection have shown that pleural tenting performed at the time of lung resection decreases chest tube duration and mean hospital stay[5]; decreases incidence of postoperative air leak[6]; and decreases air leak duration, chest tube duration, length of hospital stay, and hospital costs.[7]

### Pneumoperitoneum

Creation of pneumoperitoneum at the time of lower lobectomy or lower bilobectomy (resection of middle and lower lobes) has also been shown to decrease PAL, time of chest tube drainage, and LOS.[8,9] This step can be accomplished with a catheter placed transdiaphragmatically (through a purse-string suture) during the chest procedure or through a catheter or Veress needle, placed transabdominally in a manner similar to placing a laparoscopic port. Transient diaphragmatic paralysis via injection of the phrenic nerve with a local anesthetic has been described and can serve a similar purpose.[10]

### Surgical sealants

A Cochrane Database Review has evaluated the use of surgical sealants for the prevention or reduction of postoperative air leaks following pulmonary resection. This review included 16 randomized trials and 1642 patients.[11] Only 6 trials were able to show a significant reduction of postoperative air leaks by the use of sealants, and 3 trials showed a significant reduction in time to chest tube removal in the treatment group. These benefits (shown in a minority of trials) did not generally translate into reduced length of hospital stay, and we agree with the investigators of the Cochrane Review in not recommending routine use of these surgical sealants in patients undergoing pulmonary resection. A polymeric biodegradable hydrogel sealant (Progel) is the only sealant currently US Food and Drug Administration approved for intraoperative use during pulmonary resection. A randomized trial has suggested that intraoperative application of this product may reduce postoperative air leaks and result in 1less hospital day. However, Progel did not result in any difference in duration of chest tubes, so it is hard to attribute the reduced LOS to the product.[12]

We, and other investigators who have reviewed available data on lung sealants, have come to similar conclusions: that the current evidence does not support the routine use of these products in pulmonary resection.[13,14] However, it is possible that sealants may eventually be shown to provide some measureable benefit in patients at high risk for PAL; for example, those with moderate to severe emphysema undergoing lobectomy. However, as far as we know, this is purely theoretic, because the sealants have never been studied in this population. However, the fact that 1 study shows substantially reduced air leaks in patients after LVRS on the side treated with a sealant versus the control side not treated with sealants is suggestive.[15]

### Staple-line buttressing

The routine use of staple-line buttressing has also shown variable results. In severe emphysema (eg, LVRS), randomized data suggest that buttressing is effective for decreasing postoperative air leak and decreasing the duration of chest tube drainage and hospital stay.[16,17] Less robust data are available for patients undergoing anatomic resection. For example, one prospective randomized trial was performed in which 80 patients, undergoing lobectomy or segmentectomy, were assigned to receive staple-line buttressing with pericardial strips or standard treatment. This trial showed no advantage of buttressing with regard to time to chest tube removal or hospital stay, and there was only a trend toward reduced duration of air leak.[18] We recommend buttressing staple lines in nonanatomic pulmonary resections for patients with moderate to severe emphysema ($FEV_1$<60% of predicted) to prevent PALs.[1] In lobectomies (perhaps other than the horizontal fissure divided during right upper and middle lobectomies), the fissures are generally fairly thin and do not seem to require buttressing.

### Tissue transposition

Intrathoracic transposition of muscle flaps can function to obliterate residual spaces and, similar to a pleural tent, can be used to partition the thoracic cavity (muscle tent). Muscle transposition should be considered at the time of initial operation in cases in which complex, infected residual spaces may be created following lung resection. Serratus anterior and latissimus dorsi flaps can be transferred together or separately into the chest. Preserving the thoracodorsal vascular pedicle, both of these muscles can be transposed through a window created in the chest wall by resection of a 5-cm segment of the second or third rib.[19,20] In selected circumstances, the omentum can similarly be transposed into the thoracic cavity to fill the base of the chest,[21] either through the anterior diaphragmatic muscle or through a substernal, mediastinal tunnel.

### Other techniques

Other often-practiced, but less studied, techniques for intraoperative prevention of air leak include minimizing dissection within the fissures, minimizing inspiratory pressures when reinflating the lung, careful attention to avoid overlapping parenchymal staple lines, and closing the surgical stapler slowly in thick tissues.

Another potentially useful approach is what has been termed the fissureless technique of lobectomy, which is often performed during video-assisted thoracoscopic surgery lobectomy. In a prospective study of lobectomy, 63 patients with incomplete or fused fissures were intraoperatively randomized to receive either the traditional technique or the fissureless technique to approach the fused fissures. The incidence of PAL was significantly higher among patients with incomplete or fused fissures, and a fissureless lobectomy technique that avoided dissection of the lung parenchyma over the pulmonary artery resulted in significantly decreased PAL and reduced hospital stay.[22] Our opinion is that attention to these intraoperative details may be at least as effective as the commercially available sealants and other costly approaches.

## Postoperative Management of Air Leaks

During the initial management of a postoperative air leak, whether the leak originates from the alveoli through a peripheral tear in the visceral pleura (alveolar air leak) or from a bronchial structure (a bronchopleural fistula) can be hard to definitively determine. However, almost all postoperative air leaks are alveolar in origin, and the initial management therefore should be focused on treating this entity.

### Postoperative chest tube management

Many thoracic surgeons prefer to manage postoperative chest tubes using external suction following lung resection in efforts to improve lung expansion, minimize residual pleural spaces, and to reduce the risk of system malfunction secondary to blood clotting. Other thoracic surgeons think that suction may prevent air leaks from sealing by increasing air flow through visceral pleural defects, and that air leaks are therefore more likely to seal with no applied external suction. A traditional practice is to place chest drains to $-20$ cm $H_2O$ suction after pulmonary resection and then to convert the tubes to water seal when there is no visible air leak.

The early LVRS experience led many clinicians to question this traditional practice, with experience with these patients with severe emphysema suggesting that placing the chest tubes of patients having LVRS to the traditional $-20$ cm $H_2O$ of suction caused PALs and led to significant problems.[23,24] Surgeons who have performed substantial numbers of LVRS procedures have no doubt that this is the case. This LVRS experience stimulated

surgeons to study whether a no–external-suction algorithm can reduce air leak and PAL after non-LVRS pulmonary resections as well.

Six randomized trials have been published assessing the management of chest tubes with external suction compared with those with no external suction applied[25–30] (Table 2). Three trials showed an advantage in duration of air leak, time to chest tube removal, and/or length of hospital stay for the early water seal modality.[25,26,28] Two trials did not find a difference in these metrics.[27,29] One trial found that external suction ($-15$ cm $H_2O$) reduced the duration of persistent air leak after anatomic lung resection compared with no external suction.[30]

Significant differences in study design of these 6 trials may have resulted, to some degree, in the variability of their results. These differences included differences in the degree of external suction in the suction arm ($-10$, $-15$, $-20$ cm $H_2O$), differences in the times at which the chest drains were placed to suction (in the operating room, on postoperative day 1, or by alternating suction and no suction algorithms), definitions of PAL, drainage systems (traditional versus leak meter systems, and portable systems that may better facilitate ambulation [discussed later]), study participants (all patients vs those with visible air leak only), resection type (anatomic resection and nonanatomic resections), as well as the use of chest radiographs to evaluate pneumothorax. For example, the only study that reported a benefit to external suction followed a different algorithm from the other studies: patients were randomized to no external suction or to $-15$ cm $H_2O$ on postoperative day 1, and subsequently all patients' tubes were placed to Heimlich valve on postoperative day 3.[30]

We interpret the balance of evidence from these randomized trials to suggest that some version of reduced or part-time suction likely decreases the duration of air leak after pulmonary resection in most patients. However, the ideal algorithm remains uncertain. Although there is no high-level evidence available to date specifically in patients with severe emphysema, expert consensus and extensive clinical experience (in LVRS) suggest that patients with obstructive lung disease and an $FEV_1$ less than 45% of predicted are optimally treated with no external suction applied in the absence of a large, symptomatic, or growing pneumothorax; progressive subcutaneous emphysema; or clinical deterioration. The traditional $-20$ cm $H_2O$ of suction is clearly counterproductive in these patients. For patients without severe emphysema, we think that available evidence suggest that either alternating suction (alternating $-10$ cm $H_2O$ of

**Table 2**
**Randomized trials evaluating no external suction (NES) algorithms following pulmonary resection**

| Author | Algorithm | N | Resections | CXR Evaluation | Benefit of NES | Comments |
|---|---|---|---|---|---|---|
| Cerfolio et al,[25] 2001 | NES on POD 2 after −20 cm $H_2O$ | 33 | Lobectomy, sublobar | Yes | Yes | Greater sealing of AL by POD 3 |
| Marshall et al,[26] 2002 | NES after −20 cm $H_2O$ while in OR | 68 | Lobectomy, sublobar | Yes | Yes | Reduced duration of AL |
| Brunelli et al,[27] 2004 | NES on POD 1 after −20 cm $H_2O$ | 145 | Lobectomy | No | No | Increased complications with NES |
| Brunelli et al,[28] 2005 | Alternating −10 cm $H_2O$ (day) and NES (night) vs full-time NES, after −10 cm $H_2O$ | 94 | Lobectomy | No | Yes | Fewer PALs, shorter tube duration and LOS |
| Alphonso et al,[29] 2005 | Immediate NES | 239 | Lobectomy, sublobar | No | Yes | No differences in PAL or tube duration but increased mobilization with NES |
| Leo et al,[30] 2013 | NES or −15 cm $H_2O$ on POD 1, all tubes to Heimlich valve on POD 3 | 500 | Lobectomy, sublobar | Yes | No (there was a benefit to −15 cm $H_2O$) | Reduced PAL duration with −15 cm $H_2O$ suction in the anatomic resection subgroup |

*Abbreviations:* AL, air leak; CXR, chest radiograph; OR, operating room; PAL, prolonged air leak; POD, postoperative day.
*Data from* Refs.[25–30]

suction at night with no suction during the day) or the application of no external suction after a brief period of low suction (either in the operating room only or overnight for the first night, are reasonable).[1]

The senior author's chest tube management has evolved, for nearly all patients having lobectomy, to −10 cm $H_2O$ of suction for the first night following surgery, then full-time water seal beginning the following morning regardless of air leak, unless the air leak is subjectively large. Patients who have air leaks undergo a chest radiograph 2 to 4 hours after water seal is initiated; they return to −10 cm $H_2O$ of suction only if there is a pneumothorax more than 20% in size, increasing subcutaneous emphysema, or clinical signs of failure of water seal (eg, new atrial fibrillation, dyspnea), all of which rarely occur.

### Pleural drainage systems

In traditional chest drainage systems, air leaks are evaluated by detecting bubbles of air in the air leak chamber during forced expiratory maneuvers or cough. Using these systems, it can sometimes be difficult to differentiate a true parenchymal air leak from evacuation of a small residual pleural space in the absence of an ongoing leak, and from a momentum leak, which is the appearance of leak created by momentum of the fluid column in patients who are able to generate an unusually strong cough. Although these momentum leaks typically are present only with coughing and not with normal tidal breathing, and often are observed only during the first several coughs a patient is asked to perform, these can cause confusion and delay chest tube removal and thus discharge to home.

Different companies have produced objective systems capable of precisely measuring the amount of airflow through the chest tube. These devices express air leak in quantitative metrics collected over longer periods of time, rather than by observation of bubbles, and they have the capability to record and retrieve information that may ultimately make it possible to standardize chest tube management across different surgeons and institutions. These systems have been shown to significantly reduce the variability in deciding when to remove a chest drain[31] and to decrease the duration of chest drain and hospital stay in randomized trials.[32–34] Further, when using air leak grading systems, the amount of air leak identified in the early postoperative period can be effective in quantifying the risk of having persistent air leak in the later postoperative period and may predict which patients will not tolerate a no-external-suction algorithm.[25,35]

Traditional pleural drainage systems deliver a fixed level of suction independent from the level of intrapleural pressure, which can be variable depending on several factors, including the column of fluid in the pleural drainage system tubing. Moreover, wide oscillations in the early postoperative pleural pressures are associated with a high risk of a PAL.[36] Further, regulated pressure delivered by the digital pleural drainage devices, in which the intrapleural pressure is maintained at a consistent level within 0.1 cm $H_2O$ by a pressure sensor, is capable of stabilizing the pressure in the pleural cavity with minimal oscillations, and this may promote accelerated sealing of air leak.[37] In a single-institution randomized trial, regulated suction ($-11$ to $-20$ cm $H_2O$) compared with regulated seal ($-2$ cm $H_2O$) showed that regulated seal is effective and as safe as regulated suction, with a trend toward decreased duration of air leak in the regulated suction group.[38] A separate multicenter and international randomized trial of digital versus traditional drainage devices was recently completed. In patients undergoing anatomic resection, patients randomized to digital drainage systems had significantly shorter air leak duration, duration of chest tube placement, and postoperative lengths of stay.[32]

### Chest tube removal

Chest tubes are traditionally removed when an air leak has resolved and when the pleural fluid drainage is at an acceptable value to the thoracic surgeon, which, for many surgeons, has been estimated to be in the range of 250 to 350 mL per day. Regarding the volume of fluid drainage, there are now several studies that suggest that chest drains can be removed safely at much higher levels of effluent. Data from 2 separate institutions have recently shown that it is safe to remove chest tubes following pulmonary resection when drainage is as high as 450 to 500 mL per day, with exceedingly low rates of readmissions for symptomatic effusions.[39,40] For patients who have a persistent air leak but are otherwise ready for hospital discharge (and without large or symptomatic pneumothorax on water seal), it has been shown that these patients can be discharged

home safely on an outpatient drainage device such as a Heimlich valve as early as postoperative day 4.[39,41]

### Noninvasive Management of Prolonged Air Leak

It is rare for aggressive reinterventions to be required to treat PALs. In several published studies, the incidence of reoperation or other aggressive reinterventions to treat this complication is less than 2%.[1] The treatment strategy of watchful waiting, often as an outpatient, is largely successful. Approximately 95% of PALs that permit a no-external-suction algorithm resolve within a few weeks of operation with chest tube drainage alone, with only rare development of empyema.[1]

### Heimlich valve

For patients with no more than a small, stable, and asymptomatic pneumothorax on water seal, PALs can be managed in the outpatient setting using a 1-way valve attached to the drain. If necessary to differentiate true air leak from residual space evacuation, the patients can undergo a provocative clamping trial; most of these patients are able to safely have their chest tubes removed. A report by Cerfolio and colleagues[42] on 199 patients discharged home with a persistent air leak and chest tube placed to a suctionless portable drainage device suggested that the air leak seals in the outpatient setting in almost all patients. For 9 patients with a persistent air leak after 2 weeks of outpatient management with a Heimlich valve, all patients had their chest tubes removed without sequela, some after a provocative clamping trial.

If a period of watchful waiting for several weeks (we have waited as long as 4 weeks) is unsuccessful in treating a PAL, or if no external suction is not tolerated because of a larger leak, then the clinician must consider active interventions to mechanically seal the site of the leak. Most of these options are supported by expert consensus with variable amounts of published data.

### Pleurodesis and autologous blood patch

If the residual lung is fully expanded, chemical pleurodesis with instillation via the thoracostomy tube of tetracycline, doxycycline, or talc can promote pleural symphysis and leak closure. These treatments all seem to be effective for pleurodesis in small cases series.[43,44]

An autologous blood patch is another simple and often effective treatment of PAL. Although some reports suggest an associated increased risk of intrathoracic infection (in 1 study, 1 of 10 patients developed empyema[45]), several prospective data suggest that an autologous blood patch has superior outcomes compared with the conservative management of PAL (summarized in Ref.[46]). Two of these studies were randomized trials that suggested that intrapleural instillation of autologous blood (120 mL) decreased the duration of PAL, time to chest tube removal, and time to hospital discharge.[45]

An additional randomized trial suggested that a 100-mL instillation of autologous blood decreased the time to air leak cessation more than a 50-mL instillation.[47] We typically perform a blood patch by the sterile instillation of approximately 150 mL of blood freshly withdrawn into a 50-mL syringe from a large-bore intravenous line, and instilled immediately into the thoracostomy tube. Heparin is typically not used because it prevents the necessary intrathoracic clotting of blood that forms the patch, and we administer periprocedural antibiotics to minimize the risk of infection.

### Invasive Management of Prolonged Air Leak

More invasive procedures are indicated to treat PALs if the more conservative measures discussed earlier fail. These interventions include pneumoperitoneum placed via an abdominal catheter, as described earlier (which is reported to be effective in treating PAL in some cases[48,49]), placement of endobronchial valves, and reoperation.

### Endobronchial valves

Unidirectional endobronchial valves, originally studied for treatment of emphysema, have emerged as a useful intervention for some patients with PAL. The early experiences of several centers have shown that bronchoscopic placement of these valves can be effective in some difficult cases of PAL. The source of an air leak is typically identified by the stepwise blocking of segmental and subsegmental bronchi by a balloon catheter while monitoring the size of the air leak in the pleural drainage device. Endobronchial 1-way valves deployed in the orifice or orifices of the segment or subsegments responsible for air leak may result in the improvement or cessation of PAL.[50–52] Although these data are overall currently limited, these devices have received Humanitarian Device Exemption approval from the US Food and Drug Administration for this purpose.

### Surgical intervention

Surgical reexploration is rarely required but must be considered when other approaches have failed. The choice of operation depends on whether a residual space is present, the quality of the remaining lung, and presence or absence of pleural space infection once surgery has been decided on. A bronchoscopy should be done to rule out a bronchial rather than a parenchymal fistula. If the residual lung is sufficiently normal, the leak can be restapled or oversewn with good results, and the approach can be thoracoscopic or open. Other options include thoracoscopic applications of topical sealants,[53] with which we have no experience. Decortication of surrounding lung may be required to facilitate full lung expansion. Chemical pleurodesis or parietal pleurectomy/mechanical pleurodesis can be added when pleural apposition can be achieved.[54] If a residual space is present, that space should be obliterated with either muscle or omental transposition, although most of the data on this are derived from the bronchopleural fistula literature. Following sublobar resection, completion lobectomy is necessary on rare occasions. Thoracoplasty or the creation of an open window can be considered under extreme circumstances.

## SUMMARY

A variety of options are available to prevent and manage PALs. Intraoperative technical details are likely of greatest importance in reducing their incidence, and patients with substantial emphysema are at highest risk. Pleural tents and pneumoperitoneum created at the time of resection are helpful when residual spaces are likely; commercial buttresses and sealants have shown mixed results outside of severe emphysema and are expensive. Optimal postoperative management of chest tubes seems to include less than the traditional $-20$ cm $H_2O$ of external suction until cessation of air leak in most patients. Noninvasive approaches to resolve PALs (ie, watchful waiting with an outpatient Heimlich valve) are almost always effective, but invasive, nonsurgical interventions or surgical procedures are largely successful when required.

## REFERENCES

1. Singhal S, Ferraris VA, Bridges CR, et al. Management of alveolar air leaks after pulmonary resection. Ann Thorac Surg 2010;89(4):1327–35.
2. Brunelli A, Xiume F, Al Refai M, et al. Air leaks after lobectomy increase the risk of empyema but not of cardiopulmonary complications: a case-matched analysis. Chest 2006;130(4):1150–6.
3. Varela G, Jimenez MF, Novoa N, et al. Estimating hospital costs attributable to prolonged air leak in pulmonary lobectomy. Eur J Cardiothorac Surg 2005;27(2):329–33.
4. DeCamp MM, Blackstone EH, Naunheim KS, et al. Patient and surgical factors influencing air leak after lung

volume reduction surgery: lessons learned from the National Emphysema Treatment Trial. Ann Thorac Surg 2006;82(1):197–206 [discussion: 206–7].

5. Okur E, Kir A, Halezeroglu S, et al. Pleural tenting following upper lobectomies or bilobectomies of the lung to prevent residual air space and prolonged air leak. Eur J Cardiothorac Surg 2001; 20(5):1012–5.

6. Allama AM. Pleural tent for decreasing air leak following upper lobectomy: a prospective randomised trial. Eur J Cardiothorac Surg 2010;38(6): 674–8.

7. Brunelli A, Al Refai M, Monteverde M, et al. Pleural tent after upper lobectomy: a randomized study of efficacy and duration of effect. Ann Thorac Surg 2002;74(6):1958–62.

8. Rocco G. Intraoperative measures for preventing residual air spaces. Thorac Surg Clin 2010;20(3):371–5.

9. Toker A, Dilege S, Tanju S, et al. Perioperative pneumoperitoneum after lobectomy – bilobectomy operations for lung cancer: a prospective study. Thorac Cardiovasc Surg 2003;51(2):93–6.

10. Carboni GL, Vogt A, Kuster JR, et al. Reduction of airspace after lung resection through controlled paralysis of the diaphragm. Eur J Cardiothorac Surg 2008;33(2):272–5.

11. Belda-Sanchis J, Serra-Mitjans M, Iglesias Sentis M, et al. Surgical sealant for preventing air leaks after pulmonary resections in patients with lung cancer. Cochrane Database Syst Rev 2010;(1):CD003051.

12. Allen MS, Wood DE, Hawkinson RW, et al. Prospective randomized study evaluating a biodegradable polymeric sealant for sealing intraoperative air leaks that occur during pulmonary resection. Ann Thorac Surg 2004;77(5):1792–801.

13. Merritt RE, Singhal S, Shrager JB. Evidence-based suggestions for management of air leaks. Thorac Surg Clin 2010;20(3):435–48.

14. Malapert G, Hanna HA, Pages PB, et al. Surgical sealant for the prevention of prolonged air leak after lung resection: meta-analysis. Ann Thorac Surg 2010;90(6):1779–85.

15. Moser C, Opitz I, Zhai W, et al. Autologous fibrin sealant reduces the incidence of prolonged air leak and duration of chest tube drainage after lung volume reduction surgery: a prospective randomized blinded study. J Thorac Cardiovasc Surg 2008;136(4):843–9.

16. Stammberger U, Klepetko W, Stamatis G, et al. Buttressing the staple line in lung volume reduction surgery: a randomized three-center study. Ann Thorac Surg 2000;70(6):1820–5.

17. Hazelrigg SR, Boley TM, Naunheim KS, et al. Effect of bovine pericardial strips on air leak after stapled pulmonary resection. Ann Thorac Surg 1997;63(6): 1573–5.

18. Miller JI Jr, Landreneau RJ, Wright CE, et al. A comparative study of buttressed versus nonbuttressed staple line in pulmonary resections. Ann Thorac Surg 2001;71(1):319–22 [discussion: 323].

19. Rocco G. Pleural partition with intrathoracic muscle transposition (muscle tent) to manage residual spaces after subtotal pulmonary resections. Ann Thorac Surg 2004;78(4):e74–6.

20. Widmer MK, Krueger T, Lardinois D, et al. A comparative evaluation of intrathoracic latissimus dorsi and serratus anterior muscle transposition. Eur J Cardiothorac Surg 2000;18(4):435–9.

21. Shrager JB, Wain JC, Wright CD, et al. Omentum is highly effective in the management of complex cardiothoracic surgical problems. J Thorac Cardiovasc Surg 2003;125(3):526–32.

22. Gomez-Caro A, Calvo MJ, Lanzas JT, et al. The approach of fused fissures with fissureless technique decreases the incidence of persistent air leak after lobectomy. Eur J Cardiothorac Surg 2007;31(2):203–8.

23. Cooper JD, Patterson GA. Lung-volume reduction surgery for severe emphysema. Chest Surg Clin N Am 1995;5(4):815–31.

24. Cooper JD, Patterson GA, Sundaresan RS, et al. Results of 150 consecutive bilateral lung volume reduction procedures in patients with severe emphysema. J Thorac Cardiovasc Surg 1996;112(5):1319–29 [discussion: 1329–30].

25. Cerfolio RJ, Bass C, Katholi CR. Prospective randomized trial compares suction versus water seal for air leaks. Ann Thorac Surg 2001;71(5):1613–7.

26. Marshall MB, Deeb ME, Bleier JI, et al. Suction vs water seal after pulmonary resection: a randomized prospective study. Chest 2002;121(3):831–5.

27. Brunelli A, Monteverde M, Borri A, et al. Comparison of water seal and suction after pulmonary lobectomy: a prospective, randomized trial. Ann Thorac Surg 2004;77(6):1932–7 [discussion: 1937].

28. Brunelli A, Sabbatini A, Xiume F, et al. Alternate suction reduces prolonged air leak after pulmonary lobectomy: a randomized comparison versus water seal. Ann Thorac Surg 2005;80(3):1052–5.

29. Alphonso N, Tan C, Utley M, et al. A prospective randomized controlled trial of suction versus nonsuction to the under-water seal drains following lung resection. Eur J Cardiothorac Surg 2005; 27(3):391–4.

30. Leo F, Duranti L, Girelli L, et al. Does external pleural suction reduce prolonged air leak after lung resection? Results from the AirINTrial after 500 randomized cases. Ann Thorac Surg 2013; 96(4):1234–9.

31. Varela G, Jimenez MF, Novoa NM, et al. Postoperative chest tube management: measuring air leak using an electronic device decreases variability in

the clinical practice. Eur J Cardiothorac Surg 2009; 35(1):28–31.

32. Pompili C, Detterbeck F, Papagiannopoulos K, et al. Multicenter international randomized comparison of objective and subjective outcomes between electronic and traditional chest drainage systems. Ann Thorac Surg 2014;98(2):490–6 [discussion: 496–7].

33. Brunelli A, Salati M, Refai M, et al. Evaluation of a new chest tube removal protocol using digital air leak monitoring after lobectomy: a prospective randomised trial. Eur J Cardiothorac Surg 2010;37(1):56–60.

34. Cerfolio RJ, Bryant AS. The benefits of continuous and digital air leak assessment after elective pulmonary resection: a prospective study. Ann Thorac Surg 2008;86(2):396–401.

35. Cerfolio RJ, Bryant AS, Singh S, et al. The management of chest tubes in patients with a pneumothorax and an air leak after pulmonary resection. Chest 2005;128(2):816–20.

36. Brunelli A, Cassivi SD, Salati M, et al. Digital measurements of air leak flow and intrapleural pressures in the immediate postoperative period predict risk of prolonged air leak after pulmonary lobectomy. Eur J Cardiothorac Surg 2011;39(4):584–8.

37. Brunelli A, Beretta E, Cassivi SD, et al. Consensus definitions to promote an evidence-based approach to management of the pleural space. A collaborative proposal by ESTS, AATS, STS, and GTSC. Eur J Cardiothorac Surg 2011;40(2):291–7.

38. Brunelli A, Salati M, Pompili C, et al. Regulated tailored suction vs regulated seal: a prospective randomized trial on air leak duration. Eur J Cardiothorac Surg 2013;43(5):899–904.

39. Cerfolio RJ, Bryant AS. Results of a prospective algorithm to remove chest tubes after pulmonary resection with high output. J Thorac Cardiovasc Surg 2008;135(2):269–73.

40. Bjerregaard LS, Jensen K, Petersen RH, et al. Early chest tube removal after video-assisted thoracic surgery lobectomy with serous fluid production up to 500 ml/day. Eur J Cardiothorac Surg 2014;45(2):241–6.

41. McKenna RJ Jr, Mahtabifard A, Pickens A, et al. Fast-tracking after video-assisted thoracoscopic surgery lobectomy, segmentectomy, and pneumonectomy. Ann Thorac Surg 2007;84(5):1663–7 [discussion: 1667–8].

42. Cerfolio RJ, Minnich DJ, Bryant AS. The removal of chest tubes despite an air leak or a pneumothorax.

Ann Thorac Surg 2009;87(6):1690–4 [discussion: 1694–6].

43. Kilic D, Findikcioglu A, Hatipoglu A. A different application method of talc pleurodesis for the treatment of persistent air leak. ANZ J Surg 2006;76(8):754–6.

44. Read CA, Reddy VD, O'Mara TE, et al. Doxycycline pleurodesis for pneumothorax in patients with AIDS. Chest 1994;105(3):823–5.

45. Shackcloth MJ, Poullis M, Jackson M, et al. Intrapleural instillation of autologous blood in the treatment of prolonged air leak after lobectomy: a prospective randomized controlled trial. Ann Thorac Surg 2006;82(3):1052–6.

46. Chambers A, Routledge T, Bille A, et al. Is blood pleurodesis effective for determining the cessation of persistent air leak? Interact Cardiovasc Thorac Surg 2010;11(4):468–72.

47. Andreetti C, Venuta F, Anile M, et al. Pleurodesis with an autologous blood patch to prevent persistent air leaks after lobectomy. J Thorac Cardiovasc Surg 2007;133(3):759–62.

48. Carbognani P, Spaggiari L, Solli PG, et al. Postoperative pneumoperitoneum for prolonged air leaks and residual spaces after pulmonary resections. J Cardiovasc Surg 1999;40(6):887–8.

49. De Giacomo T, Rendina EA, Venuta F, et al. Pneumoperitoneum for the management of pleural air space problems associated with major pulmonary resections. Ann Thorac Surg 2001;72(5):1716–9.

50. Kovitz KL, French KD. Endobronchial valve placement and balloon occlusion for persistent air leak: procedure overview and new current procedural terminology codes for 2013. Chest 2013;144(2):661–5.

51. Travaline JM, McKenna RJ Jr, De Giacomo T, et al. Treatment of persistent pulmonary air leaks using endobronchial valves. Chest 2009;136(2):355–60.

52. Firlinger I, Stubenberger E, Muller MR, et al. Endoscopic one-way valve implantation in patients with prolonged air leak and the use of digital air leak monitoring. Ann Thorac Surg 2013;95(4):1243–9.

53. Thistlethwaite PA, Luketich JD, Ferson PF, et al. Ablation of persistent air leaks after thoracic procedures with fibrin sealant. Ann Thorac Surg 1999;67(2):575–7.

54. Suter M, Bettschart V, Vandoni RE, et al. Thoracoscopic pleurodesis for prolonged (or intractable) air leak after lung resection. Eur J Cardiothorac Surg 1997;12(1):160–1.

# Bronchopleural Fistula and Empyema After Anatomic Lung Resection

Giorgio Zanotti, MD[a], John D. Mitchell, MD[b],*

## KEYWORDS

- Empyema • Bronchopleural fistula • Eloesser flap • Decortication • Clagett procedure

## KEY POINTS

- Bronchopleural fistula (BPF) and empyema remain rare but serious complications after anatomic lung resection, particularly pneumonectomy.
- Careful attention to identified risk factors and proper surgical technique can minimize the risk of BPF/empyema in most cases.
- Management of BPF/empyema after surgical resection must address both issues of bronchial integrity and the infected plural space for a successful outcome.
- After pneumonectomy, resolution may require multiple, additional surgical interventions.

Empyema after anatomic pulmonary resection remains a rare but serious complication, often leading to major morbidity and increased mortality. In a modern series of 1023 patients undergoing anatomic resection, empyema occurred postoperatively in 1.1%.[1] It occurs more commonly after pneumonectomy, particularly after surgery for benign disease.[2] The reported incidence of depends in part on the postoperative surveillance protocols and diagnostic techniques used.[3,4] The associated mortality rate may exceed 10%[5]; even if the patient survives, the recurrence rate of infection can be as high as 38%.[6] Importantly, up to 80% of cases of procedure-related empyemas are associated with bronchopleural fistula (BPF)[4] and fewer than 20% of these can be expected to close spontaneously.[7] The presence or absence of BPF in the setting of postoperative pleural empyema defines 2 clinical cohorts that are distinct with respect to etiology, risk factors, and treatment algorithm.

## ETIOLOGY, RISK FACTORS, AND PREVENTION

A BPF may arise either from dehiscence or disruption of a bronchial closure after anatomic lung resection (segmentectomy, lobectomy, pneumonectomy), or from anastomotic dehiscence after bronchoplastic resection. Postoperative BPF is classified based on the time of onset after surgery as early (within the first week), intermediate (between 7 and 30 days), and late (after 30 days).[8]

There are a number of predisposing factors that may place the patient at increased risk of developing a fistula and subsequent empyema. Malnutrition, various immunosuppressive therapies (steroids, antimetabolites), prior thoracic radiation therapy, poorly controlled pulmonary or pleural infection, active smokers, and the use of induction chemotherapy have all been implicated in the development of fistula. Interestingly, induction therapy has been cited as a risk factor after pneumonectomy,[9] but not after bronchoplastic procedures.[10–12]

Disclosures: The authors have no relevant disclosures.
[a] Division of Cardiothoracic Surgery, University of Colorado School of Medicine, Academic Office 1, Room 6602, C-310, 12631 East 17th Avenue, Aurora, CO 80045, USA; [b] Section of General Thoracic Surgery, Division of Cardiothoracic Surgery, University of Colorado School of Medicine, Academic Office 1, Room 6602, C-310, 12631 East 17th Avenue, Aurora, CO 80045, USA
* Corresponding author.
E-mail address: john.mitchell@ucdenver.edu

Thorac Surg Clin 25 (2015) 421–427
http://dx.doi.org/10.1016/j.thorsurg.2015.07.006
1547-4127/15/$ – see front matter © 2015 Elsevier Inc. All rights reserved.

Early fistulas are most commonly owing to surgical technical problems. It is well-established that right pneumonectomy is associated with a greater risk (up to 13.2%) of BPF compared with left pneumonectomy (up to 5.0%).[13] There are 2 main reasons accounting for this; first, the most common anatomic variant of bronchial arterial supply is composed of 1 artery on the right, whereas a dual arterial supply is the most common configuration on the left. Second, the left main stem bronchus is protected under the aortic arch and surrounded by its vascularized mediastinal tissue, whereas the right bronchial stump has no such coverage. Overzealous mediastinal lymphadenectomy,[14] bronchial stump greater than 25 mm in diameter,[15] long bronchial stump, residual malignancy at the bronchial margin,[5] requirement for 4 or more units of intraoperative packed red blood cell transfusions,[3] completion pneumonectomy,[3] and tension along the anastomosis are associated with stump ischemia and are well-described risk factors for early failure. Stapler misfiring, improper tissue apposition, or poorly secured sutures are also common technical causes of early bronchial anastomotic breakdown.

Postoperatively, the main risk factor for BPF is positive pressure mechanical ventilation[16]; for this reason, extubation at the end of the case is typically a priority.

Late fistulas are typically secondary to patient-related factors causing poor healing: age greater than 60 years, malnutrition, ongoing pulmonary or pleural infection, and recurrence of malignancy.

Empyema after anatomic lung resection in absence of BPF is most commonly caused by intraoperative contamination by aerobic bacteria. Zaheer and colleagues[17] and Eerola and associates[18] found that *Staphylococcus aureus* is the most common organism isolated, followed by *Streptococcus pneumoniae*. Spillage of infected bronchial secretions, active plural infection at the time of surgery, and esophagopleural or gastropleural fistulas are the most common causes. Less frequently, a primary infection of pleural space, because it may occur after chest trauma with chest wall penetration or hemothorax and mycobacterial infection of the pleural cavity,[19] may lead to bronchial stump breakdown. There is scant evidence that hematogenous infection of the pleural space can occur from a distant infection site (classically osteomyelitis) without an intermediate lung infection, which in turn contaminates the pleural cavity.[20]

## PATHOLOGY

It is worth reviewing the classic time course and stages of empyema development.[21] In stage 1 (exudative, acute), exudative fluid is present, the visceral pleura remains elastic and the dimensions of the chest cavity are maintained. Stage 2 (fibrinopurulent, subacute) is characterized by the presence of infected or frankly purulent fluid, and fibrin deposition creates septations and loculations within the pleural cavity. Lung compliance may also be reduced owing to thick fibrin depositions. In stage 3 (consolidative, chronic), granulation tissue formally replaces the pleural space, and the lung becomes completely entrapped by a fibrinous peel. Late in the course, organization of the inflammatory tissue causes contraction of the affected hemithorax with ipsilateral shift of the mediastinum, elevation of the diaphragm, and narrowing of intercostal spaces.

This time course, characteristic of a common or postpneumonic empyema, is usually altered by the postoperative medical attention these patients receive, particularly with the presence of a BPF. It is imperative that the treating surgeon be acquainted with the often subtle symptoms and signs that can lead to early diagnosis and treatment.

## CLINICAL PRESENTATION AND DIAGNOSIS

Postoperative empyema of the pleural space is associated with a constellation of signs and symptoms that are dictated mainly by the presence of an infected pleural cavity and a BPF. If a BPF has indeed opened, its size and timing of formation are major determinants of the clinical picture. The duration of illness is also an important determinant of the clinical manifestations.

Minor fistulae may be occult or minimally symptomatic and are usually detected if a postoperative bronchoscopic screening for BPF is performed routinely.[22] A persistent (>7 days) air leak, especially if brisk, without a history of visceral pleural dissection or injury at the time of surgery, new evidence of pneumomediastinum, a decrease in the fluid level in the ipsilateral pleural cavity, or a new air–fluid level ("meniscus sign") at the height of the bronchial stump on chest imaging after lung resection should raise the suspicion for BPF (**Fig. 1**). In cases where the BPF is larger than a few millimeters, respiratory distress may be a prominent finding and is caused by either spillage of pleural fluid through the fistula into the contralateral lung or by "dead space" ventilation into the empty pleural space. Worsening dyspnea and productive cough with frothy or purulent sputum herald the loss of integrity of the bronchial closure. Expectoration typically worsens with the patient lying on the side opposite to the one involving the fistula. The flooding of the contralateral lung may lead to, if not overt pneumonia, an alveolar

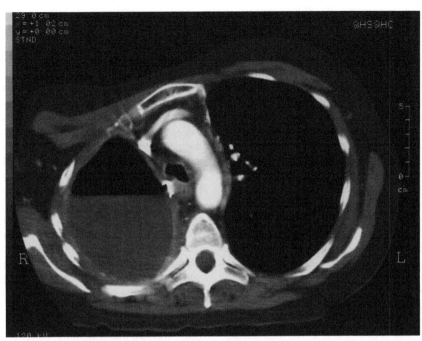

**Fig. 1.** Occurrence of an empyema associated with bronchopleural fistula after right pneumonectomy. In this supine patient, note the air–fluid interface at the level of the right mainstem stump closure.

injury similar to respiratory distress syndrome that is almost invariably a lethal condition. Fever, increasing white blood cell count, and indications of systemic inflammation are often present because of the infected pleural space; pleuritic chest pain, night sweats, and chills may also be observed and resemble symptoms of pneumonia. Interestingly, in some patients decompression of the infected contents of the pleural space into the airway may temporize some features of the systemic inflammatory response, thus making the diagnosis more difficult.

Early after surgery, the diagnosis of BPF is suggested by a combination of clinical and radiologic clues and is eventually confirmed by visualization of the fistula on bronchoscopy. Computed tomography of the chest is quite sensitive at demonstrating abnormalities related to the presence of BPF, but its sensitivity at demonstrating the presence and the location of the fistula (at least after lobectomy) is approximately 50%[23] and therefore is of little to no use in the diagnostic process. In these instances, the use of noninvasive [133]xenon ventilation scintigraphy has been used by some authors[24] to diagnose occult BPFs by visualizing equilibration of radioactive gas tracer into the empty pleural space. Alternatively, ventilation scintigraphy with other radioactive tracers such as [81]krypton and [99]technetium has also been reported. These advanced imaging techniques that use radioactive isotopes may be useful in

diagnosing selected cases of BPF but require substantial time and cooperation from a nonintubated patient and can be inconclusive in the setting of small fistulas or underlying lung disease such as chronic obstructive pulmonary disease.[25] In almost all cases, bronchoscopy is used to assess and confirm the presence of a BPF. A loss of integrity of or fine bubbling at the anastomosis after instillation of saline solution into the stump is pathognomonic. Delayed or less extensive bronchial disruptions may present diagnostic problems, even at the time of bronchoscopy. Rarely, surgical reexploration is needed as a final step to confirm or rule out the diagnosis.

## MANAGEMENT

Empyema of the chest is one of the oldest known general thoracic surgery conditions. Hippocrates (460–370 BC) first described the drainage of patients with pleural empyema more than 2000 years ago. He thought that drainage by either an intercostal incision or rib resection followed by recurrent plural irrigation was necessary.[26,27] Galenus (130–200 BC) and Celsus (25 BC-50 AD) in the Roman age devised metal tubes to drain the purulent collection, a teaching that ruled the Middle Ages, during which barber–surgeons refined the art of drainage by using solutions with mildly acidic pH (often wine).[27] The magnitude of Hippocrates's contribution to the understanding of chest empyema is underscored by the fact that few true advances in either the diagnosis or the cure of this condition were made in the following 2000 years.

In the modern era, the management of postoperative empyema of the pleural cavity depends on the etiology (including the presence or absence of a BPF), the chronicity, the state of the underlying lung (if any is left), and the patient's clinical and nutritional status. Importantly, the protean nature of the disease has made it difficult to draft evidence-based guidelines for the treatment of this condition. Therefore, the optimal treatment strategy needs to be individualized in each case based on the aforementioned evidence, the duration of illness, and the healing potential of the infected pleural cavity. To minimize morbidity and mortality, the treatment must proceed with a sense of urgency.

The initial management of an acute, post lung resection empyema consists of placement of a large-bore (32–36F) thoracostomy tube and positioning of the patient in reverse Trendelenburg position. In the case of BPF, the affected side should be "down" in the most dependent position to prevent spillage of pleural fluid into the contralateral lung. When mechanical ventilation is needed, particularly after pneumonectomy, consideration should be given to selective intubation of the uninvolved side to minimize barotrauma to the bronchial stump.

If the presence of a BPF is known or if purulent fluid is found, initiation of intravenous, broad-spectrum antibiotic therapy is undertaken. The British Thoracic Society recently published the most updated guidelines on how to direct antibiotic therapy in this complex arena.[28] Antibiotic treatment should be tailored based on the results of cultures and their sensitivity profile.

Treatment options diverge from this point depending on the presence or absence of an associated BPF. In the absence of BPF, treatment options closely mirror conventional management of simple empyema: drainage and intravenous antibiotics—and, if reoperation is deemed necessary, debridement of the pleural space and minimizing the residual pleural space. Of these, it is the residual pleural space, obligatory after anatomic lung resection, that may prove problematic. In the setting of segmentectomy, this is rarely a concern. After lobectomy, the residual intrathoracic space may be addressed with adjuncts such as temporary phrenic nerve paresis or pneumoperitoneum. In refractory (or chronic) cases, the use of muscle or omental transposition with or without thoracoplasty may be used to obliterate the infected intrathoracic space. If the options regarding tissue transposition are limited, or if the patient is significantly

debilitated, an open thoracostomy (Eloesser flap) may be used to treat the infected postlobectomy residual space. After pneumonectomy, these same options for tissue transposition or thoracostomy window are present, although these authors prefer the latter because it is much simpler and is associated with less morbidity.

If a BPF is present, concurrent management of the empyema as well as BPF repair is considered the current standard of care. The basic principles include initial drainage (described elsewhere in this article), antibiotics and optimization of nutrition; closure of the fistula, typically with autologous tissue buttressing; and appropriate management of the infected space. This is usually performed through a posterolateral thoracotomy, although a BPF after pneumonectomy may be approached preferentially via sternotomy. In poor surgical candidates, chronic empyema can be managed with a large-bore chest tube to be slowly retracted over the course of weeks, whereas a small air leak is managed expectantly or with open-window thoracostomy. Open-window thoracostomy was first described by Robinson[29] in 1916 for nontuberculous empyema and subsequently revised in 1935 by Eloesser[30] for tuberculous empyema. Several iterations of the Eloesser flap have been described since that time; the authors favor a modified "H"-type incision with underlying resection of segments of 2 to 3 ribs. The skin flaps created by the incision are then used to epithelialize the entryway into the pleural space. The opening should be placed, if possible, low and anterior in the chest to facilitate drainage. Often, this approach needs to be modified owing to prior thoracotomy incisions. Additionally, the authors preserve the serratus anterior muscle under the cephalad skin flap for use at the time of thoracostomy closure (**Fig. 2**).

At the time of thoracotomy, the bronchial stump is inspected with particular attention paid to its length. If the stump is found to be long, it should be resected back to its origin, reclosed either with suture or staples, and buttressed with autologous tissue. If flush with its origin, it needs to be reclosed using interrupted, absorbable suture and then covered with a vascularized flap. Dissection of a pneumonectomy stump for reclosure can be hazardous, given the dense fibrosis typically present and the proximity of the ligated pulmonary artery. If the stump cannot be reclosed, options include a pedicled flap that can be sewn directly to the stump and function as a plug[17] or a central bronchoplastic procedure, such as carinal resection.

The choice of the autologous tissue for coverage is important for optimal results, and in

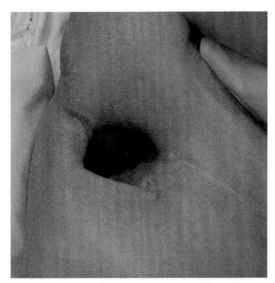

**Fig. 2.** A mature open thoracostomy before closure. Note the location just above the diaphragm; the position was modified somewhat owing to the generous prior thoracotomy. The preserved serratus is present under the cephalad skin flap.

part depends on the patient's prior surgical history. Most commonly, rotational muscle flaps are used involving the latissimus dorsi, the pectoralis major, or intercostal muscle. Free flaps are used in patients that are not candidates for pedicled tissue transfer.[31,32] The rotational muscle flaps are typically harvested before placement of the retractor. Intercostal muscle flaps are versatile, and are particularly well-suited to be combined with open thoracostomy, because the small footprint of the intercostal en route to the bronchus will not interfere with postoperative packing of the intrathoracic cavity.

Pleural flaps,[33] although being frequently used owing to their simplicity of harvest, have the disadvantage of being extremely thin and potentially lacking adequate blood supply. Their use is, therefore, questionable for more critical purposes such as buttressing a postpneumonectomy stump. Some authors reported the use of diaphragmatic[34] or omental flaps[35] with good results; these authors have found the latter particularly useful in the setting of poorly controlled infection. Brewer and associates[36] and Taghavi and colleagues[37] reported the use pericardial flaps for bronchial stump coverage with remarkable results. This, however, exposed the mediastinum to the infected milieu of the pleural cavity with inherent risk of phrenic nerve injury during the harvest.

The management of an open thoracostomy is routine, packing the space once or twice daily with gauze typically sprinkled with quarter-strength Dakin's solution. Over time, granulation of the intrathoracic cavity is noted; occasional debridement can facilitate this process. When the cavity is deemed "clean," patients are offered thoracostomy closure. Our preferred approach is a modification of the Clagett procedure, originally described by Clagett and Geraci in 1963.[38] The closure is accomplished by filling of the residual cavity with nonabsorbable antibiotics (eg, neomycin, polymyxin B) in saline, and achieving a watertight closure of the thoracostomy opening. The excessive skin lining the opening is excised, the serratus is mobilized and brought over the opening and sewn circumferentially to the fibrous pleural lining, and the skin is closed in layers. Operative mortality is less than 10% and overall success rate exceeds 80%.[17]

If the modified Clagett procedure fails, conversion to a chronic open drainage situation by means of an Eloesser flap with or without subsequent obliteration of the empty pleural space with an autologous tissue flap is the next step in management.

## SUMMARY

Postoperative empyema is a relatively rare complication after anatomic lung resection, but when present is associated with considerable morbidity. For many patients, the presence or absence of a BPF makes the difference between recovery, chronic illness, and death. Despite this, the principles underlying treatment have not changed: source control of the infection with drainage (tube thoracostomy and/or video-assisted thoracoscopic surgery vs open drainage), closure of the fistula if present, and sterilization of the pleural cavity either via decortication, filling the space with autologous tissue or with the use of the Clagett procedure. There is a lack of evidence over optimal treatment strategy because no large or randomized trials have been performed to date. The clinical scenario and surgeon's acquaintance with the various treatment techniques are the main factors influencing the treatment strategy in a case-tailored approach.

## REFERENCES

1. Allen MS, Darling GE, Pechet TT, et al. Morbidity and mortality of major pulmonary resections in patients with early-stage lung cancer: initial results of the randomized, prospective ACOSOG Z0030 trial. Ann Thorac Surg 2006;81(3):1013–9 [discussion: 1019–20].

2. Shapiro M, Swanson SJ, Wright CD, et al. Predictors of major morbidity and mortality after pneumonectomy utilizing the society for thoracic surgeons general

thoracic surgery database. Ann Thorac Surg 2010; 90(3):927–35.

3. Deschamps C, Bernard A, Nichols FC 3rd, et al. Empyema and bronchopleural fistula after pneumonectomy: factors affecting incidence. Ann Thorac Surg 2001;72(1):243–7 [discussion: 248].

4. Vallieres E. Management of empyema after lung resections (pneumonectomy/lobectomy). Chest Surg Clin N Am 2002;12(3):571–85.

5. Liberman M, Cassivi SD. Bronchial stump dehiscence: update on prevention and management. Semin Thorac Cardiovasc Surg 2007;19(4):366–73.

6. Weber J, Gräbner D, al-Zand K, et al. Empyema after pneumonectomy–empyema window or thoracoplasty? Thorac Cardiovasc Surg 1990;38(6):355–8.

7. Shields T. General thoracic surgery. Baltimore (MD): Williams and Wilkins; 1994.

8. Varoli F, Roviaro G, Grignani F, et al. Endoscopic treatment of bronchopleural fistulas. Ann Thorac Surg 1998;65(3):807–9.

9. Martin J, Ginsberg RJ, Abolhoda A, et al. Morbidity and mortality after neoadjuvant therapy for lung cancer: the risks of right pneumonectomy. Ann Thorac Surg 2001;72(4):1149–54.

10. Burfeind WR Jr, D'Amico TA, Toloza EM, et al. Low morbidity and mortality for bronchoplastic procedures with and without induction therapy. Ann Thorac Surg 2005;80(2):418–21 [discussion: 422].

11. Ohta M, Sawabata N, Maeda H, et al. Efficacy and safety of tracheobronchoplasty after induction therapy for locally advanced lung cancer. J Thorac Cardiovasc Surg 2003;125(1):96–100.

12. Rendina EA, Venuta F, De Giacomo T, et al. Safety and efficacy of bronchovascular reconstruction after induction chemotherapy for lung cancer. J Thorac Cardiovasc Surg 1997;114(5):830–5 [discussion: 835–7].

13. Darling GE, Abdurahman A, Yi QL, et al. Risk of a right pneumonectomy: role of bronchopleural fistula. Ann Thorac Surg 2005;79(2):433–7.

14. Deslauriers J, Demers P. Postpneumonectomy empyema and bronchopleural fistula. In: Yang SC, Cameron DE, editors. Current therapy in thoracic and cardiovascular Surgery. 1st. Edition. Philadelphia: Mosby; 2004. p. 304–6.

15. Hollaus PH, Setinek U, Lax F, et al. Risk factors for bronchopleural fistula after pneumonectomy: stump size does matter. Thorac Cardiovasc Surg 2003; 51(3):162–6.

16. Wright CD, Wain JC, Mathisen DJ, et al. Postpneumonectomy bronchopleural fistula after sutured bronchial closure: incidence, risk factors, and management. J Thorac Cardiovasc Surg 1996;112(5):1367–71.

17. Zaheer S, Allen MS, Cassivi SD, et al. Postpneumonectomy empyema: results after the Clagett procedure. Ann Thorac Surg 2006;82(1):279–86 [discussion: 286–7].

18. Eerola S, Virkkula L, Varstela E. Treatment of postpneumonectomy empyema and associated bronchopleural fistula. Experience of 100 consecutive postpneumonectomy patients. Scand J Thorac Cardiovasc Surg 1988;22(3):235–9.

19. Pomerantz M, Madsen L, Goble M, et al. Surgical management of resistant mycobacterial tuberculosis and other mycobacterial pulmonary infections. Ann Thorac Surg 1991;52(5):1108–11 [discussion: 1112].

20. Sherman MM, Subramanian V, Berger RL. Management of thoracic empyema. Am J Surg 1977;133(4): 474–9.

21. Sahn SA. Diagnosis and management of parapneumonic effusions and empyema. Clin Infect Dis 2007; 45(11):1480–6.

22. Bylicki O, Vandemoortele T, Orsini B, et al. Incidence and management of anastomotic complications after bronchial resection: a retrospective study. Ann Thorac Surg 2014;98(6):1961–7.

23. Westcott JL, Volpe JP. Peripheral bronchopleural fistula: CT evaluation in 20 patients with pneumonia, empyema, or postoperative air leak. Radiology 1995;196(1):175–81.

24. Pigula FA, Keenan RJ, Naunheim KS, et al. Diagnosis of postpneumonectomy bronchopleural fistula using ventilation scintigraphy. Ann Thorac Surg 1995;60(6):1812–4.

25. Gaur P, Dunne R, Colson YL, et al. Bronchopleural fistula and the role of contemporary imaging. J Thorac Cardiovasc Surg 2014;148(1):341–7.

26. Aboud FC, Verghese AC. Evarts Ambrose Graham, empyema, and the dawn of clinical understanding of negative intrapleural pressure. Clin Infect Dis 2002;34(2):198–203.

27. Miller JI Jr. The history of surgery of empyema, thoracoplasty, Eloesser flap, and muscle flap transposition. Chest Surg Clin N Am 2000;10(1): 45–53, viii.

28. Davies HE, Davies RJ, Davies CW, et al. Management of pleural infection in adults: British Thoracic Society Pleural Disease Guideline 2010. Thorax 2010;65(Suppl 2):ii41–53.

29. Robinson S. The treatment of chronic non-tuberculous chronic empyema. Surg Gynecol Obstet 1916;22:257.

30. Eloesser L. An operation for tuberculous empyema. Surg Gynecol Obstet 1935;60:1096.

31. Walsh MD, Bruno AD, Onaitis MW, et al. The role of intrathoracic free flaps for chronic empyema. Ann Thorac Surg 2011;91(3):865–8.

32. Takanari K, Kamei Y, Toriyama K, et al. Management of postpneumonectomy empyema using free flap and pedicled flap. Ann Thorac Surg 2010;89(1): 321–3.

33. Anderson TM, Miller JI Jr. Surgical technique and application of pericardial fat pad and pericardiophrenic grafts. Ann Thorac Surg 1995;59(6): 1590–1.

34. Mineo TC, Ambrogi V. Early closure of the postpneumonectomy bronchopleural fistula by pedicled diaphragmatic flaps. Ann Thorac Surg 1995;60(3): 714–5.

35. Okada M, Tsubota N, Yoshimura M, et al. Surgical treatment for chronic pleural empyema. Surg Today 2000;30(6):506–10.

36. Brewer LA 3rd, King EL, Lilly LJ, et al. Bronchial closure in pulmonary resection: a clinical and experimental study using a pedicled pericardial fat graft reinforcement. J Thorac Surg 1953;26(5): 507–32.

37. Taghavi S, Marta GM, Lang G, et al. Bronchial stump coverage with a pedicled pericardial flap: an effective method for prevention of postpneumonectomy bronchopleural fistula. Ann Thorac Surg 2005;79(1): 284–8.

38. Clagett OT, Geraci JE. A procedure for the management of postpneumonectomy empyema. J Thorac Cardiovasc Surg 1963;45:141–5.

# Management of Postoperative Respiratory Failure

Michael S. Mulligan, MD[a],*, Kathleen S. Berfield, MD[a],
Ryan V. Abbaszadeh, MD[b]

## KEYWORDS

- Postoperative pneumonia • Postpneumonectomy pulmonary edema
- Acute respiratory distress syndrome (ARDS) • Pulmonary embolism

## KEY POINTS

- Prevention of postoperative respiratory failure begins in the preoperative period.
- Postoperative respiratory failure is associated with high morbidity and mortality.
- Early recognition of signs and symptoms of postoperative respiratory failure is key to management and successful outcomes.

## INTRODUCTION

It is widely accepted that prevention of postoperative complications begins in the preoperative setting with appropriate patient selection and optimization. Such strategies include smoking cessation[1] and optimization of nutritional status and associated medical comorbidities. However, despite these efforts, respiratory failure following thoracic surgical procedures can result in significant patient morbidity and mortality in the postoperative period. This article focuses on mitigation of risk factors and management of patients with postoperative respiratory failure.

## RISK ASSESSMENT
### Preoperative Evaluation

A thorough history and physical examination are essential in identifying patients with underlying lung disease and those with a history of smoking. One study identified 5 significant independent risk factors for postoperative pulmonary complications: age greater than 75 years, body mass index greater than 30, American Society of Anesthesiologists score greater than 3, active smoking, and chronic obstructive pulmonary disease.[1] Recent respiratory infections, obesity, and a history of alcohol abuse increase the likelihood of postoperative respiratory complications, including reintubation and dependence on mechanical ventilation. Laboratory evaluation can also help identify patients at risk for postoperative pulmonary complications. For example, low serum albumin levels in the preoperative setting are associated with increased rates of pneumonia and failure to wean from mechanical ventilation. Preoperative anemia is also an independent risk factor for postoperative pulmonary complications.[1,2]

### Intraoperative Factors

Several intraoperative strategies can be implemented to reduce the likelihood of postoperative respiratory failure. Surgical approach, including the type of incision made, can influence postoperative complications. For example, a muscle-sparing thoracotomy is more likely to be better tolerated than a posterolateral approach. Additionally, minimally invasive techniques can reduce losses in postoperative impairment in respiratory muscle function, resulting in improved deep breathing and

[a] Division of Cardiothoracic Surgery, University of Washington, Seattle, WA, USA; [b] Department of General Surgery, University of Washington, Seattle, WA, USA
* Corresponding author. University of Washington Medical Center, 1959 Northeast Pacific Street, Box 356310, Seattle, WA 98195-6310.
E-mail address: msmmd@u.washington.edu

Thorac Surg Clin 25 (2015) 429–433
http://dx.doi.org/10.1016/j.thorsurg.2015.07.007

mobility. Video-assisted thoracoscopic surgery approaches are minimally invasive and do not cause the degree of respiratory muscle loss and lung function decline that open thoracotomy requires.[2]

## Postoperative Factors

Adequate pain control without causing oversedation is necessary in the postoperative period to facilitate early mobilization, clearance of secretions, and prevention of atelectasis. Use of an epidural catheter, which is placed preoperatively as a measure of preemptive pain control for use in the immediate postoperative period, is the standard of care for thoracic surgical procedures at the authors' institution. Local analgesic agents (bupivacaine or ropivacaine) and opiates can be used in combination as continuous infusions with or without additional boluses administered by nursing or directly by the patient. The epidural catheter is usually kept in place until the chest tubes are removed. In addition to effective analgesia, chest physiotherapy and aggressive pulmonary hygiene also play important roles in clearing the airway and preventing atelectasis. The judicious use of fluids, particularly in thoracic surgery, can prevent fluid overload, pulmonary edema, and eventual respiratory failure.[1–3]

## POSTOPERATIVE PNEUMONIA
### Incidence, Mortality, and Risk Factors

The incidence of postoperative pneumonia (POP) has been cited as 2.2% to 6%[4] in the literature but this is a moving target because it can be difficult to differentiate POP from the expected physiologic and radiographic responses to thoracic surgery normally seen in the postoperative period, such as fever, hypoxemia, atelectasis, and radiographic abnormalities. Regardless, POP is associated with significant mortality ranging from 20% to 50%[5,6] as well as increased hospital length of stay. Patient-specific risk factors for development of POP include preoperative hospitalization, immunocompromised state, extent of the procedure, poor underlying cardiopulmonary reserve, smoking history, and presence of atelectasis.

### Clinical Presentation

The onset of POP usually occurs within the first 5 postoperative days and there is some question whether the onset of POP is related to cessation of routine postoperative antibiotic prophylaxis, which is generally continued through the first 24 hours postoperatively.[6] Initial signs and symptoms include the development of fever, hypoxemia, leukocytosis, increased oropharyngeal secretions, dyspnea, tachypnea, and new or progressive infiltrates on chest radiography.

### Prevention

Postoperatively, an intensive pulmonary hygiene protocol, including targeted chest physiotherapy, incentive spirometry, and early ambulation, should be used to prevent atelectasis and promote clearance of secretions. Atelectasis itself is a known complication associated with pulmonary resection and most atelectasis seen in the postoperative period is subsegmental and of little clinical consequence. However, segmental atelectasis is less unlikely to improve with routine incentive spirometry and usually requires bronchoscopy. There is debate about the efficacy of bronchoscopy in patients with abundant secretions. Some studies have shown that little benefit was achieved when attempting to expel secretions with bronchoscopy, although there may be benefit for those patients whose presentation is refractory to chest physiotherapy and intensive pulmonary hygiene.[7]

### Treatment

The diagnosis and management of POP is similar to that for hospital-acquired pneumonia. When suspected, lower respiratory tract cultures should be obtained and prompt initiation of broad-spectrum antibiotics should occur. POP is often polymicrobial in nature, with Enterobacter, Staphylococcus, and Streptococcus being the most common organisms. Anaerobic coverage should also be considered following thoracoabdominal procedures. Close respiratory monitoring should be implemented in a patient with pneumonia and supplemental oxygen administered if the patient cannot appropriately oxygenate on room air. Mechanical ventilation may be required in cases of respiratory distress and respiratory failure.[8]

## POSTPNEUMONECTOMY PULMONARY EDEMA

Postpneumonectomy pulmonary edema (PPE) can occur following pulmonary resection and is defined as an acute, hypoxemic respiratory failure that is not cardiogenic in nature. It most commonly occurs following right pneumonectomy but can occur following less extensive pulmonary resections, including lobectomy. Its presentation is similar to acute respiratory distress syndrome (ARDS) and the same criteria are used for its diagnosis: bilateral infiltrates on chest radiograph, $Pao_2$, fraction of inspired oxygen less than 200, and pulmonary capillary wedge pressure less than 18.[9–11]

## Incidence, Mortality, and Risk Factors

The incidence of PPE ranges from 2.2% to 7%. More recent data suggest the average incidence following pneumonectomy is 3% to 4%, whereas lobectomy can be as low as 2%. Mortality in PPE is high and has consistently been reported as 50% to 100%. Risk factors associated with increased incidence of PPE are right pneumonectomy, perioperative fluid overload, intraoperative transfusion of fresh frozen plasma, and high intraoperative airway pressures.[10–12]

## Clinical Presentation or Pathogenesis

The onset of PPE is variable; however, most patients will present within the first 72 hours postoperatively.[13] Early indications of PPE include an increased oxygen requirement, tachypnea, tachycardia, and fever. Radiographic signs of PPE lag behind the clinical presentation and range from patchy interstitial infiltrates to frank alveolar edema. Evidence of disease progression and increasing dead space is hypercarbia and worsening hypoxemia refractory to increasing oxygen levels. Early on, signs and radiographic findings may be similar to early POP, which may delay initial diagnosis of PPE.[14] Pathophysiology of PPE has been found to mirror ARDS with initial loss of endothelial integrity followed by capillary leak and associated extravasation of proteins and inflammatory cells into the interstitial space. This inflammatory reaction eventually leads to fibroproliferative and obliterative changes at the alveolar and microvascular level. This results in interstitial fibrosis and remodeling of the pulmonary vascular bed.[14] Ongoing hypoxia and alveolar damage leads to hypoxic pulmonary vasoconstriction and development of acute pulmonary hypertension, which can lead to right ventricular strain and possible failure, which complicates the management of PPE.[14]

## Prevention

Multiple factors have been implicated in the pathogenesis of PPE and involve elements of patient management throughout the perioperative period. Perioperative volume overload has long been thought to precipitate the development of PPE, although studies have not yet demonstrated a clear causal relationship. Regardless, judicious use of intravenous fluids continues to be the rule after pneumonectomy and, certainly, volume overload can exacerbate preexisting pulmonary edema by increasing pulmonary capillary hydrostatic pressure.[12] Surgical factors, such right-sided pneumonectomy and carinal pneumonectomy, have been

associated with increased incidence of PPE as well as disruption of lymphatic drainage due to the extent of dissection.[15] Both hyperoxia and hypoxia have been implicated in the development of PPE. Hyperoxia of the contralateral lung during single-lung ventilation with the production of reactive oxygen species and reactive nitrogen species are implicated in ARDS. Additionally, hypoxic pulmonary vasoconstriction and ischemia reperfusion–type injury to the ipsilateral lung, which contribute to increased circulation of inflammatory mediators, are thought to contribute to progression of PPE or ARDS-like syndromes.[14]

## Treatment

As mentioned previously, the mortality rate of PPE is extremely high. Thus, early identification and management is essential. Inevitably, due to refractory hypoxia and hypercarbia, patients with PPE require reintubation, mechanical ventilatory support, and initiation of lung protective ventilation with low tidal volumes and high positive endexpiratory pressure.[16] Careful attention to peak airway pressures and avoidance of high pressures are key due to the risk of further barotrauma and bronchial stump dehiscence. Several small studies have also shown inhaled nitric oxide to be beneficial in the treatment of PPE due to its pulmonary vasodilatory effects and improvement in arterial oxygenation. Additionally, inhaled nitric oxide has been associated with improvement of acute pulmonary hypertension and associated right ventricular dysfunction that can be seen with ARDS.[17]

## PULMONARY EMBOLISM

Immobility and malignancy are common features seen in patients undergoing lung resection or other intrathoracic procedures, predisposing patients to the development of pulmonary embolism (PE). Therefore, PE must be considered in the differential diagnosis when evaluating a patient with new or ongoing postoperative respiratory failure.

## Incidence, Mortality, and Risk Factors

Venous thromboembolism (VTE) is a major cause of morbidity and mortality. Hospital-acquired deep vein thrombosis (DVT) is reported to be 15% to 40% among general surgical patients and is the second-most common postoperative medical complication.[18] Patient-specific risk factors include increasing patient age, history of malignancy, prior VTE, smoking, hypertension, obesity, and history of a hypercoagulable disorder. The 2012 American College of Chest Physicians (ACCP) guidelines stratifies surgical patients into

3 groups: low, moderate, and high risk for VTE. Generally, patients undergoing thoracic surgery fall into the moderate risk group and their risk of VTE in the absence of prophylaxis is estimated to be approximately 3%.[19]

## Clinical Presentation

The presentation of PE can vary widely and often presents in an atypical fashion. The most classic presentation consists of the abrupt onset of pleuritic chest pain, dyspnea, and hypoxia.[19] The timing of and progression of symptoms is unpredictable and patients may asymptomatic or present with progressive dyspnea or acute hemodynamic deterioration as the case may be for large pulmonary emboli. Additionally, atypical signs and symptoms, such as fever, wheezing, hemoptysis, abdominal pain, orthopnea, and lower extremity swelling, may be present. When PE is suspected and the patient is hemodynamically normal, computed tomography (CT) pulmonary angiogram is the imaging modality of choice. However, in the patient who is hemodynamically unstable and cannot undergo CT scan, empiric treatment with systemic anticoagulation is recommended and duplex ultrasonography of the lower extremities to look for DVT or echocardiogram to evaluate for signs of right heart strain can be used.[20]

## Prevention

Primary prevention of perioperative VTE or PE is multifaceted. Pharmacologic and mechanical prophylaxes are essential in the prevention of VTE and recommended in the postoperative setting. The 2012 ACCP guidelines recommend the use of routine pharmacologic prophylaxis with low-dose unfractionated heparin (UFH), low molecular weight heparin (LMWH), or fondaparinux.[19] The typical regimen of 5000 units of subcutaneous UFH initiated preoperatively, within 2 hours of incision and continued every 8 hours postoperatively has been shown to reduce the rate of DVT from 22.4% to 9.0%, and PE from 2.0% to 1.3%. In patients with malignancy who undergo an operation, a 4-week course of pharmacologic prophylaxis, as opposed to 1 week, was shown to reduce the incidence of VTE from 12.0% to 4.8%.[21]

## Treatment

When PE is diagnosed, anticoagulation is indicated as long as the risk of bleeding is not prohibitively high. In the hemodynamically unstable patient, without contraindication to systemic anticoagulation, thrombolysis or, in rare circumstances, embolectomy may be considered. The role for thrombolytic therapy should be considered for hemodynamically unstable patients with refractory hypoxemia, perfusion defects, refractory hypotension, and acute right ventricular dysfunction. However, there are many contraindications to thrombolytic therapy and these must be taken into account before initiation of this therapy on a case-by-case basis. Contraindications include prior intracranial hemorrhage, suspected aortic dissection, active bleeding, and ischemic stroke within 3 months of the embolism.

Treatment of PE in a hemodynamically stable patient is systemic anticoagulation with LMWH is preferred to the use of intravenous or subcutaneous UFH. Concomitantly, an oral anticoagulant such as warfarin should be initiated at the time of diagnosis. The LMWH or UFH should not be discontinued until the international normalized ratio is 2.0 for a minimum of 24 hours and not sooner than 5 days after initiation. If it is the first episode of PE and there is an identifiable and temporary risk factor such as surgery, a 3-month duration of therapy is recommended. In the case of recurrent or unprovoked PE, lifelong anticoagulation may be indicated. However, this decision must be weighed carefully and the patient's risk of bleeding and medical compliance taken into account.[22,23]

Routine placement of inferior vena cava (IVC) filter is not recommended for prevention or management of PE. However, in the presence of a contraindication, prior complication, or recurrent PE in the setting of therapeutic anticoagulation, an IVC filter should be considered.[24] In special circumstances, when ongoing thrombolytic therapy is either contraindicated or failed, or if an embolus is seen within the right atrium or proximal pulmonary artery, surgical embolectomy may be appropriate.[20]

## SUMMARY

Postoperative respiratory failure after thoracic surgery is multifactorial and is associated with significant morbidity and mortality. Early recognition and treatment of respiratory complications is key to optimizing patient outcomes. Management is labor intensive and in the setting of postpneumonectomy edema and ARDS can be protracted and resource intensive. The use of ancillary services is not discussed but is of the utmost importance in the progression of patient care. Nurses, pain management specialists, respiratory therapists, and physical and occupational therapists all play key roles in progressing patient care and preventing avoidable respiratory complications.

# REFERENCES

1. Agostini P, Cieslik H, Rathinam S, et al. Postoperative pulmonary complications following thoracic surgery: are there any modifiable risk factors? Thorax 2010;65(9):815–8.
2. Canet J, Gallart L. Postoperative respiratory failure: pathogenesis, prediction, and prevention. Curr Opin Crit Care 2014;20(1):56–62.
3. Gupta H. Development and validation of a risk calculator predicting postoperative respiratory failure. Chest 2011;140(5):1207.
4. Lee JY, Jin S-M, Lee C-H, et al. Risk factors of postoperative pneumonia after lung cancer surgery. J Korean Med Sci 2011;26(8):979–84.
5. Kollef M. Prevention of postoperative pneumonia. Hosp Physician 2007;64:47–60.
6. Schussler O, Alifano M, Dermine H, et al. Postoperative pneumonia after major lung resection. Am J Respir Crit Care Med 2006;173(10):1161–9.
7. Kazaure HS, Martin M, Yoon JK, et al. Long-term results of a postoperative pneumonia prevention program for the inpatient surgical ward. JAMA Surg 2014;149(9):914.
8. Niederman M, Craven D. Guidelines for the management of adults with hospital acquired, ventilator-associated, and healthcare-associated pneumonia. Am J Crit Care Med 2005;171:388–416.
9. Martinez F, Medina J, Ojeda D, et al. Postoperative acute respiratory distress syndrome after lung resection. Arch Bronconeumol 2007;43(11):623–7.
10. Samano M, Sancho L, Beyruti R, et al. Postpneumonectomy pulmonary edema. J bras pneumol 2005; 31(1):69–75.
11. Shapiro M, Swanson SJ, Wright CD, et al. Predictors of major morbidity and mortality after pneumonectomy utilizing the Society for Thoracic Surgeons General Thoracic Surgery Database. Ann Thorac Surg 2010;90(3):927–34.
12. Alvarez JM, Panda RK, Newman MA, et al. Postpneumonectomy pulmonary edema. J Cardiothorac Vasc Anesth 2003;17(3):388–95.
13. Turnage W, Lunn J. Postpneumonectomy pulmonary edema: a retrospective analysis of associated variables. Chest 1993;103(6):1646–50.
14. Jordan S, Mitchell JA, Quinlan GJ, et al. The pathogenesis of lung injury following pulmonary resection. Eur Respir J 2000;15(4):790–9. Available at: http://www.ncbi.nlm.nih.gov/pubmed/10780775.
15. Alvarez JM, Bairstow BM, Tang C, et al. Post-lung resection pulmonary edema: a case for aggressive management. J Cardiothorac Vasc Anesth 1998; 12(2):199–205.
16. Ventilation with lower tidal volumes as compared with traditional tidal volumes for acute lung injury and the acute respiratory distress syndrome. N Engl J Med 2000;342(18):1301–8.
17. Mathisen DJ, Kuo EY, Hahn C, et al. Inhaled nitric oxide for adult respiratory distress syndrome after pulmonary resection. Ann Thorac Surg 1998;66(6): 1894–902.
18. Venous thromboembolism: reducing the risk of venous thromboembolism (deep vein thrombosis and pulmonary embolism) in patients admitted to hospital. (n.d.). National Clinic Guideline Centre.
19. Guyatt GH, Akl EA, Crowther M, et al. Introduction to the ninth edition: Antithrombotic Therapy and Prevention of Thrombosis, 9th ed: American College of Chest Physicians Evidence-Based Clinical Practice Guidelines. Chest 2012;141(2 Suppl):48S–52S.
20. Rosenberger P, Shernan SK, Mihaljevic T, et al. Transesophageal echocardiography for detecting extrapulmonary thrombi during pulmonary embolectomy. Ann Thorac Surg 2004;78(3):862–6.
21. Zurawska U, Parasuraman S, Goldhaber SZ. Prevention of pulmonary embolism in general surgery patients. Circulation 2007;115(9):302–8.
22. Kovacs MJ, Hawel JD, Rekman JF, et al. Ambulatory management of pulmonary embolism: a pragmatic evaluation. J Thromb Haemost 2010;8(11):2406–11.
23. Nijkeuter M, Söhne M, Tick LW, et al. The natural course of hemodynamically stable pulmonary embolism: clinical outcome and risk factors in a large prospective cohort study. Chest 2007;131(2):517–23.
24. Crowther MA. Inferior vena cava filters in the management of venous thromboembolism. Am J Med 2007;120(10 Suppl 2):S13–7.

# Complications Following Carinal Resections and Sleeve Resections

Luis F. Tapias, MD, Harald C. Ott, MD, Douglas J. Mathisen, MD*

## KEYWORDS

- Carinal resection • Sleeve resection • Bronchopleural fistula • Airway anastomosis
- Airway stenosis

## KEY POINTS

- Careful patient selection is important for the success of carinal and sleeve resections.
- Attention to established technical issues is fundamental, including preservation of bronchial blood supply, proper tension-free anastomotic technique correcting size mismatch, and buttressing with vascularized tissue.
- Prevention of complications by means of adequate surgical technique is critical; once complications appear, their management is difficult.
- Bronchoscopic evaluation before discharge is useful for the early identification of potential anastomotic problems.
- Aggressive management of complications adhering to established principles should be implemented as soon as the diagnosis is made.

## INTRODUCTION

Lung-sparing bronchoplastic resection and reconstruction of the tracheobronchial tree, with and without resection of lung parenchyma, may be required and is a valid therapeutic option for patients with centrally located malignancies. Resection of the carina or main bronchi may be necessary in cases in which standard pneumonectomy or lobectomy, respectively, would not achieve complete tumor resection. Resection of the carina is most frequently performed along with a right pneumonectomy,[1] whereas bronchial sleeve resections are most frequently associated with an upper lobectomy.[2] One of the earliest reports on carinal resection was described by Belsey in 1950 and involved the lateral resection of the distal trachea and carina followed by reconstruction with a free fascial graft reinforced by stainless steel wire.[3] Likewise, Price Thomas described the performance of sleeve lobectomies as early as in 1952 for the treatment of tuberculosis and lung cancer.[4]

Historically, sleeve lung resections were generally regarded as an alternative to pneumonectomy in patients with poor cardiopulmonary reserve. However, lung-sparing procedures have shown to be beneficial in patients without cardiopulmonary limitations,[5] and must be favored over pneumonectomy whenever anatomically feasible. Therefore, sleeve lung resections have been increasingly used for patients with centrally located malignancies regardless of pulmonary function. Evidence points toward equivalent oncologic outcomes with improved survival and quality of life after sleeve resections compared with pneumonectomy.[6,7] Even though these surgical techniques have been described in the literature for

Division of Thoracic Surgery, Department of Surgery, Massachusetts General Hospital, Harvard Medical School, 55 Fruit Street, Blake 15, Boston, MA 02114, USA
* Corresponding author.
E-mail address: dmathisen@mgh.harvard.edu

Thorac Surg Clin 25 (2015) 435–447
http://dx.doi.org/10.1016/j.thorsurg.2015.07.003
1547-4127/15/$ – see front matter © 2015 Elsevier Inc. All rights reserved.

more than 60 years, recent advances in anesthetic techniques, as well as improved patient selection and postoperative care have lead to acceptable rates of postoperative morbidity and mortality, making this a valid therapeutic option in patients with involvement of the central airways.

Carinal and sleeve lung resections represent true challenges for thoracic surgeons. These patients require careful and thorough evaluation, strict attention to technical details in the operating room, a keen understanding of the principles of resection and reconstruction of the tracheobronchial tree, and dedicated postoperative care. These procedures hold great potential for significant postoperative morbidity given their impact on cardiopulmonary physiology and the risk for development of anastomotic complications.[8] Here, we aim to summarize key aspects to be considered when performing carinal or sleeve resections, and when dealing with postoperative complications.

## INDICATIONS AND CONTRAINDICATIONS
### Indications

Carinal resections and bronchoplastic procedures are most commonly indicated for the surgical treatment of centrally located tumors involving the orifice of the lobar bronchus or extending into intermediate or main bronchi or the carina. Most frequently, these are non–small cell lung cancers (NSCLC), particularly squamous cell carcinomas. However, they are also useful in the surgical treatment of centrally located low-grade malignancies, such as carcinoid tumors and salivary type tumors (eg, mucoepidermoid carcinoma and adenoid cystic carcinomas). Additionally, bronchoplastic procedures can be applied to treat benign stenosis, particularly of the mainstem bronchi, of traumatic, infectious, or idiopathic etiologies.[9]

In the case of carinal resections, a right carinal pneumonectomy is the most frequent procedure, especially in patients with NSCLC originating from the right upper lobe orifice and extending into the lateral aspect of the carina and lower trachea. The tumor length should not exceed 4 cm of trachea, as this poses anatomic limits to resection. Alternatively, carinal resections may be indicated when there is involvement of the bronchial margin after a standard pneumonectomy.

Sleeve lobectomy is indicated when tumors are located at the origin of the lobar bronchus, but do not infiltrate the remaining lobes to justify a pneumonectomy. Additionally, it may be indicated when there is direct infiltration from metastatic peribronchial nodes or a positive bronchial margin. Sleeve lobectomy is still indicated in the presence of positive N1 nodes, as it is associated with lower morbidity and mortality as well as comparable long-term results when compared with pneumonectomy.[6,7] Some conditions involve only the mainstem bronchus, including low-grade neoplasms (eg, carcinoid tumors, mucoepidermoid carcinomas, fibrous histiocytomas, and adenoid cystic carcinomas) and benign stenosis of infectious (eg, histoplasmosis), inflammatory, traumatic, iatrogenic, or idiopathic etiologies.[9] The same surgical principles hold for these bronchoplastic procedures as for sleeve lobectomy: careful technique, adjustment for size discrepancy, avoidance of devascularization, avoidance of excessive tension, and the use of pedicled vascularized tissue flaps.

### Contraindications

Absolute contraindications are related to poor surgical candidacy due to significant medical comorbidities, very low predicted postoperative pulmonary function, or extensive local invasion of the tumor precluding reconstruction. The presence of mediastinal lymph node involvement (N2 disease or greater) is considered a relative contraindication given the poor long-term results obtained in these patients. The need for resection and reconstruction of vascular structures (ie, superior vena cava or pulmonary artery) is not considered a contraindication.

### Special Situations

There are a few important special situations to carinal surgery and sleeve resections that deserve mention:

- Chronic use of corticosteroids: This can lead to impairment of airway anastomotic healing. Ideally, patients should be weaned from steroids at least 2 to 4 weeks before surgery. If necessary, coring out the obstructing tumor is beneficial until such time as resection can be done.
- Anticipated need for prolonged postoperative mechanical ventilation: Positive-pressure ventilation can put stress on the airway anastomosis. Additionally, the need for postoperative mechanical ventilation has been strongly associated with postoperative morbidity.[10] The anesthetic plan should include every effort to permit extubation at the end of the procedure.
- Neoadjuvant therapy: Patients who have received neoadjuvant therapy, particularly radiation, are at a higher risk for anastomotic complications due to relative tissue ischemia. These patients should receive an anastomotic

wrap with vascularized tissue. Coverage can be achieved with pedicled intercostal muscle flaps or omentum in these circumstances.[11,12]

## SURGICAL PRINCIPLES

Strict adherence to well-established surgical principles increases the likelihood of a successful operation while decreasing the chances for postoperative anastomotic complications. Great judgment is required in knowing the limits of resection, acceptable interruption of blood supply, and acceptable amounts of anastomotic tension.

### Tumor Resectability

Careful bronchoscopic assessment is of the upmost importance to establish quality of tissues and extent of disease. Endobronchial ultrasonography may aid in better defining bronchial or carinal infiltration. However, preoperative workup may not reliably indicate the presence or absence of bronchial or carinal involvement. Therefore, the final decision to perform a carinal or sleeve lung resection is often an intraoperative decision. The resectability of the tumor needs to be determined before any structures are divided. If resectable, a standard lobectomy or pneumonectomy should be performed, leaving the division and reconstruction of the airway last.

### Airway Dissection

Precise and careful dissection of the airway should be applied to preserve the tracheobronchial blood supply to ensure adequate healing of the anastomosis. Lateral dissection proximal and distal to the proposed lines of transection should be limited to avoid devascularization. Liberal use of frozen-section analysis will help tailor the approach so as to move forward with the most appropriate oncologic operation, as the primary goal is the complete resection of the tumor with free resection margins. The only exception is the case of adenoid cystic carcinoma, as microscopic involvement of the resection margins is frequent due to submucosal spread. This can be accepted and treated with adjuvant radiation therapy yielding acceptable long-term results.[13,14]

Anastomotic tension is the biggest contributor to anastomotic complications. Careful attention needs to be paid to the length of the airway segment to be resected. The risk for developing anastomotic complications increases with the length of resection. For carinal resections, the risk of anastomotic complications increases when the length exceeds 4 cm.[15] This is especially true in cases of right carinal pneumonectomy, as the left bronchus is restrained by the aortic arch, limiting its cephalad migration. Release maneuvers are helpful in reducing anastomotic tension for all bronchoplastic procedures.

### Size Mismatch

There is often a size mismatch when performing bronchoplastic procedures. We prefer careful placement of sutures to accommodate any discrepancies. Sutures in the larger lumen are placed slightly farther apart and slightly closer together in the smaller end. We have avoided wedge resections of the bronchus creating a "T" junction of the anastomosis or "pleating" of the bronchus as these maneuvers increase the risk of a fistula.

### Release Maneuvers

Surgeons embarking on procedures involving resection and reconstruction of the tracheobronchial tree must be familiar with available maneuvers to reduce anastomotic tension.

- Neck flexion: This is the simplest maneuver and allows the caudal motion of the trachea into the mediastinum. However, its effect is limited in alleviating tension in the distal trachea and main bronchi.
- Mobilization of the pretracheal plane: Dissection of this plane immediately anterior to the trachea provides some mobility and should be used routinely in cases of carinal resection. Blunt dissection of this plane at mediastinoscopy facilitates dissection during the operation. If indicated, mediastinoscopy should be performed at the time of proposed resection to avoid scar formation.
- Inferior pulmonary ligament: Incision of the inferior pulmonary ligament should be performed routinely.
- Inferior hilar release: This reduces anastomotic tension significantly. This release is best accomplished before starting airway resection. A U-shaped incision is made in the pericardium below the inferior pulmonary vein, with intrapericardial division of the raphe extending between the inferior pulmonary vein and the inferior vena cava (**Fig. 1**).
- Complete hilar release: Additional length may be gained by completely incising the pericardium around the hilar vessels (see **Fig. 1**).
- Laryngeal release maneuvers are not useful unless the resection extends into the midtrachea.

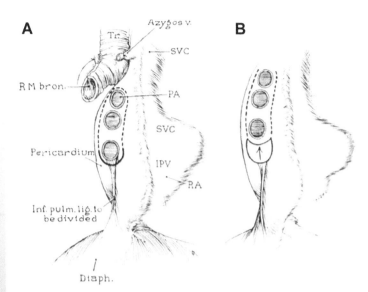

**A**

Azygos v.
Tr.
SVC
R M bron.
PA
SVC
Pericardium
IPV
R.A
Inf. pulm. lig. to
be divided
Diaph.

**B**

**Fig. 1.** (*A*) Inferior hilar (*solid line*) and full pericardial (*dotted line*) release maneuvers. (*B*) Release achieved (*arrow*).

## Anastomotic Technique

There are multiple techniques described to perform the airway anastomosis in both cases of carinal resections and sleeve resections. However, the preferred technique for airway anastomosis in the authors' institution is the sequential placement of multiple interrupted sutures at 2-mm to 3-mm intervals using absorbable material, such as 4-0 polyglactin 910 (Vicryl; Ethicon, Somerville, NJ). The use of absorbable suture material is preferred to prevent granuloma formation or stenosis at the anastomosis.[16,17] The knots are tied outside the airway lumen after all sutures have been placed, with the aid of traction sutures to decrease tension (**Figs. 2** and **3**).

Placement of vascularized tissue between the airway anastomosis and the pulmonary artery is an important principle in anastomotic technique. Wrapping of the anastomosis is typically performed with pedicled pleura or pericardial fat pad. Intercostal muscle flaps are usually used as a partial wrap given their size, which makes them too bulky to place around the anastomosis. In patients who have received neoadjuvant radiation therapy, the use of omentum or intercostal muscle should be considered.

## COMPLICATIONS OF CARINAL SURGERY AND SLEEVE RESECTIONS

Even after careful patient selection and judicious surgical technique, complications can arise in the postoperative period. Carinal resections are associated with a mortality rate of 3% to 20% and an overall morbidity rate of 11% to 50%.[8,10,18–23] Postoperative mortality can be categorized as early or late.[24] Early mortality is often related to acute respiratory distress syndrome (ARDS) or pneumonia, whereas late mortality has been almost exclusively related to anastomotic complications. Bronchial sleeve resections carry a postoperative mortality rate of 1.5% to 11.0% and an overall morbidity rate of 11.0% to 51.0%[5,8,25–44] (**Table 1**).

Procedure-specific complications after carinal and sleeve resections are mostly related to the airway anastomosis and include the development of bronchopleural fistulas, bronchovascular fistulas, benign anastomotic strictures, and local tumor recurrence at the anastomotic line. Additionally, patients undergoing carinal pneumonectomy are at risk for postpneumonectomy pulmonary edema, a catastrophic complication that deserves special mention.

In our institution, strict adherence to the aforementioned surgical principles has yielded excellent results.[39] A retrospective review of 196 patients who underwent sleeve lobectomy over a 27-year period for the surgical treatment of NSCLC or low-grade neoplasms, revealed an overall morbidity rate of 34.6% with an operative mortality of 2.0%.[39] Procedure-specific complications compared favorably with other contemporary published reports during our experience (see **Table 1**), as bronchopleural fistulas were observed in 2% of patients, and bronchovascular fistulas and anastomotic stenosis were absent. Finally, 6 (4.9%) of 123 patients operated on for NSCLC experienced recurrence at the anastomotic line.

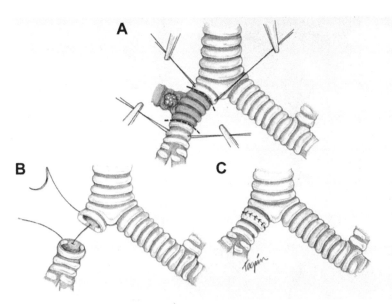

**Fig. 2.** Technique for sleeve lobectomy. (*A*) Traction sutures placed in the mid-lateral portion proximally and distally. (*B*) First anastomotic suture placed posteriorly. (*C*) Completed anastomosis.

The low rate of bronchial anastomotic complications in our institution is a direct result of routinely avoiding tension on the anastomosis by performing a hilar release maneuver whenever necessary, precise dissection with preservation of the bronchial blood supply, and placement of vascularized tissue between the bronchial anastomosis and the pulmonary artery.

## POSTPNEUMONECTOMY PULMONARY EDEMA
### Presentation

Postpneumonectomy pulmonary edema is an acute syndrome that develops within the first 72 hours after resection.[45] This syndrome represents a continuum spanning acute lung injury and ARDS based on current diagnostic criteria. It is reported to complicate 3% to 7% of all pneumonectomies, although it has been described in as many as 16% of patients. It presents more frequently after right-sided resections.[45] It has been reported in 4% to 14% of cases involving a carinal resection.[10,18,19,21,46,47] The clinical picture is that of tachypnea, hypoxia, hypercapnia, and "ground glass" infiltrates on chest imaging. Usually there is rapid deterioration mandating endotracheal intubation and mechanical ventilatory support. Multiple factors have been implicated in its pathophysiology, including fluid overload, barotrauma, disruption of lymphatic drainage, the perioperative use of blood products, occult microaspiration, systemic inflammation,

and oxidative stress leading to increased pulmonary vascular permeability.[45]

### Prevention

Every effort should be made to limit the administration of fluids and blood products intraoperatively. The anesthesiologist should be cautioned to avoid overdistension of the lung to avoid barotrauma injury. The use of a bolus of methylprednisolone before ligation of the pulmonary artery has been suggested to reduce the incidence of postpneumonectomy pulmonary edema,[48] but requires further investigation.

### Treatment

Treatment remains supportive to ensure adequate oxygen delivery by optimizing ventilator settings, hemodynamics, and pulmonary toilet, as well as nutrition and antibiotic coverage. Inhaled nitric oxide has been reported to improve oxygenation,[49,50] but these finding have not been replicated in animal studies.[51] In severe refractory cases, the use of extracorporeal membrane oxygenation should be considered.[52,53]

### Prognosis

Postpneumonectomy pulmonary edema is a catastrophic complication, as it carries a mortality risk of 50% to 100%.[45]

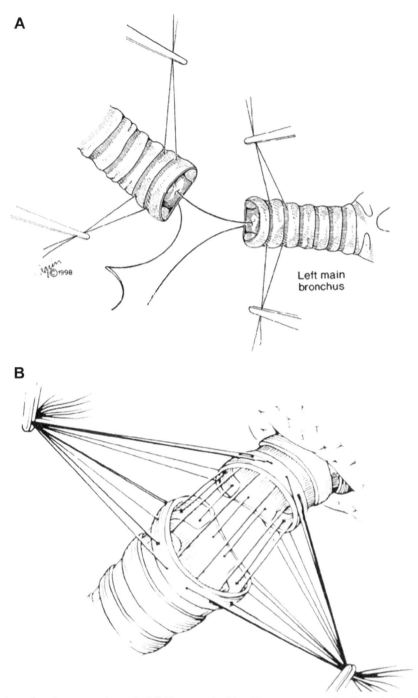

**Fig. 3.** Technique for airway anastomosis. (*A*) Placement of traction sutures proximally and distally in the mid-lateral portion and placement of the first posterior anastomotic suture. (*B*) Completed anastomotic sutures (without traction sutures) with proper spacing to control for bronchus size discrepancy.

**Table 1**
Summary of complications after carinal and sleeve resections in published surgical series with n >50

| Author, Year | n | Mortality, % | Morbidity, % | Anastomotic Complications, % | | | | Empyema, % | 5-y Survival, % |
|---|---|---|---|---|---|---|---|---|---|
| | | | | Bronchopleural Fistula/ Dehiscence/ Ischemia | Bronchovascular Fistula | Stenosis | Local Recurrence | | |
| *Carinal resection* | | | | | | | | | |
| Tedder et al,[8] 1992 | 1915 | 20.9 | — | 10.1 | 2.9 | — | 4.2 | 8.6 | — |
| Mitchell et al,[10] 1999[a] | 134 | 12.7 | 38.8 | 17.2[b] | — | — | — | 2.2 | — |
| Mitchell et al,[18] 2001[a] | 60 | 15.0 | 45.0 | 16.7[b] | — | — | 3.3 | — | 42 |
| Porhanov et al,[19] 2002 | 231 | 16.0 | 35.5 | 21.6 | — | 7.4 | 5.0 | 14.7 | 25 |
| Regnard et al,[20] 2005 | 65 | 7.7 | 50.8 | 10.8 | — | 4.6 | — | 7.7 | 27 |
| de Perrot et al,[21] 2006 | 119 | 7.6 | 47.1 | 10.1 | — | 2.5 | 4.2 | 5.0 | 44 |
| Roviaro et al,[22] 2006 | 53 | 7.5 | 11.3 | 3.8 | — | — | — | 1.9 | 33 |
| Eichhorn et al,[23] 2013 | 64 | 3.1 | 40.6 | 10.9 | — | — | — | 10.9 | 31 |
| *Sleeve lobectomy* | | | | | | | | | |
| Tedder et al,[8] 1992 | 1915 | 5.5 | — | 3.0 | 2.5 | 4.8 | 12.5 | 2.0 | 40 |
| Kawahara et al,[25] 1994 | 112 | — | — | 5.6 | 1.8 | 6.3 | 7.1 | — | — |
| Gaissert et al,[5] 1996[a] | 72 | 4.0 | 11.0 | 1.4 | — | 2.8 | 1.4 | 1.4 | 42 |
| Icard et al,[26] 1999 | 110 | 2.7 | 44.5 | 3.6 | 0.9 | 3.6 | — | — | 39 |
| Tronc et al,[27] 2000 | 184 | 1.6 | 15.8 | 1.1 | — | 2.2 | — | 2.2 | 52 |
| Fadel et al,[28] 2002 | 169 | 2.4 | 12.4 | 1.2 | 1.2 | 1.2 | 3.8 | 2.4 | 52 |
| Mezzetti et al,[29] 2002 | 83 | 3.6 | 10.8 | 3.6 | — | — | 20.0 | — | 43 |

(continued on next page)

**Table 1**
*(continued)*

| Author, Year | n | Mortality, % | Morbidity, % | Anastomotic Complications, % | | | | Empyema, % | 5-y Survival, % |
| | | | | Bronchopleural Fistula/Dehiscence/Ischemia | Bronchovascular Fistula | Stenosis | Local Recurrence | | |
|---|---|---|---|---|---|---|---|---|---|
| Terzi et al,[30] 2002 | 160 | 11.3 | 24.4 | 8.1 | 1.9 | 5.6 | — | — | 39 |
| Hollaus et al,[31] 2003 | 108 | 5.5 | 26.8 | 2.8 | — | — | — | 2.8 | — |
| Burfeind et al,[32] 2005 | 73 | 2.7 | 37.0 | 1.4 | 0.0 | 9.6 | 2.7 | — | — |
| Lausberg et al,[33] 2005 | 171 | 1.8 | — | 0.6 | — | 0.0 | — | 0.0 | 43–46 |
| Ludwig et al,[34] 2005 | 116 | 4.3 | — | 6.9 | — | 0.9 | — | 1.7 | 39 |
| Takeda et al,[35] 2006 | 62 | 4.8 | 45.2 | 3.2 | — | — | 9.7 | 9.7 | 54 |
| Yildizeli et al,[36] 2007 | 218 | 4.1 | 22.9 | 3.7 | 0.9 | 1.8 | 5.3 | 1.8 | 53 |
| Rea et al,[37] 2008 | 199 | 4.5 | 17.9 | 1.0 | 2.0 | 15.1 | — | 1.0 | 40 |
| Yamamoto et al,[38] 2008 | 201 | 1.5 | 39.8 | 2.0 | — | 1.5 | 2.5 | 3.0 | 58 |
| Merritt et al,[39] 2009[a] | 196 | 2.0 | 34.6 | 2.0 | 0.0 | 0.0 | 4.8 | 2.0 | 44 |
| Milman et al,[40] 2009 | 64 | 3.1 | 45.3 | 0.0 | 1.6 | 1.6 | 4.7 | — | 41–48 |
| Gómez-Caro et al,[41] 2011 | 58 | 3.4 | 34.5 | 0.0 | 1.7 | 0.0 | 1.7 | 3.4 | 62 |
| Storelli et al,[42] 2012 | 103 | 2.9 | 23.3 | 0.0 | 0.0 | 1.0 | 7.8 | — | 63 |
| Gonzalez et al,[43] 2013 | 99 | 3.0 | 50.5 | 2.0 | — | 3.0 | — | — | 28–45 |
| Bylicki et al,[44] 2014 | 108 | — | — | 9.3 | — | 12.0 | — | — | — |

[a] Experience at Massachusetts General Hospital.
[b] Includes all anastomotic complications.

## ANASTOMOTIC COMPLICATIONS
### Bronchopleural Fistula

#### Presentation

Bronchopleural fistulas (BPFs) occur when there is disruption of the anastomotic line and direct communication to the pleural space. They develop as a result of ischemia or excessive tension at the anastomosis. Clinical manifestations are temporally related to the surgical procedure. Early presentations are characterized by large air leaks with significant and progressive subcutaneous emphysema and varying degrees of hemodynamic and respiratory compromise. BPFs occurring later in the postoperative period manifest with a productive cough, fever and air-fluid levels on chest imaging. BPFs develop in 3.8% to 21.6% of patients undergoing carinal resections[8,19–23] and in 0% to 8.1% of patients after sleeve resections[5,8,25–44] (see **Table 1**). Bronchoscopy is fundamental to confirm the diagnosis.

#### Management

Treatment of BPFs should be directed toward effectively draining the pleural space, antibiotic coverage, and management of the contaminated residual pleural space. Small fistulas may close with these measures. Persistent BPFs may require anastomotic revision.

- Drainage of the pleural space: Thoracostomy tube placement is usually the initial step. This must be performed promptly after pneumonectomy to prevent aspiration of potentially infected pleural fluid into the contralateral lung. Depending on the presentation, complete drainage usually benefits from debridement and lysis of loculations.
- Antibiotic therapy: Broad-spectrum antibiotic coverage is necessary, including antifungals.
- Revision of airway anastomosis: BPFs occurring within 30 days of operation are referred to as early, whereas BPFs beyond 30 days are referred to as late. Both will ultimately require revision of the airway anastomosis. However, an early BPF in the absence of infection may be amenable to a single-stage repair, whereas a late BPF is more likely to require a multistage approach including drainage, debridements, and repair. In both instances, successful repair will depend on removal of necrotic airway tissue and buttressing of the compromised anastomosis with healthy tissue, such as muscle or omentum. If repair is attempted, it is imperative that well-vascularized muscle be used to buttress the repair and separate it from any nearby vascular structures. Endobronchial techniques have been championed by some but have limited applicability. Successful closure of BPF may result in anastomotic stricture requiring dilation or revision. A careful assessment of risk of repair versus completion pneumonectomy and limited pulmonary reserve must be made.
- Management of contaminated residual space: Continuous drainage of the pleural space may require chronic management with an open thoracostomy or the obliteration of the pleural space with the interposition of muscle flaps or thoracoplasty.

### Bronchovascular Fistula

#### Presentation

Bronchovascular fistulas are rare but almost invariably carry a very poor prognosis. These patients typically manifest with massive hemoptysis and severe acute respiratory and hemodynamic compromise and may die precipitously. The massive bleed is often preceded by a "sentinel bleed." This should prompt emergent evaluation and intervention. Bronchovascular fistulas have been reported in 2.9% of patients undergoing carinal resections,[8] although most reports did not specifically mention the presence or absence of this complication (see **Table 1**). They occur in 0% to 2.5% of patients after sleeve resections.[8,25,26,28,30,32,36,37,39–42] Patients undergoing combined airway and vascular resections and reconstructions may be at a particularly higher risk for the development of bronchovascular fistulas. Mortality is close to 100%, with very few reported cases describing an early diagnosis and emergent surgical correction.

#### Management

Prevention of any fistula is paramount. Careful attention to technique, preservation of blood supply, minimizing anastomotic tension, and viable tissue coverage to buttress and separate the anastomosis from nearby vascular structures is essential. There should be a high index of suspicion for this complication in the postoperative period. It is good practice to bronchoscope all patients who have had a bronchoplastic procedure before discharge. This may identify impending problems that may prompt prolonged observation or intervention as needed. When hemoptysis occurs in a patient who has had a carinal or sleeve resection, a bronchovascular fistula should be suspected immediately, and bronchoscopy performed on an emergency basis. If confirmed, the patient should be taken immediately to the operating room. In cases of sleeve resections, a completion pneumonectomy may be necessary.

In their classic review in 1992, Tedder and colleagues[8] reported 16 cases of bronchovascular fistula yielding an incidence of 2.6% after bronchoplastic procedures. According to this review, the result was invariably fatal whenever the outcomes were specified. After this review, we found 11 surgical series with a sample size of more than 50 patients that specifically stated the occurrence of bronchovascular fistulas after sleeve lobectomies.[25,26,28,30,32,36,37,39–42] Among 1462 patients included in these reports, there were 16 (1.1%) cases of bronchovascular fistula, resulting in the death of 14 patients (mortality: 88%). Specific management was detailed for 3 patients.[28,36,40] All underwent completion pneumonectomy (2 carinal pneumonectomies). One patient developed ARDS after the reintervention leading to death. The remaining 2 patients survived. Although infrequent, these results stress the severity of this complication and the need to avoid it.

## Anastomotic Stricture/Stenosis

### Presentation

Benign strictures or stenosis, including suture granuloma formation, have an insidious onset and are the result of ischemia at the anastomosis leading to scar formation. Most frequently, stenosis is diagnosed during routine postoperative surveillance bronchoscopy. If bronchoscopy reveals the bronchial anastomosis appears ischemic but intact, the patient should be kept in hospital until the bronchus declares itself. If it starts to break down, surgical intervention is warranted to avoid a fistula or separation. If the bronchus remains intact, the patient can be observed with frequent bronchoscopies. However, patients may present with postobstructive pneumonitis, pneumonia, dyspnea, hemoptysis, coughing, or wheezing,[54] which may prompt further interventions. Routine surveillance imaging studies may also suggest narrowing of the bronchial lumen or may show postobstructive pneumonia. Anastomotic strictures have been described to occur in 2.5% to 7.4% of patients after carinal resections[19–21] and in 0% to 15.1% of patients undergoing sleeve resections[5,8,25–28,30,32–34,36–44] (see **Table 1**). The occurrence of suture granulomas has reportedly decreased with the decreased use of silk or nonabsorbable sutures when constructing the airway anastomosis.[8,16,17] Also, a continuous suture technique using nonabsorbable material has been associated with benign circumferential stenosis.[17]

### Management

Surveillance bronchoscopy is necessary to monitor the anastomosis, aspirate secretions, remove granulation tissue, and obtain tissue to rule out tumor recurrence as the etiology. Bronchoscopic resection of granulomas at the suture line is usually curative. Patients with benign anastomotic strictures are best managed initially with bronchoscopic balloon dilation.[55] If the stricture recurs, repeated bronchoscopic dilations can be performed. However, if the patency of the anastomosis cannot be practically sustained by dilation, the use of endobronchial silicone stents should be considered, but this could be difficult after sleeve lobectomy, given that the remaining mainstem bronchus is generally very short and segmental bronchi are very close to the anastomosis inferiorly. Indications for intervention are repeated infections, shortness of breath, or collapse of the remaining lung. Patients should be evaluated with pulmonary function tests and ventilation perfusion scans. If symptoms are absent, watchful waiting may be prudent. In cases of severe anastomotic strictures, segmental resection of the stricture with reanastomosis is favored,[9] but this decision must be balanced with the structural integrity of the remaining lung parenchyma. These operations are quite difficult secondary to scarring between the airway and vascular structures. Therefore, completion pneumonectomy may be necessary if segmental resection is not possible or when the remaining lung is structurally compromised by postobstructive effects.[25] One series reported that the most common indication for completion pneumonectomy after bronchial sleeve resections was the occurrence of benign anastomotic stenosis.[56]

## Local Recurrence

### Presentation

Tumor recurrence at the anastomotic suture line is usually discovered during surveillance bronchoscopy. It is to be expected in cases with positive tracheobronchial margins. The liberal use of intraoperative frozen-section analysis of the resected specimen should minimize the risk of residual malignancy. Some series have reported tumor recurrence at the anastomosis even when negative margins were confirmed on permanent section analysis.[25] Local tumor recurrence has been reported in fewer than 5% to 10% of cases of carinal and sleeve resections (see **Table 1**), with isolated reports of very high rates up to 20%.[29]

### Treatment

Recurrence at the anastomosis after a sleeve lobectomy in patients without evidence of extensive nodal or metastatic disease may be treated with completion pneumonectomy.[8,25,56] The same is true for patients who are found to have a positive bronchial margin on the final histologic evaluation.[56] The limitation usually lies in the fitness of the patients to withstand further resection of lung parenchyma. Poor surgical candidates for completion pneumonectomy can be treated with radiation therapy. The use of lasers, brachytherapy, photodynamic therapy, or expandable metallic stents may be required as palliation of airway obstruction.

## SUMMARY

Careful patient selection and attention to technical details should minimize postoperative complications following bronchoplastic procedures. Complications when they do occur are often devastating, and require early detection and aggressive treatment. Unsuccessful management of complications often leads to death.

## REFERENCES

1. Lanuti M, Mathisen DJ. Carinal resection. Thorac Surg Clin 2004;14:199–209.
2. Predina JD, Kunkala M, Aliperti LA, et al. Sleeve lobectomy: current indications and future directions. Ann Thorac Cardiovasc Surg 2010;16(5):310–8.
3. Belsey R. Resection and reconstruction of the intrathoracic trachea [Internet]. Br J Surg 1950;38(150): 200–5. Available at: http://www.ncbi.nlm.nih.gov/pubmed/14791963. Accessed February 15, 2015.
4. Thomas C. Conservative resection of the bronchial tree [Internet]. J R Coll Surg Edinb 1956;1(3):169–86. Available at: http://www.ncbi.nlm.nih.gov/pubmed/13307666. Accessed February 15, 2015.
5. Gaissert HA, Mathisen DJ, Moncure AC, et al. Survival and function after sleeve lobectomy for lung cancer. J Thorac Cardiovasc Surg 1996;111:948–53.
6. Ferguson MK, Lehman AG. Sleeve lobectomy or pneumonectomy: optimal management strategy using decision analysis techniques. Ann Thorac Surg 2003;76(03):1782–8.
7. Deslauriers J, Grégoire J, Jacques LF, et al. Sleeve lobectomy versus pneumonectomy for lung cancer: a comparative analysis of survival and sites or recurrences. Ann Thorac Surg 2004;77:1152–6.
8. Tedder M, Anstadt MP, Tedder SD, et al. Current morbidity, mortality, and survival after bronchoplastic procedures for malignancy [Internet]. Ann Thorac Surg 1992;54(2):387–91.
9. Bueno R, Wain JC, Wright CD, et al. Bronchoplasty in the management of low-grade airway neoplasms and benign bronchial stenoses [Internet]. Ann Thorac Surg 1996;62(3):824–9.
10. Mitchell JD, Mathisen DJ, Wright CD, et al. Clinical experience with carinal resection. J Thorac Cardiovasc Surg 1999;117:39–53.
11. Muehrcke DD, Grillo HC, Mathisen DJ. Reconstructive airway operation after irradiation. Ann Thorac Surg 1995;59(94):14–8.
12. Shrager JB, Wain JC, Wright CD, et al. Omentum is highly effective in the management of complex cardiothoracic surgical problems. J Thorac Cardiovasc Surg 2003;125(3):526–32.
13. Gaissert HA, Grillo HC, Shadmehr MB, et al. Long-term survival after resection of primary adenoid cystic and squamous cell carcinoma of the trachea and carina. Ann Thorac Surg 2004;78:1889–97.
14. Honings J, Gaissert HA, Weinberg AC, et al. Prognostic value of pathologic characteristics and resection margins in tracheal adenoid cystic carcinoma [Internet]. Eur J Cardiothorac Surg 2010;37(6):1438–44.
15. Wright CD, Grillo HC, Wain JC, et al. Anastomotic complications after tracheal resection: prognostic factors and management. J Thorac Cardiovasc Surg 2004;128(5):731–9.
16. Frist WH, Mathisen DJ, Hilgenberg AD, et al. Bronchial sleeve resection with and without pulmonary resection [Internet]. J Thorac Cardiovasc Surg 1987;93(3):350–7. Available at: http://www.ncbi.nlm.nih.gov/pubmed/3821144. Accessed February 15, 2015.
17. Hsieh CM, Tomita M, Ayabe H, et al. Influence of suture on bronchial anastomosis in growing puppies [Internet]. J Thorac Cardiovasc Surg 1988;95(6):998–1002. Available at: http://www.ncbi.nlm.nih.gov/pubmed/3374164. Accessed February 15, 2015.
18. Mitchell JD, Mathisen DJ, Wright CD, et al. Resection for bronchogenic carcinoma involving the carina: long-term results and effect of nodal status on outcome. J Thorac Cardiovasc Surg 2001;121:465–71.
19. Porhanov VA, Poliakov IS, Selvaschuk AP, et al. Indications and results of sleeve carinal resection. Eur J Cardiothorac Surg 2002;22:685–94.
20. Regnard JF, Perrotin C, Giovannetti R, et al. Resection for tumors with carinal involvement: technical aspects, results, and prognostic factors. Ann Thorac Surg 2005;80:1841–6.
21. De Perrot M, Fadel E, Mercier O, et al. Long-term results after carinal resection for carcinoma: does the benefit warrant the risk? J Thorac Cardiovasc Surg 2006;131(1):81–9.
22. Roviaro G, Vergani C, Maclocco M, et al. Tracheal sleeve pneumonectomy: long-term outcome. Lung Cancer 2006;52:105–10.
23. Eichhorn F, Storz K, Hoffmann H, et al. Sleeve pneumonectomy for central non-small cell lung cancer: indications, complications, and survival [Internet]. Ann Thorac Surg 2013;96(1):253–8.
24. Ruffini E, Parola A, Papalia E, et al. Frequency and mortality of acute lung injury and acute respiratory

distress syndrome after pulmonary resection for bronchogenic carcinoma. Eur J Cardiothorac Surg 2001;20:30–6 [discussion: 36–7].

25. Kawahara K, Akamine S, Takahashi T, et al. Management of anastomotic complications after sleeve lobectomy for lung cancer [Internet]. Ann Thorac Surg 1994;57(6):1529–32 [discussion: 1532–3].

26. Icard P, Regnard JF, Guibert L, et al. Survival and prognostic factors in patients undergoing parenchymal saving bronchoplastic operation for primary lung cancer: a series of 110 consecutive cases. Eur J Cardiothorac Surg 1999;15:426–32.

27. Tronc F, Grégoire J, Rouleau J, et al. Long-term results of sleeve lobectomy for lung cancer. Eur J Cardiothorac Surg 2000;17:550–6.

28. Fadel E, Yildizeli B, Chapelier AR, et al. Sleeve lobectomy for bronchogenic cancers: factors affecting survival. Ann Thorac Surg 2002;74:851–9.

29. Mezzetti M, Panigalli T, Giuliani L, et al. Personal experience in lung cancer sleeve lobectomy and sleeve pneumonectomy. Ann Thorac Surg 2002;73:1736–9.

30. Terzi A, Lonardoni A, Falezza G, et al. Sleeve lobectomy for non-small cell lung cancer and carcinoids: results in 160 cases. Eur J Cardiothorac Surg 2002;21:888–93.

31. Hollaus PH, Wilfing G, Wurnig PN, et al. Risk factors for the development of postoperative complications after bronchial sleeve resection for malignancy: a univariate and multivariate analysis. Ann Thorac Surg 2003;75:966–72.

32. Burfeind WR, D'Amico TA, Toloza EM, et al. Low morbidity and mortality for bronchoplastic procedures with and without induction therapy. Ann Thorac Surg 2005;80:418–22.

33. Lausberg HF, Graeter TP, Tscholl D, et al. Bronchovascular versus bronchial sleeve resection for central lung tumors. Ann Thorac Surg 2005;79:1147–52.

34. Ludwig C, Stoelben E, Olschewski M, et al. Comparison of morbidity, 30-day mortality, and long-term survival after pneumonectomy and sleeve lobectomy for non-small cell lung carcinoma. Ann Thorac Surg 2005;79:968–73.

35. Takeda SI, Maeda H, Koma M, et al. Comparison of surgical results after pneumonectomy and sleeve lobectomy for non-small cell lung cancer. Trends over time and 20-year institutional experience. Eur J Cardiothorac Surg 2006;29:276–80.

36. Yildizeli B, Fadel E, Mussot S, et al. Morbidity, mortality, and long-term survival after sleeve lobectomy for non-small cell lung cancer. Eur J Cardiothorac Surg 2007;31:95–102.

37. Rea F, Marulli G, Schiavon M, et al. A quarter of a century experience with sleeve lobectomy for non-small cell lung cancer. Eur J Cardiothorac Surg 2008;34:488–92.

38. Yamamoto K, Miyamoto Y, Ohsumi A, et al. Sleeve lung resection for lung cancer: analysis according to the type of procedure [Internet]. J Thorac Cardiovasc Surg 2008;136(5):1349–56.

39. Merritt RE, Mathisen DJ, Wain JC, et al. Long-term results of sleeve lobectomy in the management of non-small cell lung carcinoma and low-grade neoplasms [Internet]. Ann Thorac Surg 2009;88(5):1574–82.

40. Milman S, Kim AW, Warren WH, et al. The incidence of perioperative anastomotic complications after sleeve lobectomy is not increased after neoadjuvant chemoradiotherapy [Internet]. Ann Thorac Surg 2009;88(3):945–51.

41. Gómez-Caro A, García S, Jiménez MJ, et al. Lung sparing surgery by means of extended bronchoangioplastic (sleeve) lobectomies. Arch Bronconeumol 2011;47(2):66–72.

42. Storelli E, Tutic M, Kestenholz P, et al. Sleeve resections with unprotected bronchial anastomoses are safe even after neoadjuvant therapy. Eur J Cardiothorac Surg 2012;42:77–81.

43. Gonzalez M, Litzistorf Y, Krueger T, et al. Impact of induction therapy on airway complications after sleeve lobectomy for lung cancer [Internet]. Ann Thorac Surg 2013;96(1):247–52.

44. Bylicki O, Vandemoortele T, Orsini B, et al. Incidence and management of anastomotic complications after bronchial resection: a retrospective study [Internet]. Ann Thorac Surg 2014;98:1961–7. Available at: http://linkinghub.elsevier.com/retrieve/pii/S0003497514015082.

45. Villeneuve PJ, Sundaresan S. Complications of pulmonary resection: postpneumonectomy pulmonary edema and postpneumonectomy syndrome. Thorac Surg Clin 2006;16:223–34.

46. Rea F, Marulli G, Schiavon M, et al. Tracheal sleeve pneumonectomy for non small cell lung cancer (NSCLC): short and long-term results in a single institution. Lung Cancer 2008;61:202–8.

47. Roviaro G, Varoli F, Romanelli A, et al. Complications of tracheal sleeve pneumonectomy: personal experience and overview of the literature. J Thorac Cardiovasc Surg 2001;121:234–40.

48. Cerfolio RJ, Bryant AS, Thurber JS, et al. Intraoperative solumedrol helps prevent postpneumonectomy pulmonary edema. Ann Thorac Surg 2003;76:1029–35.

49. Mathisen DJ, Kuo EY, Hahn C, et al. Inhaled nitric oxide for adult respiratory distress syndrome after pulmonary resection. Ann Thorac Surg 1998;66(98):1894–902.

50. Rabkin DG, Sladen RN, DeMango A, et al. Nitric oxide for the treatment of postpneumonectomy pulmonary edema. Ann Thorac Surg 2001;72(01):272–4.

51. Filaire M, Fadel E, Decante B, et al. Inhaled nitric oxide does not prevent postpneumonectomy pulmonary edema in pigs. J Thorac Cardiovasc Surg 2007;133:770–4.

52. Dünser M, Hasibeder W, Rieger M, et al. Successful therapy of severe pneumonia-associated ARDS after pneumonectomy with ECMO and steroids [Internet]. Ann Thorac Surg 2004;78(1):335–7. Available at: http://www.ncbi.nlm.nih.gov/pubmed/15223462. Accessed March 3, 2015.

53. Verhelst H, Vranken J, Muysoms F, et al. The use of extracorporeal membrane oxygenation in postpneumonectomy pulmonary oedema [Internet]. Acta Chir Belg 1998;98(6):269–72. Available at: http://www.ncbi.nlm.nih.gov/pubmed/9922817. Accessed March 3, 2015.

54. Farkas EA, Detterbeck FC. Airway complications after pulmonary resection. Thorac Surg Clin 2006;16:243–51.

55. Sheski FD, Mathur PN. Long-term results of fiberoptic bronchoscopic balloon dilation in the management of benign tracheobronchial stenosis. Chest 1998;114:796–800.

56. Van Schil PE, Brutel de la Rivière A, Knaepen PJ, et al. Completion pneumonectomy after bronchial sleeve resection: incidence, indications, and results. Ann Thorac Surg 1992;53:1042–5.

# Anastomotic Leakage Following Esophagectomy

Carolyn E. Jones, MD, Thomas J. Watson, MD*

## KEYWORDS

- Anastomotic leaks • Esophagectomy • Esophagogastrostomy • Esophageal stents
- Esophageal cancer

## KEY POINTS

- Anastomotic leaks following esophagectomy remain a major source of morbidity.
- Esophagogastric anastomotic leaks are associated with a spectrum of clinical presentations, leading to multiple treatment options tailored to the specific needs.
- Systemic, local, and technical factors may contribute to the cause of leaks following esophagectomy with esophagogastrostomy.
- Esophageal stenting has been successful at managing a significant number of anastomotic leaks following esophagectomy and has decreased the need for reoperation.
- When reoperation is necessary to treat an esophagogastric anastomotic leak, techniques to maintain esophagogastric continuity should be considered and usually are successful.

## INTRODUCTION

Esophagectomy is a major surgical procedure with the potential for significant perioperative morbidity and mortality. Recent data suggest that the number of esophagectomies performed in the United States is increasing at an annual rate of 4%, with approximately 18,000 cases in 2013.[1] Anastomotic leakage following esophageal resection and reconstruction has been one of the most common, feared, morbid, and potentially mortal complications faced by the patient and esophageal surgeon. Such leaks have been associated not only with the septic sequelae of mediastinitis, peritonitis, or cervical wound infection, but also with the development of atrial fibrillation, pneumonia, respiratory failure, and the need for reoperation or reintubation, leading to increased length of stay in the hospital and the risk of postoperative death.[2,3] Mortality has been reported in up to 20% of patients when an anastomotic leak has occurred, although this percentage seems to be decreasing.[4,5] An overall leak rate of 12% was reported from a collective review of series from the 1980s,[6] with cervical anastomoses being associated with a higher incidence of leak (10%–25%) than those performed in the chest (<10%).[7–12] A literature review from 1995 found postesophagectomy leak rates of 30% when reconstruction was performed via primary esophagogastrostomy, depending on how vigorously the diagnosis of a leak was pursued and how it was defined.[13] Contemporary reports do not reveal a sharp decline in anastomotic leak rates compared with the results from past decades. A recent analysis of the Society of Thoracic Surgeons General Thoracic Database found an overall leak rate of 10.6% among 7595 esophagectomies, with rates of 12.3% and 9.3% for cervical and intrathoracic anastomoses, respectively.[14]

A leak can lead to significant sequelae not only in the early postoperative period, but also in the long term because of the potential for a

Division of Thoracic and Foregut Surgery, Department of Surgery, University of Rochester Medical Center, 601 Elmwood Avenue, Box Surgery, Rochester, NY 14642, USA
* Corresponding author.
E-mail address: Thomas_watson@urmc.rochester.edu

Thorac Surg Clin 25 (2015) 449–459
http://dx.doi.org/10.1016/j.thorsurg.2015.07.004
1547-4127/15/$ – see front matter © 2015 Elsevier Inc. All rights reserved.

subsequent anastomotic stricture leading to dysphagia. Given the frequency and morbidity of anastomotic leaks, an understanding of their cause and predisposing factors, techniques for prevention, and management principles are of primary importance to the surgical team. Anastomotic leakage can occur following foregut reconstruction with any of the commonly used conduits, including stomach, colon, or jejunum. Because the stomach is the most frequent esophageal substitute, this article is limited to data concerning esophagogastric anastomotic leaks. Many of the principles underlying the cause and treatment of such leaks, however, can be extrapolated to other esophageal replacement organs.

## DIAGNOSIS

Issues fundamental to the understanding of esophagogastric anastomotic leaks, their clinical relevance, and their optimal management strategy are the manner in which they are detected (**Box 1**) and how they are defined (**Box 2**). Leaks often first present with postoperative fever or leukocytosis. The surgeon must have a high index of suspicion for an anastomotic disruption whenever the patient demonstrates a septic decline in the early postoperative period. In cases of a cervical anastomosis, the development of erythema, induration, or fluctuance along the neck incision may be a harbinger of an underlying leak. For either cervical or intrathoracic anastomoses, the presence of bile, enteric content, saliva, or air in a surgically placed drain adjacent to the site signifies a likely anastomotic breakdown. In such cases, the diagnosis may be obvious, although the underlying contributors may require further investigation. The development of a new pleural effusion within the first days following esophagectomy, especially if in the vicinity of an intrathoracic anastomosis, should be considered a leak until proved otherwise, realizing that other causes, such as chylothorax, are in the differential diagnosis.

Contrast esophagography has been a commonly used test for the detection of

---

> **Box 1**
> **Methods to diagnose esophageal leak**
>
> - Clinical signs and symptoms
> - Contrast esophagogram
> - Flexible upper endoscopy
> - Computed tomography scan (with or without oral contrast)
> - Analysis of amylase level in drain fluid
> - Measurement of serum C-reactive protein

---

> **Box 2**
> **Grading of esophagogastric anastomotic leaks**
>
> - Grade I: Radiologically or endoscopically detected without clinical signs
> - Grade II: Minor leak
> - Grade III: Major leak with overt sepsis
> - Grade IV: Gastric conduit necrosis

---

anastomotic or conduit leakage following esophagectomy. In addition to providing an assessment of anastomotic integrity, the study provides information on the contour and emptying of the esophageal replacement conduit and the integrity and patency of a pyloroplasty, if performed. The examination is most commonly ordered on postoperative day 5 to 7, because that is the time period during which most leaks are likely to develop.

The traditional approach has been to commence the study using a water-soluble contrast agent, such as Gastrografin (diatrizoate meglumine and diatrizoate sodium solution; Bracco Diagnostics Inc, Monroe Township, NJ) out of fear that leaked barium could exacerbate cervical, mediastinal, pleural, or abdominal sepsis. Gastrografin, however, can cause a severe chemical pneumonitis if aspirated. Extreme caution is necessary in the postesophagectomy setting to prevent aspiration. This patient cohort is often elderly may have neck swelling when a cervical incision has been performed, and may have vocal cord dysfunction from recent intubation or iatrogenic recurrent laryngeal nerve injury during surgery, each factor adversely affecting swallowing function. An esophagogram may not be feasible in the patient who is septic, intubated, or otherwise unable to swallow oral contrast. A normal study with a water-soluble agent should be followed with thin barium to improve the sensitivity for detection of a leak.[15] Even a negative barium study does not exclude a leak, however, because a false-negative rate of 57% has been reported.[16]

Given the limitations, risks, and inaccuracies associated with contrast esophagography, other methods for assessing esophagogastric anastomotic integrity have been advocated. Computed tomography with or without orally administered contrast allows visualization of the neck, thorax, and abdomen on a single examination, and facilitates not only detection of an anastomotic leak, but also helps determine the extent and location of extraluminal fluid collections in need of drainage.

Some surgeons have advocated routine use of postoperative flexible esophagogastroduodenoscopy as an alternative to radiographs. Endoscopy avoids the need for orally administered contrast and can be performed expeditiously at the bedside, even on a patient who is having difficulty swallowing or is intubated and on mechanical ventilator support. In addition, endoscopy allows assessment of anastomotic and fundic tip perfusion and integrity, facilitating identification of subtle degrees of mucosal ischemia or anastomotic disruption not discernible on imaging studies, and areas of more severe gastric conduit necrosis or breakdown (**Fig. 1**). Despite concerns about anastomotic trauma with such an approach, flexible endoscopy has proved safe even in the early postoperative period. One potential complication is that an intrathoracic anastomotic disruption can predispose to tension pneumothorax from insufflation during the endoscopic procedure. Appropriate chest drainage should be in place, or immediately available, to manage this problem if it arises.

Other methods for assessing anastomotic leaks include determination of amylase levels from the effluent of adjacent drains, and serial measurements of serum C-reactive protein.[17]

## CAUSE AND PREVENTION

As with all wounds, the propensity for esophageal and other enteric anastomoses to heal is impacted by several systemic, local, and technical factors (**Box 3**). Some of these factors are modifiable and should be optimized before, during, or after surgery. Other factors are fixed and inherent to the patient, although they should be considered in the process of risk-stratification before esophagectomy.

### Systemic Factors

Multiple systemic factors are known to impair esophagogastric anastomotic healing, in particular malnutrition.[10,15] Many patients undergoing esophagectomy are nutritionally depleted because of the presence of dysphagia or anorexia from an

---

**Box 3**
**Factors impacting esophagogastric anastomotic healing**

I. Systemic
- Severe malnutrition
- Hypovolemia/hypotension
- Heart failure
- Hypertension
- Renal insufficiency
- Coronary disease
- Vascular disease
- Steroid use
- Diabetes mellitus
- Tobacco use
- Systemic chemotherapy

II. Local
- Arterial insufficiency
- Venous compromise
- Gastric trauma/inflammation/fibrosis
- Extrinsic compression
- Gastric distention
- Infection
- Radiation therapy

III. Technical
- Tension
- Anastomotic location
- Anastomotic technique
- Anastomotic buttressing
- Errors

---

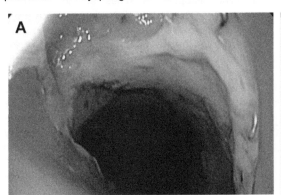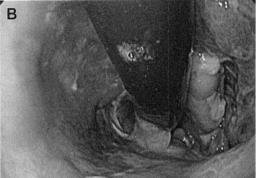

**Fig. 1.** Endoscopic views of an esophagogastric anastomosis revealing subtle ischemic changes without a gross leak. (*A*) Antegrade view. (*B*) Retrograde view also demonstrating the gastric fundic tip.

underlying esophageal cancer or motility disorder, or the effects of recent chemotherapy or radiation. The value of preoperative nutritional support is debated, with most studies supporting its use only in cases of severe nutritional depletion.[17] Although the definition of severe malnutrition is not exact, a loss of greater than 20% of usual body weight or a serum albumin less than 3.0 g/dL are commonly accepted criteria.[18]

The duration of nutritional therapy, when indicated, is also a matter of controversy. In theory, preoperative enteral or parenteral nutritional supplementation should improve healing and lower anastomotic leak rates, although this must be balanced against the urgency of surgical intervention, particularly for malignancy, the likelihood of successful repletion, and the potential for complications, such as sepsis, especially when the parenteral route is used. Preoperative nutrition is aided by placement of an esophageal stent in cases of bulky tumors causing luminal obstruction and dysphagia, although concerns exist regarding the negative impact such stents may have on subsequent tumor resectability. Anorexia may limit oral intake even when esophageal luminal patency has been re-established with a stent. Feeding gastrostomy or jejunostomy tubes may be placed to provide enteral nutrition in cases when an oral diet is inadequate. Total parenteral nutrition, on occasion, may be necessary before esophagectomy.

Of major importance in the perioperative period is the prevention of hypotension and hypovolemia.[18–21] Although the definition of hypotension and the assessment of hypovolemia are not precise, many surgeons are liberal with the administration of fluids during and immediately after surgery to maximize splanchnic perfusion and minimize vasoconstriction within the gastric vasculature. A retrospective review of 137 patients with anastomotic leaks following gastrointestinal surgery (pancreatectomy, esophagectomy, or colectomy) found low serum albumin (<3.5 g/dL), anemia (hemoglobin <8 g/dL), hypotension, the use of inotropes, and blood transfusion to be independent predictors of their occurrence.[22] The risk of anastomotic leak was four times greater in patients who required inotropic support in the perioperative period, and three times higher in patients who developed hypotension.

The recent Society of Thoracic Surgeons Thoracic database analysis of anastomotic leak following esophagectomy found obesity, heart failure, coronary disease, vascular disease, hypertension, steroids, diabetes, renal insufficiency, tobacco use, procedure duration greater than 5 hours, and type of procedure to be associated with leak ($P<.05$) on univariate analysis. On multivariate analysis, heart failure, hypertension, renal insufficiency, and type of procedure were predictive of leak.[14] Another retrospective, population-based review from the United Kingdom found low body mass index and neoadjuvant chemotherapy to be significantly associated with esophagogastric anastomotic leak.[23] In addition, a study assessing patients undergoing transhiatal esophagectomy for esophageal cancer found weight loss, low forced expiratory volume, and low preoperative albumin to be associated with postoperative anastomotic leak.[3]

## Local Factors

The most important local factor impacting esophagogastric anastomotic integrity is the adequacy of the perfusion to the gastric conduit and esophageal remnant. The blood supply to the esophagus is not usually a concern, given the segmental nature of its arterial inflow and venous drainage, the extensive submucosal vascular plexus within the esophageal wall, and the short length of esophagus typically remaining after esophageal resection. On occasion, particularly if the inferior thyroid arteries have been ligated previously (eg, as part of a thyroidectomy) and a long portion of the esophagus has been mobilized, the vasculature of the esophagus may be impaired, predisposing to anastomotic leak.

The rich blood supply to the stomach makes it a suitable esophageal substitute. After gastric mobilization for esophageal replacement, the perfusion of the fundus is compromised, because it is a watershed zone of blood flow from the short gastric, left gastric, and right gastroepiploic arteries, the former two typically being ligated as part of the procedure. Because the fundus is the most common site for anastomosis to the residual esophagus, the ischemia inherent to gastric mobilization is a major risk factor for poor anastomotic healing. Similarly, venous obstruction from any of a variety of causes, including disrupted tributaries, scarring, extrinsic compression, twisting, or distention, may adversely impact anastomotic integrity.

Care must be exercised in mobilization of the gastric conduit to preserve the blood supply, derived mainly from the right gastroepiploic vessels with lesser contributions from the right gastric artery and vein, and to minimize trauma to the smaller vessels comprising the intramural collaterals within the gastric wall. Prior gastric surgery with resultant chronic inflammation and disruption of the gastric blood supply, both macroscopic and microscopic, also may adversely impact esophagogastric anastomotic healing.

Gastric distention likely is a factor compromising esophagogastric anastomotic integrity. Many esophageal surgeons routinely decompress the stomach with a nasogastric tube for several days after an esophagectomy to prevent aspiration of retained gastric contents and to minimize gastric distention that might impair anastomotic healing. In addition, local cervical, mediastinal, or abdominal infection, which can result from intraoperative soilage of spilled esophageal or gastric contents, can prevent healing if in the vicinity of the anastomosis. Finally, an esophagogastric anastomosis placed in a preoperative radiation field has been found to be a strong predictor of anastomotic leakage in patients with esophageal cancer treated with neoadjuvant chemoradiation.[24,25]

## Technical Factors

Tension is detrimental to the healing of any wound, particularly an anastomosis. Adequate mobilization and proper construction of the gastric tube are critical to the success of esophagogastric anastomotic healing. An appropriately prepared gastric conduit should reach to the cervical level without excessive tension. The narrower the gastric conduit, the longer its length, although excessive narrowing can lead to an impaired blood supply from disruption of submucosal collaterals. Balancing conduit length and perfusion, some surgeons have recommended a gastric tube transverse diameter of 4 to 5 cm as being optimal.

Cervical esophageal anastomoses are thought to be more prone to leakage than those performed in the chest, because of the greater length of the gastric conduit necessary to reach the neck, the resultant anastomotic tension, and the decreased blood supply at the fundic tip (used for cervical anastomoses) compared with a more distal location along the gastric body (used for intrathoracic anastomoses). The difference in final position between cervical and intrathoracic anastomoses, however, may only be a few centimeters. Thus, factors other than conduit length may be important. Extrinsic compression by the relatively rigid spine, sternum, and trachea at the level of the thoracic inlet may impair healing of anastomoses created in the neck. In addition, increased esophageal motion during flexion and extension of the neck also has been theorized to negatively impact cervical anastomoses, especially when the esophageal remnant is short.

An extensive body of literature has evolved regarding leak rates depending on the location of the esophagogastric anastomosis (**Table 1**). The available data support the contention that rates are higher in the neck than in the chest, although recent reports suggest the gap may be narrowing.[14] The consequences of leakage in the neck, however, tend to be less than for leakage into the chest. Cervical leaks usually can be managed adequately with a previously placed surgical drain or with opening and packing of the neck wound, whereas intrathoracic leaks may require placement of image-guided percutaneous tubes or reoperation for drainage, closure, containment, or diversion. Anastomotic leakage into the chest has the potential for unilateral or bilateral pleural contamination, mediastinitis, and erosion into the membranous airway, pulmonary parenchyma, or major vascular structures, such as the aorta, with lethal consequences. Although intrathoracic leakage traditionally has been associated with significant morbidity and mortality, the ability to rescue the patient from the consequences of such leaks has improved in recent years.[26]

## Anastomotic Technique

Methods of constructing the esophagogastric anastomosis vary and include hand-sewn (continuous or interrupted, single- or double-layer, and absorbable or nonabsorbable sutures), stapled (circular or linear), and hybrid approaches combining sutures and staples. In addition, the anastomosis can be performed in an end-to-end, end-to-side, or side-to-side fashion. Whichever technique is used, the anastomosis needs to be constructed carefully, incorporating all layers of the esophageal and gastric walls while avoiding excessive tissue

**Table 1**
**Population-based analyses of esophagogastric anastomotic leak rates based on anastomotic location**

| Author, Year | # | Study Design | Leak Rate |
| --- | --- | --- | --- |
| Hulscher et al,[29] 2001 | 5662 | Systematic review and meta-analysis | Cervical = 13.6%<br>Intrathoracic = 7.2% |
| Markar et al,[30] 2013 | 298 | Systematic review and meta-analysis | Cervical = 13.6%<br>Intrathoracic = 3% |
| Kassis et al,[14] 2013 | 7595 | Retrospective database review | Cervical = 12.3%<br>Intrathoracic = 9.3% |

*Data from Refs.[14,29,30]*

strangulation, and creating a "watertight" closure not under excessive tension. A mastery of several approaches is optimal for the surgeon to be able to apply the best one in any specific situation.

Multiple reports have compared anastomotic leak rates among various techniques. A recent meta-analysis[27] found lower leak rates with a linear stapled esophagogastric anastomosis compared with a completely hand-sewn technique. A separate meta-analysis by the same authors found no difference in leak rates between linear stapled and circular stapled esophagogastric anastomoses.[28] Regardless of the technique, the incidence of leaks is higher for anastomoses performed in the neck compared with those in the chest, as confirmed in two recent meta-analyses.[29,30]

The route of transposition of the gastric conduit also is a factor in the propensity for an anastomotic leak to occur. Out of 1030 patients undergoing transhiatal esophagectomy at the University of Michigan in whom the stomach was positioned in the posterior mediastinum, the anastomotic leak rate was 13%, whereas out of seven patients undergoing a retrosternal gastric pull-up, the leak rate was 86%.[31] Several factors potentially contribute to the higher leak rate with the retrosternal route, including the longer distance the stomach must traverse, and the relative lack of surrounding soft tissue divestments. With a retrosternal conduit, the anastomosis sits in a subcutaneous position and is unsupported during a cough or Valsalva maneuver. When the conduit is within the posterior mediastinum, the anastomosis is buttressed posteriorly by the prevertebral fascia, laterally by the carotid sheath, and anteriorly by the membranous trachea. These surrounding structures not only aid healing, but also support the anastomosis during internal pressurization.

## ADJUNCTS FOR PREVENTION

Despite an awareness of the factors predisposing to esophagogastric anastomotic leakage following esophagectomy, and efforts to optimize modifiable risks, the incidence of leaks remains significant. As a result, various adjunctive measures have been introduced to help prevent or control anastomotic leaks and their sequelae.

Ischemia of the mobilized and partially devascularized gastric fundus is an important cause of esophagogastric leaks. Ischemic preconditioning is based on the hypothesis that the vascularity of the gastric fundus can be improved, and anastomotic leaks reduced, by partial devascularization in advance of esophagectomy to improve the gastric microcirculation (the "delay phenomenon").

The concept of division of the left gastric and short gastric vessels at the time of laparoscopic staging before esophagectomy holds appeal, in that such an approach would not necessarily increase the cost or morbidity to the overall treatment paradigm for an esophageal malignancy if such staging already were being contemplated. The timing between partial devascularization and subsequent esophagectomy is a matter of debate, with one animal study showing increased gastric neovascularity 30 days, but not 7 days, after division of the left, right, and short gastric vessels.[32] The optimal extent of devascularization also remains a subject for further investigation. A separate animal study found relative preservation of gastric blood flow to the fundic tip with preoperative ligation of both the short gastric and left gastric vessels, although not with ligation of the short gastric vessels alone.[33] A recent review article assessed the published literature regarding ischemic preconditioning before esophagectomy and concluded that the available evidence does not support its use outside of a clinical research protocol.[34]

Another surgical adjunct for decreasing leak rates following esophagectomy is the use of a pedicled omental flap for wrapping the esophagogastric anastomosis. Several reports, including one systematic review of randomized control trials, have assessed outcomes with this technique and have shown lower leak rates compared with unbuttressed anastomoses.[5,35–37]

Biocompatible sealants have been used during various types of operations, such as lung resections or vascular procedures. No approved sealants are currently on the market for prevention or treatment of esophageal perforations or anastomotic leaks, and there are no studies assessing their utility in adults. Two studies of fibrin glue for the prevention of esophagogastric anastomotic leaks in children suggested a benefit to its use.[38,39] The efficacy of various sealants following esophagectomy is a topic in need of further investigation.

Other adjuncts for prevention of esophagogastric anastomotic leaks include pleural tenting after Ivor Lewis esophagectomy,[40] intraoperative assessment of gastric graft perfusion using laser-assisted fluorescent-dye angiography,[41] and planned delay of oral intake following surgery.[42] Perhaps a combination of preventative measures will lead to a meaningful decrease in leak rates over time.

## MANAGEMENT

The management of an esophagogastric anastomotic leak requires considerable clinical judgment and depends on the location of the anastomosis; the extent of the anastomotic disruption; the adequacy of conduit perfusion; the involvement of adjacent structures, such as the airway or lung; the degree of sepsis; and the hemodynamic stability of the patient. The principles governing treatment of anastomotic leakage are the same as those for esophageal perforation in general (**Box 4**).

## Nonoperative Approaches

Occult anastomotic leaks (grade I) occurring in patients not exhibiting clinical signs or symptoms, and detected as part of routine postoperative endoscopy or imaging studies, can be managed with a delay in institution of oral feeding and enteral nutritional support via a jejunostomy or nasogastric/nasoduodenal feeding tube. Signs of infection should prompt the early administration of broad-spectrum antibiotics. Spillage of saliva or gastric secretions are controlled with previously placed surgical drains, if present, or the introduction of percutaneous drains into the involved areas of the pleural space and mediastinum.

## Surgical Options

Leaks associated with cervical anastomoses generally are treated by wound opening and packing. The risk of extensive mediastinitis is less compared with intrathoracic leaks, because the contamination is generally confined to the cervical soft tissues. Leaks in the chest, although less common than those in the neck, can result in severe sepsis and mediastinitis requiring additional closed drainage with chest tubes or surgical washout.

The percentage of circumferential disruption of the anastomosis and the extent of conduit necrosis also determine management options. Small disruptions are managed with delayed oral intake, enteral or parenteral nutritional support, drainage of adjacent fluid collections, antibiotics, and time.

Moderate to large disruptions are more challenging. Surgical repair in such cases is fraught with difficulties because the factors resulting in the initial leak, such as compromised blood flow and anastomotic tension, are usually still present at the time of a reoperation. Additional factors, such as contamination of the surgical field, hemodynamic or respiratory compromise, and the effects of systemic sepsis, further complicate reintervention. Repair of the anastomosis, when undertaken, should include buttressing with viable tissue, such as omentum, pericardial fat, or muscle flap around the suture line.

If repair is not feasible at the time of re-exploration, management options include wide local drainage, placement of a large, exteriorized T-tube across the defect, or takedown of the anastomosis with cervical/cervicothoracic esophagostomy (with or without resection of the remaining intrathoracic stomach). The latter commits the patient to a subsequent foregut reconstruction, a sizable undertaking with associated morbidity and the potential for mortality, assuming sufficient recovery to allow reoperation.

A single institution, retrospective review of 761 patients undergoing esophagectomy over a 10-year time period (1993–2003) found 48 patients (6.3%) with anastomotic leak.[43] Of the 47 patients available for analysis, 27 (57%) were managed nonoperatively and 20 (43%) required operative intervention. Primary anastomotic repair was possible in 14 patients, reinforcement of the anastomosis with viable tissue was possible in six patients, and esophageal diversion was necessary in two patients. Median hospitalization was 20 days in the nonoperative group and 31 days in the operative group ($P = .0037$). The authors concluded that contained leaks could be managed nonoperatively and that esophagogastric continuity could be preserved in most cases.

---

**Box 4**
**Principles of management of esophageal perforations**

- Systemic antibiotics
- Close or occlude the defect as soon as possible
- Drain associated fluid collections
- Prevent distal obstruction
- Ensure lack of factors keeping perforation open (eg, tumor, foreign body, persistent infection)
- Esophageal diversion or resection if sepsis poorly controlled with more conservative measures

## Stenting

Esophageal stenting has been introduced in recent years as an option for treatment of clinically significant esophageal perforations and esophagogastric anastomotic leaks.[44–50] Stents can be placed expeditiously, even in an intensive care setting, avoiding many of the issues associated with surgical reintervention. The goal of stenting is closure of the anastomotic defect, realizing that associated fluid collections may require additional image-guided percutaneous or operative drainage. If endoscopy reveals significant gastric ischemia, stenting may not be appropriate because conduit excision may be required.

Anastomotic leaks involving less than 30% of the circumference have been shown to be appropriate for stent placement. Properly positioned, stents can seal the area of disruption and allow for healing. A fully covered self-expanding metal, plastic, or hybrid stent of a large diameter is the ideal choice, because subsequent removal is necessary (**Fig. 2**). Uncovered or partially covered stents are not appropriate, because they may be difficult to remove at a later date. Larger-diameter stents typically are used to seal perforations compared with stents placed for palliation of obstructing esophageal cancers.

A common problem with stents placed across esophagogastric anastomoses is migration. Stent placement into a gastric conduit with a relatively large diameter prevents adherence of the stent to the gastric wall; the stent is seated mainly via its interface with the esophageal mucosa. Because fully covered stents are necessary for anastomotic leaks, adherence to the mucosa is further compromised compared with stents with an uncovered proximal portion, which permits tissue ingrowth. Adjuncts to stent placement, such as endoscopic clipping or suturing, have been advocated to assist in the prevention of stent migration in this scenario. Other complications associated with stents include inadequate coverage of the leak; plugging; and erosion into surrounding structures, such as the airway or major blood vessels, particularly if the stent is left in place for a prolonged period of time.

A study of 17 patients undergoing stent placement for acute intrathoracic anastomotic leaks following esophagectomy found successful leak occlusion in all.[48] Fourteen patients (82%) were able to resume an oral diet within 72 hours of stent placement. Stent migration occurred in three patients (18%), requiring repositioning in two and replacement in one. All stents were subsequently removed at a mean of 17 ± 9 days.

A separate study assessed 18 (11.3%) anastomotic leaks out of 160 minimally invasive esophagectomies performed at a single institution.[51] Leaks were managed with a variety of techniques including neck drainage (N = 4), esophageal diversion (N = 2), thoracoscopic drainage with or without T-tube placement (N = 3), or endoscopic stenting with or without percutaneous drainage (N = 9). Leaks were successfully controlled in 89% of the patients treated surgically, and 100% of the patients treated with stenting. No 60-day or in-hospital mortality was noted in either group. The authors noted a shift over time to endoscopic management of leaks at their institution.

### Aerodigestive Fistula Management

The close proximity of the esophagogastric anastomosis and the gastric conduit to the lung parenchyma and membranous airway when the

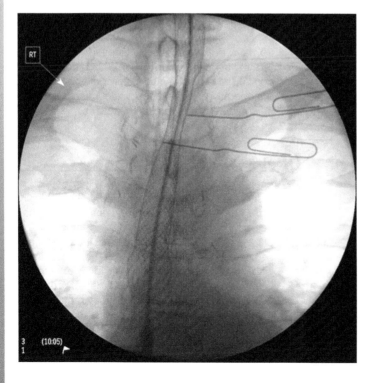

Fig. 2. Intraoperative radiograph of a fully covered self-expanding metal esophageal stent positioned across an esophagogastric anastomotic leak with associated stenosis. Note the paper clips placed to identify the location of the anastomosis.

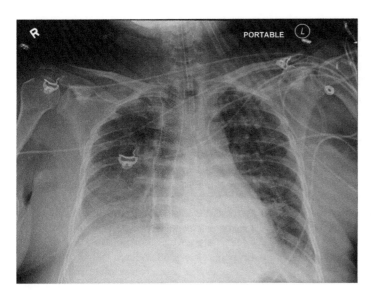

**Fig. 3.** Chest radiograph of a patient referred with multiple, covered, self-expanding metal esophageal stents placed to occlude an esophagogastric anastomotic fistula to the membranous trachea following esophagectomy. The fistula was later closed via right thoracotomy with extrusion of the stents, takedown of the esophagogastric anastomosis, cervical esophagostomy, primary repair of the trachea, and buttressing of the trachea and gastric closure with intercostal muscle flaps. Because the patient had significant respiratory compromise at the time of surgical repair, the operation was performed under venovenous extracorporeal membrane oxygenation support.

stomach is positioned within the posterior mediastinum predisposes to aerodigestive fistula formation. Such fistulization often requires emergent intervention because of the associated aspiration of pharyngeal and gastric secretions into the lungs, leading to pneumonia/pneumonitis and respiratory compromise. In these cases, a temporary endoesophageal stent may be placed across the anastomosis to control contamination (**Fig. 3**). Stenting, however, is a poor long-term solution, because the fistula requires eventual operative intervention.

The principles behind surgical management of anastomotic fistulae to the airway include primary repair of the anastomosis, if possible, and closure of the defect in the airway. The latter may be aided by the use of pericardium or aortic homograft as a buttress or patch (Dr Doug Mathisen, Massachusetts General Hospital, Boston, MA, personal communication, 2015). Vascularized soft tissue, such as omentum or a muscle flap, should be interposed between the esophagogastric and airway suture lines to prevent refistulization. If the patient requires a thoracotomy to complete the repair and single-ventilation is not tolerated, the procedure can be performed under venovenous extracorporeal membrane oxygenation support.

The degree of anastomotic disruption and associated gastric ischemia is often extensive enough to require conduit excision and the creation of a cervical or cervicothoracic esophagostomy. If the patient survives, delayed reconstruction can be considered after a full recovery, usually months later. At the time of subsequent reconstruction, a conduit other than the stomach is necessary. Options include of a substernally transposed colon or jejunal interposition with or without "supercharging," depending the vascularity of the conduit and the length needed to reach the remnant esophagus.[52,53]

## SUMMARY

Anastomotic leaks remain a significant clinical challenge following esophagectomy with foregut reconstruction. Despite an increasing understanding of the multiple contributing factors, advancements in perioperative optimization of modifiable risks, and improvements in surgical, endoscopic, and percutaneous management techniques, leaks remain a source of major morbidity associated with esophageal resection. Fortunately, the mortality resulting from anastomotic leaks seems to be improving. As with most disease processes, prevention is best, although even a perfectly executed esophageal resection in an otherwise healthy individual can result in anastomotic leakage. The surgeon should be well versed in the principles underlying the cause of leaks and strategies to minimize their occurrence. Similarly, when confronted with a leak, the surgeon must exercise sound judgment in deciding on a treatment paradigm that is best for the circumstances of the individual. Appropriately diagnosed and managed, most anastomotic leaks following esophagectomy can be brought to a successful resolution.

## REFERENCES

1. Jancin B. Esophagectomy cases have been steadily rising. Thorac Surg News 2013;9(1):6.

2. Conners RC, Reuben BC, Neumayer LA, et al. Comparing outcomes after transthoracic and transhiatal esophagectomy: a 5-year prospective cohort of 17,395 patients. J Am Coll Surg 2007;205:735–40.

3. Tabatabai A, Hashemi M, Mohajeri G, et al. Incidence and risk factors predisposing anastomotic leak after transhiatal esophagectomy. Ann Thorac Med 2009;4:197–200.

4. Ben-David K, Sarosi GA, Cendan JC, et al. Decreasing morbidity and mortality in 100 consecutive minimally invasive esophagectomies. Surg Endosc 2012;26:162–7.

5. Dai JG, Zhang ZY, Min JX, et al. Wrapping of the omental pedicle flap around esophagogastric anastomosis after esophagectomy for esophageal cancer. Surgery 2011;149:404–10.

6. Muller JM, Erasmi H, Stelzner M, et al. Surgical therapy of oesophageal carcinoma. Br J Surg 1990;77:845–57.

7. Vigneswaran WT, Trastek VF, Pairolero PC, et al. Transhiatal esophagectomy for carcinoma of the esophagus. Ann Thorac Surg 1993;56:838–46.

8. Chasseray VM, Kiroff GK, Buard JL, et al. Cervical or thoracic anastomosis for esophagectomy for carcinoma. Surg Gynecol Obstet 1989;169:55–62.

9. Tilanus HW, Hop WC, Langenhorst BL, et al. Esophagectomy with or without thoracotomy: is there any difference? J Thorac Cardiovasc Surg 1993;105:898–903.

10. Patil PK, Patel SG, Mistry RC, et al. Cancer of the esophagus: esophagogastric anastomotic leak: a retrospective study of predisposing factors. J Surg Oncol 1992;49:163–7.

11. Shahian DM, Neptune WB, Ellis FH Jr, et al. Transthoracic versus extrathoracic esophagectomy: mortality, morbidity and long-term survival. Ann Thorac Surg 1986;41:237–46.

12. King RM, Pairolero PC, Trastek VF, et al. Ivor Lewis esophagogastrectomy for carcinoma of the esophagus: early and late functional results. Ann Thorac Surg 1987;44:119–22.

13. Urschel JD. Esophagogastrostomy anastomotic leaks complicating esophagectomy: a review. Am J Surg 1995;169:634–40.

14. Kassis ES, Kosinski AS, Ross P Jr, et al. Predictors of anastomotic leak after esophagectomy: an analysis of the Society of Thoracic Surgeons General Thoracic Database. Ann Thorac Surg 2013;96:1919–26.

15. Swanson JO, Levine MS, Redfern RO, et al. Usefulness of high-density barium for detection of leaks after esophagogastrectomy, total gastrectomy, and total laryngectomy. AJR Am J Roentgenol 2003;181:415–20.

16. Solomon DG, Sasaki CT, Salem RR. An evaluation of the routine use of contrast radiography as a screening test for cervical anastomotic integrity after esophagectomy. Am J Surg 2012;203:467–71.

17. Dutta S, Fullarton GM, Forshaw MJ, et al. Persistent elevation of C-reactive protein following esophagogastric cancer resection as a predictor of postoperative surgical site infectious complications. World J Surg 2011;35:1017–25.

18. Dewar L, Gelfand G, Finley RJ, et al. Factors affecting cervical anastomotic leak and stricture formation following esophagogastrectomy and gastric tube interposition. Am J Surg 1992;163:484–9.

19. Perracchia A, Bardini R, Ruol A, et al. Esophagovisceral anastomotic leak: a prospective statistical study of predisposing factors. J Thorac Cardiovasc Surg 1988;95:685–91.

20. Buzby GP, Blouin G, Colling CL, et al. Perioperative total parenteral nutrition in surgical patients. N Engl J Med 1991;325:525–32.

21. Baker JP, Detsky AS, Wesson DE, et al. Nutritional assessment: a comparison of clinical judgment and objective measurements. N Engl J Med 1982;306:969–72.

22. Choudhuri AH, Uppal R, Kumar M. Influence of non-surgical risk factors on anastomotic leakage after major gastrointestinal surgery: audit from a tertiary care teaching institute. Int J Crit Illn Inj Sci 2013;3:246–9.

23. Escofet X, Manjunath A, Twine C, et al. Prevalence and outcome of esophagogastric anastomotic leak after esophagectomy in a UK regional cancer network. Dis Esophagus 2010;23:112–6.

24. Juloori A, Tucker SL, Komaki R, et al. Influence of preoperative radiation field on postoperative leak rates in esophageal cancer patients after trimodality therapy. J Thorac Oncol 2014;9:534–40.

25. Hulscher JB, van Sandick JW, de Boer AG, et al. Extended transthoracic resection compared to limited transhiatal resection for adenocarcinoma of the esophagus. N Engl J Med 2002;347:1662–9.

26. Martin LW, Swisher SG, Hofstetter W, et al. Intrathoracic leaks following esophagectomy are no longer associated with increased mortality. Ann Surg 2005;242:392–402.

27. Deng XF, Liu QX, Zhou D, et al. Hand-sewn vs linearly stapled esophagogastric anastomosis for esophageal cancer: a meta-analysis. World J Gastroenterol 2015;21:4757–64.

28. Zhou D, Liu QX, Deng XF, et al. Comparison of two different mechanical esophagogastric anastomosis in esophageal cancer patients: a meta-analysis. J Cardiothorac Surg 2015;10:67.

29. Hulscher JB, Tijssen JG, Obertop H, et al. Transthoracic versus transhiatal resection for carcinoma of the esophagus: a meta-analysis. Ann Thorac Surg 2001;72:306–13.

30. Markar SR, Arya S, Karthikesalingam A, et al. Technical factors that affect anastomotic integrity following esophagectomy: systematic review and meta-analysis. Ann Surg Oncol 2013;20:4274–81.

31. Orringer MB, Marshall B, Iannettoni MD, et al. Transhiatal esophagectomy for treatment of benign and malignant disease. World J Surg 2001;25: 196–203.

32. Perry KA, Banarjee A, Liu J, et al. Gastric ischemic conditioning increases neovascularization and reduces inflammation and fibrosis during gastroesophageal anastomotic healing. Surg Endosc 2013;27:753–60.

33. Beck SM, Malay MB, Gagne DJ, et al. Experimental model of laparoscopic gastric ischemic preconditioning prior to transhiatal esophagectomy. Surg Endosc 2011;25:2470–7.

34. Yuan Y, Duranceau A, Ferraro P, et al. Vascular conditioning of the stomach before esophageal reconstruction by gastric interposition. Dis Esophagus 2012;25:740–9.

35. Yuan Y, Zeng X, Hu Y, et al. Omentoplasty for oesophagogastrostomy after oesophagectomy. Cochrane Database Syst Rev 2014;(10):CD008446.

36. Sepesi B, Swisher SG, Walsh GL, et al. Omental reinforcement of the thoracic esophagogastric anastomosis: an analysis of leak and reintervention rates in patients undergoing planned and salvage esophagectomy. J Thorac Cardiovasc Surg 2012;144: 1146–50.

37. Yoshida N, Baba Y, Watanabe M, et al. Triangulating stapling technique covered with the pedicled omental flap for esophagogastric anastomosis: a safe anastomosis with fewer complications. J Am Coll Surg 2015;220:e13–6.

38. Saldana-Cortes JA, Larios-Arceo F, Prieto-Diaz-Chavez E, et al. Role of fibrin glue in the prevention of cervical leakage and strictures after esophageal reconstruction of caustic injury. World J Surg 2009; 33:986–93.

39. Upadhyaya VD, Gopal SC, Gangopadhyaya AN, et al. Role of fibrin glue as a sealant to esophageal anastomosis in cases of congenital esophageal atresia with tracheo-esophageal fistula. World J Surg 2007;31:2412–5.

40. Asteriou C, Barbetakis N, Lalountas M, et al. Modified pleural tenting for prevention of anastomotic leak after Ivor Lewis esophagogastrectomy. Ann Surg Oncol 2011;18:3737–42.

41. Zehetner J, DeMeester SR, Alicuben ET, et al. Intraoperative assessment of perfusion of the gastric graft and correlation with anastomotic leaks after esophagectomy. Ann Surg 2014;262(1):74–8.

42. Bolton JS, Conway WC, Abbas AE. Planned delay of oral intake after esophagectomy reduces the cervical anastomotic leak rate and hospital length of stay. J Gastrointest Surg 2014;18:304–9.

43. Crestanello JA, Deschamps C, Cassivi SD, et al. Selective management of intrathoracic anastomotic leak after esophagectomy. J Thorac Cardiovasc Surg 2005;129:254–60.

44. Freeman RK, Van Workom JM, Ascioti AJ. Esophageal stent placement for the treatment of iatrogenic intrathoracic esophageal perforation. Ann Thorac Surg 2007;83:2003–8.

45. Hunerbein M, Stroszczynski C, Moesta KT, et al. Treatment of thoracic anastomotic leaks after esophagectomy with self-expanding plastic stents. Ann Surg 2004;240:801–7.

46. Chak A, Singh R, Linden PA. Covered stents for the treatment of life-threatening cervical esophageal anastomotic leaks. J Thorac Cardiovasc Surg 2011;141:834–44.

47. D'Cunha J, Rueth NM, Groth SS, et al. Esophageal stents for anastomotic leaks and perforations. J Thorac Cardiovasc Surg 2011;142:39–46.

48. Freeman RK, Vyverberg A, Ascioti AJ. Esophageal stent placement for the treatment of acute intrathoracic anastomotic leak after esophagectomy. Ann Thorac Surg 2011;92:204–8.

49. Wilson JL, Louie BE, Farivar AS, et al. Fully covered self-expanding metal stents are effective for benign esophagogastric disruptions and strictures. J Gastrointest Surg 2013;17:2045–50.

50. Eizaguirre E, Larburu S, Asensio JI, et al. Treatment of anastomotic leaks with metallic stent after esophagectomies. Dis Esophagus 2015. [Epub ahead of print].

51. Nguyen NT, Rudersdorf PD, Smith BR, et al. Management of gastrointestinal leaks after minimally invasive esophagectomy: conventional treatments vs. endoscopic stenting. J Gastrointest Surg 2011; 11:1952–60.

52. Kesler KA, Pillai ST, Birdas TJ, et al. "Supercharged" isoperistaltic colon interposition for long-segment esophageal reconstruction. Ann Thorac Surg 2013; 95:1162–8.

53. Blackmon SH, Correa AM, Skoracki R, et al. Supercharged pedicled jejunal interposition for esophageal replacement: a 10 year experience. Ann Thorac Surg 2012;94:1104–11.

# Management of Conduit Necrosis Following Esophagectomy

Karen J. Dickinson, MBBS, BSc, MD, FRCS,
Shanda H. Blackmon, MD, MPH*

## KEYWORDS

- Esophagectomy • Conduit • Complication • Necrosis • Reconstruction

## KEY POINTS

- Prevention of conduit ischemia or necrosis is better than conduit loss and esophageal diversion.
- Intraoperative assessment of conduit ischemia by the surgeon clinically is poor; specialized techniques, for example, Doppler fluorescence, may be useful.
- Intraoperative suspicion of conduit ischemia should always be acted on, and an alternative conduit may be necessary.
- Primary esophageal defunctioning may be necessary for intraoperative graft necrosis (with venting gastrostomy and feeding jejunostomy).
- Vigilance is required to detect postoperative gastric conduit necrosis as clinical signs may be nonspecific.

## INTRODUCTION

Restoration of intestinal continuity following esophagectomy for benign and malignant conditions can be performed using gastric, jejunal, and colonic conduits. In most cases, the stomach is used for reconstruction with other grafts held in reserve. Conduit necrosis is a devastating complication of esophagectomy. Fortunately, this is rare and is only reported in less than 2% of primary resections with reconstruction.[1,2] The first strategy should be prevention; the authors discuss identification of high-risk patients, operative techniques used to improve conduit vascularity, and methods for the intraoperative and postoperative monitoring of vascularity of these intestinal grafts. The authors discuss strategies to deal with intraoperative conduit ischemia and necrosis. Early identification of this serious complication is key to achieving a good outcome for patients; identification of suspicious clinical signs, investigation of potential conduit necrosis, and timely management are crucial. A multidisciplinary approach is key to the management of these patients. The role of the thoracic surgeon is complimented by the critical care team, gastroenterologists, dieticians, microbiologists, and, in some cases, plastic surgeons. The authors also discuss the options and challenges of delayed reconstruction after conduit loss.

## DEFINITION AND CONSEQUENCES
### Definition

Conduit necrosis after esophagectomy is defined as death of the conduit used for reconstruction of the esophagus. The necrotic organ may be stomach, jejunum (pedicled or free graft, with or without supercharging), or colon (with or without supercharging). Conduit ischemia after esophagectomy is defined as inadequate blood supply to the conduit used for reconstruction of the

Disclosure for Financial Support: No disclosures.
Department of Thoracic Surgery, Mayo Clinic, MA-12-00-1, 200 First Street, Rochester, MN 55905, USA
* Corresponding author.
E-mail address: Blackmon.shanda@mayo.edu

Thorac Surg Clin 25 (2015) 461–470
http://dx.doi.org/10.1016/j.thorsurg.2015.07.008
1547-4127/15/$ – see front matter © 2015 Elsevier Inc. All rights reserved.

esophagus. An ischemic conduit may progress to necrosis and may present early in the postoperative course with an anastomotic leak or weeks to months after surgery with a stricture.

### Consequences

The consequences of conduit necrosis are grave, both for the patients in terms of potential mortality but also in terms of quality of life. Mortality after conduit necrosis can exceed 90%.[3–6] Focal necrosis of the conduit is most likely to occur in the region of the anastomosis, as this has the most tenuous blood supply. It is essential that any gastrointestinal anastomosis should be created without tension and with a good blood supply. Focal ischemia of the anastomosis is, therefore, likely to cause an anastomotic leak. Anastomotic leaks occur in around 10% of esophagectomies nationally[7] and can be graded from I to IV (grade I, radiological leak only; grade II, minor contained leak; grade III, major leak with evidence of sepsis; grade IV, conduit necrosis).[8,9] Leaks without significant clinical sequelae can be managed conservatively or endoscopically, for example, with a covered stent and endoscopically sutured in place to prevent migration.[10,11] Necrosis of the entire conduit or a large section will require reoperation for resection and an end esophagostomy for diversion, in combination with a venting gastrostomy (where applicable), drainage of collections, and feeding jejunostomy. The patients' clinical status must then be optimized before reconstruction can be considered.[12–14] The consequences for patients are significant. Although an end esophagostomy on the chest rather than the neck can be hidden under clothes and patients will still be able to eat, there is no denying the physical and psychological effects of being dependent on jejunostomy feeding and the anticipation of further major surgery for reconstruction.

A late consequence of conduit ischemia is the development of a stricture, either in the conduit itself or at the anastomosis. Conduit ischemia, anastomotic leak, and stricture are intertwined clinical entities.[15] Strictures will present with dysphagic symptoms and will affect patients' quality of life. Multiple dilatations will often be required in these patients.

### PREVENTION
#### Preoperative: Individual Risk Assessment

Of key importance to the management of conduit necrosis is the identification of risk factors and high-risk patients. Preoperative and intraoperative strategies can be used to optimize patients, their anatomy, and physiology. In some cases the risks of conduit necrosis and morbidity/mortality from surgery will be prohibitive, and patients and families should be counseled accordingly. Patients with significant comorbidity have been shown to have an odds ratio (OR) of 2.2 (1.1–4.3, $P = .023$) for the development of conduit ischemia.[15] Additionally, conduit ischemia was associated with an OR of 5.5 (2.5–12.10) for anastomotic leak and 4.4 (2.0–9.6) for stricture development.[15] Patient factors, such as smoking, neoadjuvant therapy, and preoperative weight, were not, however, associated with increased ischemia. Intuitively, when contemplating esophageal reconstruction, the authors are concerned about patients with diabetes, hypertension, and peripheral arterial disease. In comorbid patients a strategy to deal with this is to perform delayed conduit formation. Of the 37 patients in whom this was used, 6 had diabetes, 18 hypertension, 16 coronary artery disease, 10 were obese (body mass index >30), and 2 had undergone previous pneumonectomy.[16] Preoperative risk assessment of any patient undergoing esophageal resection is essential and should include a full history and examination including assessment of cardiorespiratory function (ie, supervised exercise in clinic, cardiopulmonary exercise testing, pulmonary function testing, echocardiography, coronary angiography where indicated). For hypertensive patients control should be assessed and end organ damage identified, for diabetic patients assessment of diabetic control is critical (hemoglobin $A_{1c}$) and, in the presence of previous abdominal surgery or where colonic interposition is considered mesenteric angiography should be performed.

### Intraoperative: Ischemic Preconditioning, Assessment of Conduit, Blood Pressure Support

#### Ischemic preconditioning
Ischemic preconditioning of the gastric conduit before esophageal reconstruction has been proposed in an attempt to reduce conduit necrosis and anastomotic leak rates. Urschel and colleagues[17,18] first described this in 1997. Subsequently Schröder and colleagues[19,20] demonstrated that the gastric conduit microcirculation takes 4 days to return to preoperative levels after esophagectomy. The mechanism of effect is unclear, but neovascularization of the stomach and release of humoral factors to improve the blood supply to the fundal area have both been proposed. The basis for this concern is related to studies in cadaveric specimens after esophagectomy in which it has been shown that 20% of the blood flow to the top of the gastric conduit is

derived from the mucosal capillary network rather than a named vessel.[21]

Preconditioning may take the form of radiological embolization of the arterial supply of the stomach or involve preresection laparoscopic ligation of the left gastric artery and/or short gastric arteries. Initial experience with preoperative arterial embolization was not successful and complicated by high rates of pancreatitis and splenic infarction.[22] However, this was likely because the splenic and short gastric arteries were embolized in addition to the left gastric artery. When preresectional laparoscopy is performed, a celiac lymph node dissection and inspection for omental, peritoneal, and liver metastases are also possible. To elucidate the mechanism by which preconditioning may reduce anastomotic complications, one group monitored vascular endothelial growth factor (VEGF) levels in patients undergoing laparoscopic ligation of the left gastric artery compared with those without.[23] No significant difference was observed between the two groups, which may be because of an early increase in VEGF levels or because neoangiogenesis is not the mechanism responsible. A recent systematic review of factors affecting anastomotic integrity following esophagectomy demonstrated that in 12 studies with 1215 patients, no difference in anastomotic leak rates was observed in those being preconditioned (8.83%) compared with those not (14.11%) (pooled OR = 0.73, 95% confidence interval 0.5–1.06, $P = .1$).[24] There was no evidence of statistical heterogeneity or bias. When sensitivity analysis was performed for studies comparing preoperative vessel embolization, no difference between leak rates was seen in those patients with and without intervention. The same was true for studies comparing laparoscopic vessel ligation with no ligation. The present clinical evidence does not favor preoperative preconditioning of the gastric conduit. In fact, this may be associated with increased cost given the additional surgery and hospital admission.

### Intraoperative assessment of conduit vascularity

The intraoperative clinical impression of conduit perfusion is not particularly accurate.[25–27] Techniques exist to assess blood supply to the conduit and can be applied to gastric, jejunal, and colonic reconstructions. These techniques include fluorescence angiography (eg, Woods lamp), handheld Doppler, laser Doppler flowmetry and spectrophotometry, transmucosal oxygen saturation measurement, hydrogen clearance, visible light spectroscopy, single-photon emission computed tomography (SPECT), esophagogastroduodenoscopy (EGD), CT angiography,

conventional angiography, and laser-induced fluorescence of indocyanine green[28] (**Tables 1** and **2**).

Arguably the most commonly used intraoperative assessment of conduit perfusion, when used, are Doppler ultrasound and intravenous (IV) fluorescent dye; they have reported sensitivity of up to 60%.[29] These techniques are easily used in the operating room, with a handheld Doppler or with the SPY system (Fluorescence Imaging System [Novadaq, USA]) in which a fluorescent agent (indocyanine green) enables visualization of the perfusion of the proposed conduit.[30] Murawa and colleagues[31] were the first to publish use of the SPY system in the assessment of the gastric conduit; several other studies have suggested utility of this technique.[28,32,33] These studies are all small, however, and not powered to detect a clinically significant difference in anastomotic leak rates. The SPY system may be particularly useful when a complex esophageal reconstruction is considered to assess the adequacy of supercharging the conduit and to assess jejunal or colonic blood supply (**Fig. 1**).

Although not all intraoperative assessments give real-time information with regard to the adequacy of conduit blood flow (eg, SPECT), information gained from these studies can be used to guide intraoperative decision making. The authors recommend using these tools in conjunction with clinical acumen to decide whether the conduit blood supply is suitable or whether another conduit must be sought.

### Perfusion pressure

Patients undergoing esophagectomy are predisposed to hemodynamic changes, secondary to fluid shifts, intraoperative fluid loss, epidural anesthesia, IV fluid administration, and the potential use of vasopressor agents. It is common for patients undergoing esophagectomy to have a thoracic epidural for analgesia. It can be postulated that epidural anesthesia causes increased blood flow in the gastric conduit by way of sympathetic block; in fact, a small human study has demonstrated increased gastric conduit blood flow 1 hour and 18 hours following thoracic epidural anesthesia.[34] Despite this, administration of an intraoperative thoracic epidural bupivacaine bolus has been shown to reduce blood flow at the tip of the gastric conduit during esophagectomy.[35] Administration of IV adrenaline reversed this reduced blood flow. Many surgeons have reservations with regard to the intraoperative administration of vasopressor agents and are concerned about reducing perfusion to the conduit. In animal models, the administration of vasopressors, noradrenaline in swine,[36] has been associated with reduced perfusion to

**Table 1**
**Comparison of technologies used to assess perfusion of the gastric conduit in esophageal reconstructive surgery**

| Technology | Advantages | Disadvantages |
|---|---|---|
| Fluorescence angiography/ Wood lamp | Cost-efficient<br>Availability<br>Familiarity<br>Microvasculature/macrovasculature | 1-Time injection<br>Renal clearance<br>Dye leaks into extracellular space |
| Conventional angiography | Cost-efficient<br>Familiarity<br>Microvasculature/macrovasculature | Inconvenient in the operating room<br>Time inefficient |
| Handheld Doppler | Cost-efficient<br>Familiarity<br>Difficulty visualizing microvasculature | Limited to microvasculature<br>No big-picture view |
| Laser Doppler flowmetry and spectrophotometry | Ease of use<br>Time efficient<br>Highly reproducible | Limited to microvasculature<br>No big-picture view |
| Transmucosal oxygen saturation | Correlates with tissue fluorescein studies<br>Allows postoperative monitoring | Limited to microvasculature<br>No big-picture view |
| Hydrogen clearance | Has been reported | Time-consuming<br>Unstable electrode placement<br>Questionable reproducibility |
| Visible light spectroscopy | Ease of use | Representation of perfusion<br>No big-picture view |
| SPECT | Noninvasive<br>Reproducible results | Time-consuming data acquisition<br>Postacquisition images are reformatting<br>No use in the operating room |
| EGD | Availability<br>Familiarity | Risks damage to anastomosis<br>After-the-fact diagnosis<br>No direct visualization of the vasculature |
| CT angiography | Availability<br>Image quality | Inability to perform intraoperatively<br>Expensive<br>Radiation exposure |
| Laser-induced fluorescence of indocyanine green | Ease of use<br>Intraoperative assessments<br>Time efficient<br>Visualizes both microvasculature and microvasculature<br>No renal clearance<br>Software analysis of perfusion (research aid)<br>Reproducible results | High start-up costs<br>No postoperative assessment |

*From* Pacheco PE, Hill SM, Henriques SM, et al. The novel use of intraoperative laser-induced fluorescence of indocyanine green tissue angiography for evaluation of the gastric conduit in esophageal reconstructive surgery. Am J Surgery 2013;205:350; with permission.

the conduit. However, in a small human study, the administration of IV phenylephrine following a bupivacaine bolus via thoracic epidural increased the flux (as measured in perfusion units) to the anastomotic end of the gastric conduit.[37] Intraoperative use of vasopressors has, however, been associated with increased incidence of adult respiratory distress syndrome.[38] This may be a surrogate marker of patient comorbidity and perioperative instability.

An alternative strategy to maintain perfusion pressure to the tip of the gastric conduit is

**Table 2**
**Esophageal tube conduits**

| Conduit | Blood Supply | Selection/Placement |
|---|---|---|
| Stomach | Gastroepiploic | First choice for total esophageal replacement |
| Colon | Marginal artery of Drummond | Second choice for total esophageal replacement |
| Long-segment supercharged pedicled jejunum | *Superior:* mesenteric anastomosis to LIMA/LIMV or cervical vessels<br>*Inferior:* SMA | Second choice for total esophageal replacement |
| Free jejunum | Mesenteric anastomosis to LIMA/LIMV or cervical vessels | Isolated short-segment cervical esophageal reconstruction |
| Pedicled jejunum | SMA | Optimal for vagal-sparing jejunal interposition (Merendino procedure) resection (vagus-sparing resection) or short segmental resection |
| Skin/forearm | Radial artery anastomosis to LIMA/LIMV or cervical vessels | Optimal for segmental neck resection, small area patch |
| Myocutaneous flap | Flap artery anastomosis to LIMA, LIMV, cervical vessels, or AV loop | Last choice when no other options remain |

*Abbreviations:* AV, arteriovenous; LIMA, left internal mammary artery; LIMV, left internal mammary vein; SMA, superior mesenteric artery.
*From* Blackmon SH, Dickinson KJ. Atlas of esophageal intervention. New York: Springer; 2015; with permission.

aggressive fluid resuscitation. The administration of intraoperative volume allows the patients' blood pressure and, hence, conduit perfusion pressure to be maintained. This strategy may, however, necessitate a large volume of fluid, which may have implications in terms of pulmonary edema and bowel edema responsible for postoperative ileus. It has been shown that a restrictive intraoperative fluid regimen coupled with

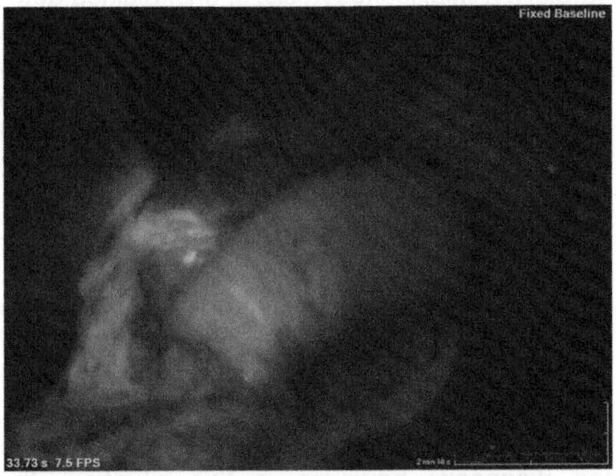

**Fig. 1.** SPY imaging of jejunal conduit demonstrating perfusion after it has been tunneled.

norepinephrine to maintain a mean arterial pressure of 65 mm Hg or greater reduced the incidence of pneumonia and respiratory complications with no increase in anastomotic leak or incidence of conduit ischemia.[39]

With regard to conduit perfusion, current evidence does not support one approach over the other when fluid resuscitation or vasopressor administration are used to correct the decrease in blood pressure seen in 40% to 60% with general anesthetic agent administration. This is similar to the current evidence regarding free flaps in plastic surgery.[40–43] Recently, however, it has been shown that intraoperative vasopressor use is not uncommon during free tissue transfer flaps and this did not seem to adversely affect patient outcomes.[44] Although care should be taken extrapolating these results to the often-pedicled gastrointestinal reconstructions after esophagectomy, it may be that judicious use of vasopressors during esophageal resections is not always harmful. In fact, hypotension with concomitant reduced conduit perfusion is not benign. Clear communication between the surgical and anesthetic team is required to form a management strategy tailored to each patient.

## Management of Acute Intraoperative Conduit Loss

Intraoperative conduit loss is dreaded. This loss may occur because of injury to the right gastroepiploic artery (GEA) during dissection, inadequate perfusion from the right GEA caused by previous surgery, or because of patient factors, such as arterial disease or intraoperative hemodynamic instability. The key factor in appropriate management is timely recognition of intraoperative conduit loss. Conduit loss can be occult. In this situation methods of assessing conduit perfusion may suggest inadequate blood flow, or clinically the conduit may look hypoperfused. If action is not taken at this point, definite and irreversible conduit loss will occur. Supercharging the conduit and enabling adequate arterial supply and venous drainage should be considered if feasible (ie, for jejunal or colonic conduits). Gastric conduits are not usually supercharged. If supercharging of the conduit can be performed and perfusion improves, that is, peristalsis and pulsatile blood flow in the mesenteric arcade, the intestinal anastomosis can be completed. If there is any doubt as to the viability of the conduit, anastomosis should not be performed. When this is the case, or in the case of frank conduit ischemia or even necrosis, a damage-control strategy should be used. If hemodynamic instability in patients has contributed to or resulted from the conduit failure, it may be appropriate to simply resect the ischemic/necrotic area and close the patients. This approach allows transfer to an intensive care facility and optimization. This solution is not durable, and patients must be appropriately drained before closure (ie, nasogastric [NG], gastrostomy when appropriate) and brought back to the operating room within 24 to 48 hours for definitive management. The definitive surgical approach would be defunctioning esophagostomy, venting gastrostomy, feeding jejunostomy, and preserving as much of the conduit as possible while resecting all ischemic/necrotic tissue.

Intraoperative conduit loss in stable patients may be approached differently. In the case of loss of the gastric conduit as a consequence of local anatomy or vascular injury, other conduits should be considered. Patient factors and length of surgery should be taken into consideration. If, for example, the surgery has already taken many hours, it may be better to formally defunction patients (esophagostomy, venting gastrostomy, and feeding jejunostomy). If the operative time is relatively short and there is minimal edema of the bowel, reconstruction can be performed at the same time as resection of the ischemic/necrotic conduit. The jejunum and the colon should be assessed for suitability. The jejunum is preferred in this situation as the colon is unlikely to be prepped. Consideration should be given to supercharging the graft, and intraoperative consultation with plastic surgical colleagues should be arranged. Reconstruction with the jejunum or colon can proceed in the usual fashion after resection of the ischemic stomach conduit. The authors advocate preserving as much of the stomach conduit as possible as this can then be used in the reconstruction.

When there is concern for the viability of the conduit, particularly in patients with significant comorbidity, an alternative option to an end esophagostomy and gastrostomy has been described. Oezcelik and colleagues[16] describe the technique of delayed esophagogastrectomy for patients with conduit ischemia intraoperatively. A cervical esophagostomy was performed and the gastric conduit brought to the neck either through the posterior mediastinum or retrosternally. The conduit was then secured in the neck, but no anastomosis was performed. At 90 days postoperatively, by reopening the cervical incision, the gastric conduit was identified by locating a marker suture. When the conduit looked healthy, anastomosis was performed, in some cases requiring resection of the left half of the manubrium, left sternoclavicular joint, and the medial portion of the first rib. This technique was used in 37 out of 554 patients over a 7-year period; 35 patients were reconstructed, and 9% experienced dysphagia postoperatively.

## Management of Delayed Conduit Loss

The key principle to managing delayed conduit ischemia/necrosis is to identify this early. Patients with conduit necrosis may be extremely unwell and deteriorate suddenly. More often there is an insidious course. Patients may develop a tachycardia, pyrexia, leukocytosis, or unexplained deterioration in condition in the absence of pneumonia or an anastomotic leak. In these patients, it is important to consider and aggressively investigate conduit ischemia to enable this to be managed appropriately. Even with this in mind, mortality of this condition approaches 90%.

If patients are systemically unwell and the diagnosis apparent, for example, bloody NG aspirate, lactic acidosis, hemodynamic instability, it is appropriate to proceed to the operating room. Patients should be resuscitated aggressively and broad-spectrum IV antibiotics commenced. Before incision, EGD can be performed to confirm the diagnosis; however, in this situation, the authors would argue video-assisted thoracic surgery/thoracotomy/reopening of the neck incision (depending on esophagectomy approach) is required to visualize the conduit. If the conduit is unsalvageable, this should be resected. An end esophagostomy should be performed, with a venting gastrostomy (if some stomach is salvageable) and feeding jejunostomy.

### Investigation of conduit ischemia after surgery

In patients in whom diagnosis is in doubt, investigation is required to determine the viability of the conduit. Several studies have been used to evaluate conduits following esophagectomy and include meglumine diatrizoate (Gastrografin) swallow, CT, and EGD. Early detection is critical to survival in these patients.

More traditionally, upper gastrointestinal contrast swallows have been used in order to assess the esophageal conduit postoperatively for anastomotic leak. Gastrografin, barium, and iohexol (Omnipaque) can all be used. Barium can persist for some time and interfere with subsequent imaging, whereas Gastrografin is water soluble and does not. Gastrografin, however, can cause pneumonitis; Omnipaque may be preferred in this situation as it is less caustic if aspirated.

It can be argued that a leak is only significant if there is evidence of clinical deterioration. Up to 40% of anastomotic leaks are detected using Gastrografin swallow in asymptomatic patients.[45] In addition, the mucosa cannot be adequately visualized during contrast swallow. It is possible to see ischemic-appearing changes (cobblestoning surface changes or change to a dark color) of the mucosa with conduit ischemia, but at this point patients are likely to be critically unwell. The administration of oral contrast is also associated with a risk of aspiration and is not possible in intubated patients.[46,47] Contrast could be cautiously administered through an NG tube but again is associated with aspiration risk. For these reasons, several studies have shown routine esophageal contrast swallow to have potential dangers and suggested their use should be limited.[46–49]

CT with oral contrast may be considered more sensitive than contrast swallow and is able to give added information with regard to pneumonia, pleural effusion, and other thoracic or abdominal abnormality. Despite this, aspiration risk persists; it has been demonstrated that a normal CT examination does not exclude ischemia of the gastric conduit.[50]

The use of EGD to assess the conduit after esophagectomy has been viewed with caution because of the concern of disrupting the fresh anastomosis. Subtle mucosal ischemia that would not be radiologically apparently can be seen on EGD. In a manner similar to the grading of anastomotic leaks following esophagectomy, a grading system for ischemic changes and leak apparent on EGD has been proposed.[50] Grade I ischemia represents 'dusky bluish colored mucosa in the vicinity of the anastomosis covered with tenacious metallic appearing mucous that could not be washed off'; grade II 'partial anastomotic breakdown with equivocal viability of normal pink mucosa margins'; grade III 'complete circumferential breakdown with pink mucosal margins'; and grade IV 'complete conduit ischemia manifested by necrotic black mucosa throughout the gastric conduit with the anastomosis still intact.' The degree of ischemia observed on EGD can guide management. For example, those patients with milder ischemic changes, which may be associated with a small anastomotic leak, may be managed successfully with stenting, venting, enteral feeding, and antibiotics. Page and colleagues[51] have described how all patients undergoing esophagectomy safely underwent routine endoscopy in the first postoperative week to detect anastomotic leakage after esophagectomy. In these patients, clinical care was guided by the EGD findings and postoperative conduit perfusion problems were preempted.

### Optimization of Patients Before Reconstruction

Having survived the necrotic conduit and subsequent surgical intervention, it is essential for patients to recuperate before considering reconstruction. During the in-hospital postoperative course, sepsis should be managed appropriately, with IV antibiotics depending on culture results and drainage of collections as appropriate. During this time, enteral nutrition should be established. Dietician and physiotherapy input are essential during this period. Patient education with regard to their esophagostomy is critical. Patients should be taught how to care for their skin and their appliance. They should be educated as to when to re-present to their physician, for example, stenosis of the esophagostomy, cellulitis.

### Reconstruction Options

There are several ways to create a neo-esophagus when resection of the esophagus is required. The stomach is always the first choice of esophageal reconstruction, when available. In order to ensure adequate blood flow to the conduit and reduce the risk of conduit necrosis, careful mobilization of the stomach is required, paying attention not to damage the gastroepiploic vessels and use minimal handling of the conduit to protect the submucosal arcade.

When the gastric conduit is not suitable or frankly ischemic/necrotic, the esophagus can be reconstructed using jejunum[14] or colon.[52] Short jejunal grafts can be used (eg, the Merendino procedure for a gastrointestinal junction gastrointestinal stromal tumor resection and reconstruction) but are not suitable for reconstruction after gastric conduit necrosis. When using the jejunum to reconstruct the esophagus, this can be done in a roux-en-Y fashion if the esophageal remnant is of sufficient length and vascularity. If the esophagus is shorter and the reconstruction must travel a greater distance, a supercharged jejunal graft can be used to reconstruct the esophagus. Supercharging the jejunum was first described in 1947, but it only recently has been more widely used.[53] The authors recommend supercharging the jejunal graft, and this surgery should be performed in collaboration with plastic surgical colleagues. The microvascular arterial and venous anastomoses are critical to the survival of this graft, which is often run on the second jejunal branch of the superior mesenteric artery, the first preserved to ensure adequate blood supply to the biliopancreatic jejunal limb. An indicator flap is left exteriorized so that in the postoperative course of the surgery the blood supply to the conduit can be inferred and monitored. The principles of management of plastic surgical flaps are applied in the perioperative period with avoidance of hypotension and most advocate avoidance of vasopressor agents. The perioperative risk in these patients is more than those undergoing a primary esophagectomy with gastric conduit reconstruction. Early complications have been reported with pneumonia in 30% of patients and a higher anastomotic leak rate of 32% and a 5% incidence of graft necrosis.[13] The 90-day mortality was 10% in this series. This finding is a reflection of the more tenuous blood supply to the graft, even with supercharging, and the complex nature of this surgery. Despite this, postoperative quality of life and graft function is generally good. Eighty-three percent of patients were able to return to eating their regular diet, and segmental peristalsis was observed on follow-up manometry.

When colonic conduits are used to reconstruct the esophagus after ischemia or necrosis of the gastric conduit, the left or the right colon may be used. Advocates of the left colon for esophageal reconstruction suggest that the smaller diameter allows less distension and redundancy and less variation in the blood supply and the conduit ultimately can be a longer length.[1,5,54] Kesler and colleagues[52] suggest that the right colon can be used if the right colon is less than 8 cm in diameter, the right colonic artery is not dominant over the ileocolic artery, and preoperative mesenteric angiography does not demonstrate a dominant ascending branches of the inferior mesenteric artery. The substernal route is often preferred for colonic interposition, and the conduit may also be supercharged. As with the supercharged jejunal grafts, resection of the left hemi-manubrium, clavicle, and first rib is required to allow space for the conduit, to perform the vascular anastomoses, and to avoid obstruction and venous engorgement of the conduit caused by entrapment. At long-term follow-up in expert hands, the quality of life as assessed by the RAND 36-Item Short Form Health Survey and assessment of gastrointestinal function demonstrated that 89% of patients experienced no dysphagia, 84% were free of regurgitation, and 84% free of heartburn. Importantly, 90% of patients were within normal body mass index limits.[55] In this series, 7 of the 79 patients underwent reoperation for colonic redundancy.

### Postreconstruction Management

Careful follow-up of patients in whom esophageal reconstruction has been necessary for conduit necrosis is essential. This follow-up is not only to detect any evidence of tumor recurrence for those who underwent esophageal resection for malignancy. Quality-of-life assessment is critical to provide the best outcomes for these patients. Medical management, for example, of reflux symptoms, is often all that is necessary to improve functional outcomes. However, in some, revision surgery will be required, for example, if redundancy of the conduit is encountered. Complex esophageal reconstruction is not commonplace, and patient support groups provide an invaluable source of empathy and advice to these patients.

## REFERENCES

1. DeMeester TD, Johansson K-E, Franze I, et al. Indications, surgical technique, and long-term functional results of colon interposition or bypass. Ann Surg 1988;208:460–74.
2. Wang LS, Huang MH, Huang BS, et al. Gastric substitution for resectable carcinoma of the esophagus: an analysis of 368 cases. Ann Thorac Surg 1992;53:289–94.
3. Horvath OP, Lukacs L, Cseke L. Complications following esophageal surgery. Recent Results Cancer Res 2000;155:161–73.
4. Gaissart HA, Mathisen DJ. Short segment colon and jejunal interposition. Semin Thorac Cardiovasc Surg 1992;4:328–35.

5. Cerfolio RJ, Allen MS, Deschamps C, et al. Esophageal replacement by colon interposition. Ann Thorac Surg 1995;59:1382–4.

6. Fujita H, Yamana H, Sueyoshi S, et al. Impact on outcome of additional microvascular anastomosis-supercharge-on colon interposition for esophageal replacement: comparison and multivariate analysis. World J Surg 1997;21:998–1003.

7. Kassis ES, Kosinski AS, Ross P Jr, et al. Predictors of anastomotic leak after esophagectomy: an analysis of the society of thoracic surgeons general thoracic database. Ann Thorac Surg 2013;96:1919–26.

8. Lerut T, Coosemans W, Decker G, et al. Anastomotic complications after esophagectomy. Dig Surg 2002; 19:92–8.

9. Low DE, Alderson D, Cecconello I, et al. International consensus on standardization of data collection for complications associated with esophagectomy: esophagectomy complications consensus group (ECCG). Ann Surg 2015;262(2):286–94.

10. Schaheen L, Blackmon SH, Nason KS. Optimal approach to the management of intrathoracic esophageal leak following esophagectomy: a systematic review. Am J Surg 2014;208:536–43.

11. Stephens EH, Correa AM, Kim MP, et al. Classification of esophageal stent leaks: leak presentation, complications and management. Ann Thorac Surg 2014;98:297–303.

12. Baker CR, Forshaw MJ, Gossage JA, et al. Long-term outcome and quality of life after supercharged jejunal interposition for oeosphageal replacement. Surgeon 2014;13(4):187–93.

13. Blackmon SH, Correa AM, Skoracki R, et al. Supercharged pedicled jejunal interposition for esophageal replacement: a 10-year experience. Ann Thorac Surg 2012;94:1104–11.

14. Gaur P, Blackmon SH. Jejunal graft conduits after esophagectomy. J Thorac Dis 2014;6(Suppl 3): S333–40.

15. Briel JW, Tamhanker AP, Hagen JA, et al. Prevalence and risk factors for ischemia, leak, and stricture of esophageal anastomosis: gastric pull up versus colon interposition. J Am Coll Surg 2004; 198:536–42.

16. Oezcelik A, Banki F, DeMeester SR, et al. Delayed esophagogastrectomy: a safe strategy for management of patients with ischemic gastric conduit at time of esophagectomy. J Am Coll Surg 2009;208: 1030–4.

17. Urschel JD, Antkowiak JG, Delacure MD, et al. Ischemic conditioning (delay phenomenon) improves esophagogastric anastomotic healing in the rat. J Surg Oncol 1997;66:254–6.

18. Urschel JD. Ischemic conditioning of the stomach may reduce the incidence of esophagogastric anastomotic leaks complicating esophagectomy: a hypothesis. Dis Esophagus 1997;10:217–9.

19. Schröder W, Beckurts KT, Stahler D, et al. Microcirculatory changes associated with gastric tube formation in the pig. Eur Surg Res 2002;34:411–7.

20. Schröder W, Holscher AH, Bludau M, et al. Ivor-Lewis esophagectomy with and without laparoscopic conditioning of the gastric conduit. World J Surg 2010;34:738–43.

21. Liebermann-Meffert DMI, Meier R, Siewert JR. Vascular anatomy of the gastric tube used for esophageal reconstruction. Ann Thorac Surg 1992; 54:1110–5.

22. Akiyama S, Ito S, Sekiguchi H, et al. Preoperative embolization of gastric arteries for esophageal cancer. Surgery 1996;120:542–6.

23. Bludau M, Holscher AH, Vallbohmer D, et al. Vascular endothelial growth factor expression following ischemic conditioning of the gastric conduit. Dis Esophagus 2013;26:847–52.

24. Markar SR, Arya S, Karthikesalingam A, et al. Technical factors that affect anastomotic integrity following esophagectomy: systematic review and meta-analysis. Ann Surg Oncol 2013;20:4274–81.

25. Bulkley GB, Zuidema GD, Hamilton SR, et al. Intraoperative determination of small intestinal viability following ischemia injury: a prospective, controlled trial of two adjuvant methods (Doppler and fluorescein) compared with standard clinical judgment. Ann Surg 1981;93:628–37.

26. Karliczek A, Benaron DA, Bass PC, et al. Intraoperative assessment of microperfusion with visible light spectroscopy in esophageal and colorectal anastomoses. Eur Surg Res 2008;41:303–11.

27. Karliczek A, Harlaar NJ, Zeebregts CJ, et al. Surgeons lack predictive accuracy for anastomotic leakage in gastrointestinal surgery. Int J Colorectal Dis 2009;24:569–76.

28. Pacheco PE, Hill SM, Henriques SM, et al. The novel use of intraoperative laser-induced fluorescence of indocyanine green tissue angiography for evaluation of the gastric conduit in esophageal reconstructive surgery. Am J Surg 2013;205:349–52.

29. Ballard JL, Stone WM, Hallett JW, et al. A critical analysis of adjuvant techniques used to assess bowel viability in acute mesenteric ischemia. Am Surg 1993;59:309–11.

30. Gurtner GC, Jones GE, Neligan PC, et al. Intraoperative laser angiography using the SPY system: review of the literature and recommendations for use. Ann Surg Innov Res 2013;7:1.

31. Murawa D, Hunerbein M, Spychala A, et al. Indocyanine green angiography for the evaluation of gastric conduit perfusion during esophagectomy – first experience. Acta Chir Belg 2012;122:275–80.

32. Kumagi Y, Ishiguro T, Haga N, et al. Hemodynamics of the reconstructed gastric tube during esophagectomy: assessment of outcomes with indocyanine green fluorescence. World J Surg 2014;38:138–43.

33. Rino Y, Yukawa N, Sato T, et al. Visualization of bloody supply route to the reconstructed stomach by indocyanine green fluorescence imaging during esophagectomy. BMC Med Imaging 2014;22:14–8.

34. Michelet P, Roch A, D'Journo XB, et al. Effect of thoracic epidural anesthesia on gastric blood flow after oesophagectomy. Acta Anaesthesiol Scand 2007;51:587–94.

35. Al-Rawi OY, Pennefather SH, Page RD, et al. The effect of thoracic epidural bupivacaine and an intravenous adrenaline infusion on gastric tube flow during esophagectomy. Anesth Analg 2008;106:884–7.

36. Theodorou D, Drimousis PG, Larentzakis A, et al. The effect of vasopressors on perfusion of the gastric graft after esophagectomy. An experimental study. J Gastrointest Surg 2008;12:1497–501.

37. Pathak D, Pennefather SH, Russell GN, et al. Phenylephrine infusion improves blood flow to the stomach during oesophagectomy in the presence of thoracic epidural anesthesia. Eur J Cardiothorac Surg 2013;44:130–3.

38. Paul DJ, Jamieson GG, Watson DI, et al. Perioperative risk analysis for acute respiratory distress syndrome after elective oesophagectomy. ANZ J Surg 2011;81:700–6.

39. Buise M, Van Bommel J, Mahra M, et al. Pulmonary morbidity following esophagectomy is decreased after introduction of a multimodal anesthetic regimen. Acta Anaesthesiol Belg 2008;59:257–61.

40. Monroe MM, McClelland J, Swide C, et al. Vasopressor use in free tissue transfer surgery. Otolaryngol Head Neck Surg 2010;142:169–73.

41. Cordeiro PG, Santamaria E, Hu GY, et al. Effects of vasoactive medications on the blood flow of island musculocutaneous flaps in swine. Ann Plast Surg 1997;39:524–31.

42. Massey MF, Gupta DK. The effects of systemic phenylephrine and epinephrine on pedicle artery and microvascular perfusion in a pig model of myoadipocutaneous rotational flaps. Plast Reconstr Surg 2007;120:1289–99.

43. Harris L, Goldstein D, Hofer S, et al. Impact of vasopressors on outcomes in head and neck free tissue transfer. Microsurgery 2012;32:15–9.

44. Kelly DA, Reynolds M, Crantford C, et al. Impact of intraoperative vasopressor use in free tissue transfer for head, neck and extremity reconstruction. Ann Plast Surg 2014;72:S135–8.

45. Schaible A, Sauer P, Hartwig W, et al. Radiologic versus endoscopic evaluation of the conduit after esophageal resection: a prospective, blinded intra-individually controlled diagnostic study. Surg Endosc 2014;28:2078–85.

46. Sauvanet A, Baltar J, Le Mee J, et al. Diagnosis and conservative management of intrathoracic leakage after oesophagectomy. Br J Surg 1998;85:1446–9.

47. Griffin S, Lamb P, Dresner S, et al. Diagnosis and management of a mediastinal leak following radical oesophagectomy. Br J Surg 2001;88:1346–51.

48. Fan S, Lau W, Yip W, et al. Limitations and dangers of Gastrografin swallow after esophageal and upper gastric operations. Am J Surg 1988;160:322–3.

49. Page R, Shackcloth M, Russell G, et al. Surgical treatment of anastomotic leaks after oesophagectomy. Eur J Cardiothorac Surg 2005;27:337–43.

50. Oezcelik A, Banki F, Ayazi S, et al. Detection of gastric conduit ischemia or anastomotic breakdown after cervical esophagogastrectomy: the use of computed tomography scan versus early endoscopy. Surg Endosc 2010;24:1948–51.

51. Page RD, Asmat A, McShane J, et al. Routine endoscopy to detect anastomotic leakage after esophagectomy. Ann Thorac Surg 2013;95:292–8.

52. Kesler KA, Pillai ST, Birdas TJ, et al. 'Supercharged' isoperistaltic colon interposition for long-segment esophageal reconstruction. Ann Thorac Surg 2013; 95:1162–9.

53. Longmire WP. A modification of the roux technique for antethoracic esophageal reconstruction: an anastomosis of the mesenteric and internal mammary blood vessels. Surgery 1947;22:94–100.

54. Thomas P, Fuentes P, Guidicelli R, et al. Colon interposition for esophageal replacement: current indications and long-term function. Ann Thorac Surg 1997; 64:757–64.

55. Greene C, De Meester SR, Augustin F, et al. Long-term quality of life and alimentary satisfaction after esophagectomy with colon interposition. Ann Thorac Surg 2014;98:1713–20.

# Functional Conduit Disorder Complicating Esophagectomy

Kamran Mohiuddin, MD[a], Donald E. Low, MD, FRCS(C)[b],*

## KEYWORDS

- Esophagectomy • Disorders • Functional conduit disorder • Esophageal cancer

## KEY POINTS

- Multimodality therapy as well as early detection of esophageal cancer has increased long-term survival, making postoperative quality of life an important issue in a larger portion of patients following esophagectomy.
- Functional problems after esophagectomy can dramatically affect quality of life.
- Anastomosis placed in the mid and lower chest can increase the incidence of delayed gastric emptying and reflux.
- Delayed gastric emptying, anastomotic stricture, dumping, and reflux are common sequelae of esophagectomy.
- Surgeons should be committed to long-term follow-up of these patients and develop strategies for treating these functional disorders.

## INTRODUCTION

In the United States, esophagectomy is performed for a wide spectrum of conditions but predominantly for cancer. Approximately 85% of the 18,170 patients diagnosed annually with esophageal cancer in the United States will die of their disease.[1] The early detection and resection of esophageal cancer provides the best chance of cure.[2] The most common esophageal cancer surgical procedures are (1) open transhiatal esophagectomy, (2) open transthoracic or Ivor Lewis esophagectomy (ILE), (3) open 3-hole or McKeown esophagectomy, and (4) hybrid or full minimally invasive esophagectomy.[3–5] All these procedures are complex, technically challenging, and require advanced surgical skill and training. The optimum approach to resection depends on individual patient and tumor characteristics, body habitus,

patient comorbidities, history of previous surgery, individual surgeon biases, and surgeon preferences. The advantages of various technical approaches and the incidence of morbidity and mortality associated with esophageal resection, as well as postoperative quality of life, remain controversial issues in thoracic surgery and thoracic oncology.

Outcomes from surgical approaches for esophageal cancer have significantly improved. In the early 1940s, perioperative mortality of 72% was associated with esophagectomy.[6] In 1946, introduction of the standardized Ivor Lewis approach for esophagectomy helped to reduce this mortality.[3] Modern case series estimate that perioperative mortality ranges from 5% to 10%, with morbidity rates greater than 50%,[7–10] although high-volume centers have demonstrated a mortality rate less than 2%.[11–13] Currently, overall 5-year

[a] Virginia Mason Medical Center, 1100 Ninth Avenue, Seattle, WA 98101, USA; [b] Digestive Disease Institute Esophageal Center of Excellence, Ryan Hill Research Foundation, Virginia Mason Medical Center, 1100 Ninth Avenue, Seattle, WA 98101, USA
* Corresponding author.
E-mail address: donald.low@virginiamason.org

Thorac Surg Clin 25 (2015) 471–483
http://dx.doi.org/10.1016/j.thorsurg.2015.07.009
1547-4127/15/$ – see front matter © 2015 Elsevier Inc. All rights reserved.

survival rate in patients amenable to definitive treatment ranges from 19% to 30%.[14] Barrett's surveillance programs have increased detection of early-stage cancer, increasing the potential for cure and making the maintenance of quality of life increasingly important. Esophagectomy has the potential to be a life-altering operation. Patients can lose up to 15% to 20% of their body weight from the time of diagnosis through the first 6 months after the surgery, but this trend typically stabilizes after 6 months. Most patients adapt to smaller, more frequent, meals. Simple sugars and fluids at mealtime may need to be avoided until the function of the conduit is established. It is important to match the surgical approach according to the tumor and physiologic issues. Other factors that can affect functional outcome include choice of reconstructive conduit, and location, as well as technique of anastomosis. Short-term conduit function will vary but can be impacted by timing of nasogastric (NG) tube removal, timing of resumption of oral diet, and utilization of postoperative jejunostomy feeding tubes.

The reconstructive method of choice for most surgeons after esophagectomy is gastric interposition (>90% of the cases). Colon interposition is an appropriate alternative but in many centers the colon is used when the stomach is unavailable due to tumor extension or previous surgery.[15,16] According to the Society of Thoracic Surgeons (STS) guidelines, the gastric tube is the preferred esophageal substitute. Alternatively, in some cases, the small intestine, pedicled Roux-en-Y reconstruction (typically appropriate to the level of the inferior pulmonary vein), free graft (requires microvascular anastomosis), or pedicled skin-muscle flaps, can be selectively used. Either thoracic or cervical anastomoses are applied for gastric tube reconstruction. The creation of the gastric neo-esophagus is associated with substantial alteration to the stomach blood supply. Ligation of left gastric, short gastric, and left gastroepiploic arteries typically results in significant potential for ischemia at the tip of the conduit, which is typically the location of the anastomosis.[17] Anastomotic methods can include hand-sewn anastomoses (continuous and interrupted sutures, single-layer or double-layer sutures, absorbable or nonabsorbable stitches), stapling (circular and linear), and combined hand-sewn and stapled anastomoses.[18,19]

Delayed gastric emptying (DGE), dumping syndrome, anastomotic stricture/leak, and reflux are recognized postoperative complications that can contribute to nutritional problems and impact postoperative quality of life. There is no one surgical approach that can eliminate any one of these complications, but certain techniques have the potential to reduce conduit dysfunction. The restoration of foregut function after esophagectomy greatly affects patient satisfaction and continues to challenge esophageal surgeons. This review focuses specifically on functional conduit disorders after esophagectomy.

## DELAYED GASTRIC EMPTYING

After esophagectomy, the stomach is commonly used to restore the continuity of the upper gastrointestinal tract.[20,21] However, functional conduit disorders, such as DGE, can occur, which significantly impacts postoperative nutrition and quality of life. DGE puts patients at increased risk of aspiration pneumonia, malnutrition, decreased patient satisfaction, prolonged hospital stay, and readmissions.[22,23] The current literature reports the incidence of DGE as ranging between 10% and 50%.[24–27] However, documenting the actual incidence is complex because the definition of DGE varies among institutions. Most of the time patients complain of reflux, regurgitation, early satiety, pain, and bloating while eating.

DGE may result from a number of causes: vagotomy, torsion of the stomach in the right chest, compression of distal gastric conduit at the hiatus, gastric conduit redundancy, and pyloric obstruction. The incidence of DGE appears to be higher in patients with intrathoracic anastomosis due to the increased potential of gastric conduit redundancy above the level of the diaphragm. Early satiety after esophagectomy is common, and results from diminished motor function and loss of gastric reservoir. Immediately after esophagectomy, the gastric conduit functions as a nonmotile tube, and ingested food must empty by gravity alone (**Fig. 1**). Patients should be routinely advised to initiate oral nutrition with multiple (5–6) small portions throughout the day, rather than attempt to consume 3 regular meals in the first month after reconstruction. Gastric contractility is not completely lost after esophagectomy and the denervated stomach may recover some motor function over time. This is one of the issues that surgeons use to support a stepwise resumption of oral intake following esophagectomy and the use of temporary jejunostomy tubes. The motor activity of the gastric tube is affected by the size, shape, and location of the neo-esophagus. The gastric conduit can be placed in 3 locations: (1) the original esophageal bed in posterior mediastinum, (2) retrosternal space, or (3) tunneled subcutaneously anterior to the sternum. There have been no studies to date that show significant differences in conduit emptying between these various pathways.[28–30]

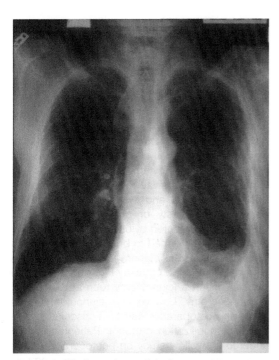

**Fig. 1.** Air-filled gastric conduit that encourages gravity drainage of fluids and food as long as no pyloric obstruction is present.

In an effort to promote gastric emptying, many surgeons perform pyloric drainage procedures, such as pyloroplasty or pyloromyotomy. Both procedures are generally considered simple procedures; however, they may be complicated by stricture, leak, and an increased incidence of dumping. As a result of these issues, and the limited evidence-based documentation of benefit, many surgeons do not routinely perform an emptying procedure during esophagectomy. In a prospective randomized trial of 72 patients who underwent transthoracic esophagectomy with or without pyloroplasty, Cheung and colleagues[31] found no complications resulting from pyloroplasty and no statistically significant difference in symptoms at 6 months and at 2 years. Similarly, in a meta-analysis of 9 randomized controlled trials encompassing 553 patients, Urschel and colleagues[32] found no difference in mortality, leak rate, or pulmonary complications in patients who did or did not undergo pyloric drainage. These trials, notwithstanding the STS, recommend drainage of the gastric conduit by pyloroplasty or myotomy after esophagectomy to decrease the incidence of DGE and the potential of pulmonary complications due to aspiration.

The realization is that none of these studies specifically assesses the postoperative quality of life. There has been some concern that pyloric drainage procedure may predispose to dumping syndrome. Gastric emptying continues to improve up to a year after surgery. The incidence of early DGE can be decreased by use of a structured approach to the reintroduction of oral intake. This approach is the reason many surgeons advocate the routine insertion of a jejunostomy at the time of esophagectomy. This allows most nutrition immediately after surgery to be supplied through the enteral feeding tube, with the patient taking limited oral liquids or pureed diet in the 2 to 3 weeks after surgery.

DGE can be classified as either immediate or persistent. Immediate DGE usually occurs within 10 to 14 days and may be due to mucosal edema, loss of gastric motility, or conduit redundancy. Persistent DGE occurs more than 14 days after surgery, is typically associated with pyloric obstruction or stricture or conduit redundancy, and may respond to prokinetic agents, such as metoclopramide or erythromycin. Erythromycin therapy can significantly aid in the function and emptying of the gastric conduit.[33] Recently, botulinum toxin and endoscopic pyloric dilation also have been used as an effective and safe treatment for both immediate and DGE.[34] Cerfolio and colleagues[35] evaluated the use of Botox injection into the pylorus at the time of esophagogastrectomy and found that it is safe and decreases the operative time when compared with pyloroplasty or pyloromyotomy. In addition, it can improve the incidence of early DGE, and may decrease respiratory complications, shorten hospital stay, and reduce late bile reflux. On the contrary, Eldaif and colleagues[36] performed a retrospective review of all patients who underwent an open esophageal resection. They divided 322 patients into 3 groups for analysis: botulinum injection (n = 78), pyloromyotomy (n = 45), and pyloroplasty (n = 199). It was discovered that patients receiving botulinum injections demonstrated similar rates of DGE on postoperative radiologic evaluation compared with patients undergoing pyloromyotomy and pyloroplasty. However, patients receiving botulinum experienced more postoperative reflux symptoms, increased use of promotility agents, increased requirement for postoperative endoscopic interventions, and increased incidence of irreversible postoperative dumping syndrome. Recently, Salameh and colleagues[37] described the use of gastric electrical stimulation to treat gastroparesis in intractable delayed emptying of the vagally denervated intrathoracic stomach after esophagectomy by using a battery-powered neuro-stimulator connected to the gastric antrum. The results were promising but the data are in a very early stage and require thoracotomy.

The stomach has historically been the preferred conduit for esophageal replacement. The most desirable width of gastric conduit has been debated. Every effort should be made to construct the gastric conduit to provide a direct route through the hiatus and into the small bowel. Most surgeons strongly recommend avoiding placement of the anastomosis in the lower chest. Conduit redundancy above the diaphragm allows food to accumulate above the diaphragm. This accumulation can result in retention of food and fluids within the conduit, promoting reflux, regurgitation, and ultimately dilation of the conduit. Patients who present with DGE and are found on radiologic examination to have significant redundancy and food retention, should undergo esophagogastroduodenoscopy (EGD) to assess the pylorus with consideration of dilatation and Botox injection. Patients should be advised to eat in small volumes and a "witnessed" upper gastrointestinal series (member of the surgical team is present during the upper gastrointestinal study to direct positioning of the patient to discover which orientation best promotes conduit emptying) can be used to determine the optimal postprandial positioning for promoting the gastric emptying. Revision surgery may be required, which can involve mobilization of the distal gastric conduit to place additional length below the diaphragm. If significant conduit dilation is present, the gastric conduit may need revision to remove the supradiaphragmatic redundancy and improve conduit emptying. This revisional surgery must be done with careful attention paid to the preservation of the conduit blood supply (**Fig. 2**). According to Wormuth and colleagues,[38] during esophageal reconstruction, the greatest challenge is the preparation of the esophageal conduit, completion of the esophageal anastomosis, and revisional conduit ischemia. The risk of ischemia is related to conduit type, length of conduit, comorbidities, and/or operative technique.

Our current approach involves producing a relatively narrow 3 to 4 cm conduit, targeting anastomosis in the upper chest 3 to 4 cm above the azygous vein or in the cervical region. Special attention is paid toward producing a straight (nonredundant) pathway for the conduit into the abdomen (**Figs. 3** and **4**). We do not routinely perform pyloroplasty or pyloromyotomy unless there is a documented pyloric stricture. A Kocher maneuver is performed to bring the pylorus up to 2 to 4 cm from the diaphragmatic hiatus, which also straightens the pathway into duodenum. We routinely insert a jejunostomy tube at the time of esophagectomy. Low-volume jejunostomy feeds begin on postoperative day 1, in association with an early mobilization protocol. Patients typically undergo a swallow study on postoperative day 3 or 4 to examine the anastomosis and, equally importantly, to assess gastric emptying (**Figs. 5** and **6**). The findings of these studies are categorized into 2 groups: (1) gastric emptying is immediate, which results in the NG tube being removed and limited oral intake being initiated the next morning, or (2) gastric emptying is delayed, which results in the NG tube remaining in place and the patient is placed on erythromycin. After 48 hours, we repeat the swallow study and, if gastric emptying is still delayed, the NG tube is removed and we perform endoscopy with pyloric dilation (to 1.5 cm maximum diameter) and also inject

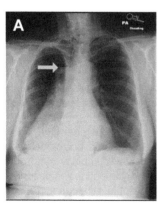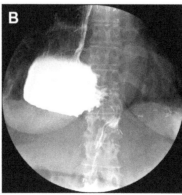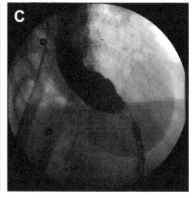

**Fig. 2.** (*A*) A 68-year-old female patient 2 years after Ivor Lewis esophagectomy for cancer. Severe problem with early satiety, regurgitation, and weight loss. Chest radiograph shows a dilated redundant conduit with an air fluid level high (see *arrow*) in the right chest. (*B*) Contrast study of the same patient showing supradiaphragmatic reservoir in a redundant gastric conduit. (*C*) Patient did not respond to prokinetic agents, pyloric dilation, and Botox injection. She ultimately underwent repeat right thoracotomy with resection of gastric conduit redundancy with repeat contrast study showing more regular conduit contour and improved emptying.

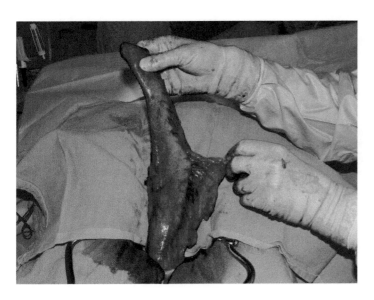

**Fig. 3.** Narrow conduit with blood supply maintained through right gastro-epiploic and right gastric artery.

Botox. Our current target day for discharge is day 7. At time of hospital discharge, patients are on liquid or pureed oral intake (1 cup per hour) along with nocturnal jejunostomy feeds. We provide structured dietary advancement for the next 6 weeks with decreasing jejunostomy feeds.

## Dumping

One of the common clinical complications of altered gastric function postesophagectomy is dumping syndrome. It is estimated that 5% to 68% of patients show some manifestation of dumping syndrome after esophagectomy.[39–42] However, 5% to 10% of patients show symptoms with moderate severity, and 1% to 5% of patients experience severe symptoms.[33] Patients typically report feeling dizzy, nauseated, and diaphoretic, while having episodes of abdominal cramping and bloating, flushing, and explosive diarrhea. Based on the presentation of symptoms, dumping syndrome can be divided into Early (10–30 minutes after eating) and Late (1–3 hours after eating), with the patients experiencing a combination of both presentations. Early symptoms of dumping syndrome postesophagectomy are more common, most frequently in women and in a younger age group. Decreased capacity of the gastric conduit and changes in pyloric orientation and function can increase the tendency for dumping, especially in the months after esophagectomy. Most cases are mild and controlled with dietary modification.

The pathophysiology of dumping syndrome is multifactorial. Dumping syndrome manifests as a variety of gastrointestinal and vasomotor symptoms. It is usually a clinical diagnosis but can be

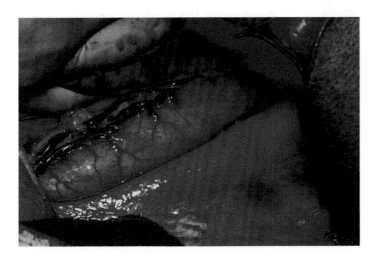

**Fig. 4.** Conduit positioned in bed of the esophagus in patient undergoing left thoraco-abdominal resection, demonstrating direct pathway into abdominal cavity and no conduit redundancy.

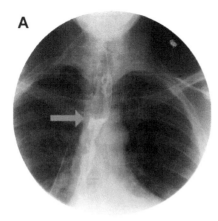
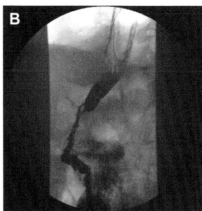

**Fig. 5.** A 72-year-old-male patient 3 days after Ivor Lewis esophagectomy undergoing "witnessed" upper gastrointestinal study (water-soluble contrast followed by thin barium) showing (*A*) intact anastomosis in the upper chest (*arrow*) and (*B*) immediate emptying through the pylorus, which allows NG tube removal and initiation of oral intake.

confirmed by documenting symptoms of hypoglycemia after oral glucose challenge test. Early dumping, 10 to 30 minutes after ingestion, is typically due to the rapid transit of hyperosmolar gastric contents into the upper gastrointestinal tract.[43] Late dumping is diagnosed by symptoms occurring 1 to 3 hours after eating.[44] The rapid transport of carbohydrate to the small intestine triggers the release of insulin and leads to subsequent hypoglycemic symptoms.[45,46] Although effective gastric emptying is the preferred goal after esophagectomy, no current strategy has been developed to standardize the objective assessment of gastric emptying after esophageal resection.

Eating small, frequent meals, avoiding liquids with meals, and avoiding eating foods containing sugar and other simple carbohydrates can decrease the incidence of dumping. Separating liquids and solids during meals can prevent, and may also decrease, the severity of dumping. To meet daily caloric needs, intake of protein and fat should be increased.[47–49] Most dumping syndromes improve over time. Nonsurgical options for management include administration of pharmacologic therapy. In severe cases, drugs include tincture of opium, diphenoxylate, beta blockers, methysergide, acarbose, and octreotide. Although they have not demonstrated conclusive benefit in previous reports, they can be considered.[50–53] Patients with severe dumping syndrome are rarely unable to attain adequate nutrition orally. In these patients, placement of jejunostomy tube or central venous access for total parenteral nutrition can be required.

### Anastomotic Stricture/Dysphagia

Anastomotic stricture after esophagectomy is an important postoperative event that impacts quality of life and the ability to resume a normal pattern of eating. Anastomotic stricture causes dysphagia; however, dysphagia after esophagectomy may not necessarily be associated with an anastomotic stricture. Most postoperative dysphagia can be classified as anastomotic or functional due to oropharyngeal dysfunction. Similarly, strictures can be classified into scar contracture and/or stricture associated with localized leak or ischemia. Anastomotic strictures are reasonably common after esophagectomy, with a mean reported prevalence of 30% (range, 9%–48%).[54–56] Previous reports have identified several risk

**Fig. 6.** Another patient showing delayed gastric emptying on day 3, which delays NG tube removal and treatment with erythromycin.

factors for developing anastomotic strictures, including postoperative anastomotic leakage, poor vascularization of the gastric tube, and a stapled rather than a hand-sewn anastomosis, and in patients with preoperative cardiac disease, hypoalbuminemia, increased intraoperative blood loss, hypotension, hypoxemia, and diabetes mellitus.[57] In recent years, the incidence of complications after esophagectomy has decreased, but the rate of occurrence of anastomotic stricture has remained relatively stable.

Endoscopy and barium swallow examinations are the initial assessments for investigating early and late dysphagia after esophagectomy. The esophagus is a muscular tube with elastic walls. In the resting state, the lumen is in a collapsed state, whereas during the swallowing process, the muscles of the esophagus relax to accommodate the food bolus (anterior-posterior diameter, up to 2 cm; lateral diameter, up to 3 cm). However, esophagogastric anastomotic healing produces a scar resulting in an inelastic segment associated with the scar around the anastomosis. The size of the anastomosis varies depending on the diameter of the stapler, the anastomotic method, and an individual's degree of scar contraction. Therefore, patients who consume solid food that forms a bolus exceeding the diameter of the anastomosis will experience periodic dysphagia and the potential for bolus obstruction. If the patient is masticating the food adequately, an anastomotic luminal diameter of 1 cm should be adequate to consume a diversified diet.

One-layer hand-sewn anastomosis has lower rates of stricture formation than 2-layer hand-sewn anastomosis.[58] Similarly, end-to-end circular stapler anastomosis has a higher rate of stricture formation versus side-to-side longitudinal semimechanical anastomosis, which creates a larger cross-sectional anastomotic area.[55] It is recommended to use at least a 25-mm load when using a circular stapler. Most cases with anastomotic stricture respond to early dilation, and when performed by an experienced endoscopist, dilation can be safely done as early as postoperative day 3 to 5. Early anastomotic strictures are a major contributor to the occurrence of anastomotic leak. Strictures are also common sequelae of anastomotic leak and there is evidence to suggest that elective dilation in patients who have experienced an anastomotic leak after esophagectomy can decrease the incidence and severity of anastomotic stricture.

Trentino and colleagues[59] reported that after a mean of 3.6 dilations, there was an 83% success rate. However, several studies have also suggested that the anastomosis continues to mature and the moderate stricture can resolve spontaneously. Early treatment of strictures consists of dilation using a through-the-scope balloon or wire-directed bougie. The use of bougie dilators involves 2 mechanisms of dilation: a shearing force and a radial force; whereas, balloon dilation involves only a radial force. For stricture dilation, it is essential to first assess the luminal diameter, and then dilate up to 3 levels at a time. For example, if the stricture diameter is 0.8 cm, initial dilatation should involve sequential 27, 30, and 33 French dilation.

For strictures that do not respond to an initial dilation, subsequent dilations can be done with synchronous injection of steroids. The esophageal dilation is routinely performed in an outpatient setting and intralesional steroid injection is combined with the esophagogastric dilation procedure. Triamcinolone acetate or acetonide 10 mg/mL is the most common dose used, and it can be increased up to 40 mg/mL.[60–62] The volume of corticosteroid used per injection has varied from 0.5 to 2.8 mL. In a randomized study, Ramage and colleagues[61] standardized the dosage to 0.5-mL aliquots of 20 mg each of 40 mg/mL triamcinolone acetonide. Ramboer and colleagues[63] used a betamethasone preparation: one 1-mL vial containing 5 mg betamethasone as a dipropionate suspension diluted into usually 5 mL, and sometimes 10 mL, of normal saline solution and injected as 0.5-mL to 1.0-mL aliquots. Miyashita and colleagues[64] used a total of 8 mg dexamethasone (2 mL) injected endoscopically into 4 sites (2 mg/ 0.5 mL per site) at the anastomotic site immediately after dilation. However, there were no differences among the reported studies with regard to the response outcome after using different steroid formulations. The number of injection sessions in the reported series also varies from only 1, to as many sessions as the number of dilations. Kochhar and Makharia[60] used a maximum of 4 sessions, whereas Rupp and colleagues[65] carried out a maximum of 5 sessions and Gandhi and colleagues[66] conducted as many as 13 sessions. The number of sessions is an issue that has not yet been settled and requires standardization. Our approach is to use steroid injection in no more than 2 dilations and, if unsuccessful in restoring normal swallowing, move to other treatment approaches.

Electroincision is an alternative option to dilation in patients with refractory or recurrent esophagogastric anastomotic strictures. The optimal stricture for this procedure is short and membranous, rather than long and tapered. This treatment option is safe and effective, with reports showing results superior to dilation alone.[67] Historically, patients with refractory strictures have been taught to self-dilate. Although still an acceptable option, it requires extensive time for patient instruction and not all patients are suitable.

Approximately 50% of strictures are resolved with a single dilation.[68] If strictures are refractory to dilation and corticosteroid injection, the next option is to consider use of a removable self-expandable metallic (SEMS) or plastic (SEPS) stent. Stents are not considered first-line treatment for early strictures. They are reserved only for patients who have failed previous therapy (usually multiple sessions of dilation).[69] In rare cases, the dilation does not open the stricture at all, or the stricture opens but then closes within a short period of time. In those cases in which the stricture closes within a short period of time, the goal is to place the stent to hold the stricture open for an extended prolonged period of time, causing the scar tissue to remodel around the stent to decrease the incidence of recurrence. We currently recommend leaving the stent in place for 2 to 3 weeks (**Fig. 7**).

There are 2 major types of esophageal stents: SEMS and SEPS. The metal stents are used for palliation of malignant conditions, and plastic stents are used for the management of benign esophageal conditions, such as tracheoesophageal fistulas, esophageal strictures, esophageal perforations, and also for postoperative esophagectomy leaks. Until recently, there were no SEMS approved for use in benign conditions by the US Food and Drug Administration (FDA), although there are published reports of SEMS being used in benign strictures. There are multiple types of prostheses that are available from various manufacturers. The metal stents are made of nitinol (alloy of nickel and titanium) and plastic stents are made of polyester. There are 3 types of SEMS: fully covered, partially covered, and uncovered. There is evidence that covered SEMS are better than uncovered stents in benign conditions. A fully covered nitinol stent has recently been approved by the FDA (Niti-S; TaeWoong Medical, Seoul, Korea) to be used in benign and malignant esophageal strictures. Recently, SEPS have been increasingly used in the treatment of benign esophageal diseases that include esophageal strictures, fistulas, perforation, and anastomotic leaks.[70] The SEPS are made of polyester netting embedded in a silicone membrane, creating a polyester mesh outer cover with a smooth silicone inner lining that is present for the entire length of the stent. The middle and distal portions are of the same diameter, whereas the proximal end of the stent is flared in an attempt to prevent distal migration. There are potential advantages of SEPS over SEMS, which include ease of retrieval, limited local tissue reaction, and lower cost.[71–78]

The self-expandable plastic stent Polyflex (Boston Scientific, Natick, MA) is a silicone device with an encapsulated monofilament braid made of polyester and can be used to manage difficult stricture after esophagectomy. The mesh is completely covered by a silicone layer with a smooth inner surface and a more structured outer surface to decease the incidence of migration.[79] The edges are protected with silicone to avoid impaction and/or tissue damage at the proximal and distal ends. The radiopaque markers are located at the proximal, midpoint, and distal ends of the stent to help in positioning at the time of insertion. Potential complications include stent migration, airway compression, aspiration, pain, nausea, and vomiting. There have also been several cases of stricture development at the end of the stent flare, especially in partially covered stents. These strictures are most commonly due to granulation tissue proliferation. The granulation tissue and stricture typically resolve on stent removal. The introduction of proton pump inhibitors, improved stent technology, and the development of better and safer endoscopy and dilation techniques, has resulted in a major decrease in the complications secondary to the treatment of anastomotic stricture.

Our approach in early dysphagia is to perform a swallow study to assess for swallowing mechanism disorder, anastomotic leak, or stricture. If a stricture is identified, we perform EGD 2 to 8 weeks after esophagectomy with balloon dilation up to 1.0 cm. In late dysphagia secondary to stricture, we perform EGD and, depending on degree of stenosis, we perform wire-directed bougie dilation. If the stricture is 0.5 cm in diameter, we dilate to 18, 21, and 24, and then repeat the EGD in 2 weeks to assess the stricture. If recurrence persists after 2 dilations, we use steroid injection of triamcinolone acetate 10 mg/mL into 4 quadrants (total dose 40 mg/mL). If stricture persists, we consider either needle-knife electroincision or will insert an expandable removable stent with elective removal plan 2 to 3 weeks later (see **Fig. 7**).

## Reflux

Esophageal resection and reconstruction results in removal of the gastroesophageal antireflux mechanism, increasing the risk for prolonged exposure to gastric acid and duodenal juice. Reflux is a common problem after esophagectomy, occurring in 60% to 80% of patients and impacts quality of life.[80] Clinical manifestations may include cervical heartburn or with regurgitation,

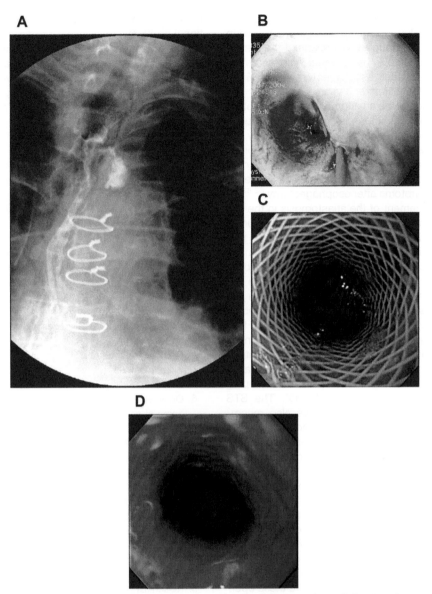

**Fig. 7.** A 60-year-old female patient discovered to have localized leak on day 5 following thoraco-abdominal resection with cervical anastomosis. (*A*) A Gastrografin swallow study confirming localized anastomotic leak which was treated with antibiotics and holding oral intake with resolution. (*B*) Endoscopy of the same patient demonstrating a tight anastomotic stricture that had been treated with multiple dilations. (*C*) Endoscopy following the insertion of a Polyflex stent across the stricture (Boston Scientific). (*D*) Endoscopic picture immediately after stent removal 4 weeks after insertion showing widely patent anastomosis.

aspiration, bile-induced and gastric acid-induced laryngitis, vomiting, chronic cough, hoarseness, inability to lie in a supine position, choking, and recurrent pneumonias. DGE also can increase the severity of reflux symptoms.

Symptoms after esophagectomy are typically more troublesome when patients are supine. In some cases this can lead to sleep deprivation. The negative intrathoracic pressure in the chest and the positive intra-abdominal pressure work

together to promote reflux across the anastomosis. The pyloric drainage procedures may promote duodenogastric reflux, leading in turn to bile reflux into the proximal esophagus.

It has been assumed that gastric acid secretion typically decreases after esophagectomy due to vagal interruption. Gutschow and colleagues[81] studied 91 patients who had undergone tubular stomach reconstruction associated with esophageal resection by monitoring intraluminal gastric pH and bile. There were 3 groups based on the length of follow-up (group 1 ≤1 year, group 2 = 1–3 years, group 3 ≥3 years) and the results showed that 32.3% had normal acid secretion within 1 year after esophagectomy, 81.5% by 2 years, and 97.6% after 3 years.

The location of the anastomosis, as well as other technical conduit factors, is an important issue in the prevention of reflux after esophagectomy. An anastomosis below the aortic arch, utilization of whole stomach, and having a significant portion of the gastric conduit in the abdomen can increase the reflux symptoms after esophagectomy.[82,83] As a result, placement of the anastomosis in the upper chest (above the aortic arch), tubulization of gastric conduit, and mobilizing of the pylorus to a position within 2 to 8 cm of the diaphragmatic hiatus is recommended. Also, patients should be encouraged to change eating habits, which will lead to less chance of reflux, especially in the early stages after esophagectomy. These should include eating 6 small nutritious meals a day, taking small bites, chewing food well, sitting in an upright position for 45 to 60 minutes after eating, avoiding lying in the supine position immediately after meals, walking after meals, and sleeping with their head elevated 20° to 30°. The STS evidence-based surgical guidelines also recommend a high intrathoracic anastomosis above the azygous vein or a cervical anastomoses as the preferred anastomotic location, and avoiding a low intrathoracic anastomosis.

Some surgeons routinely keep patients on H2 blocker or proton pump inhibitors after esophagectomy. There are surgical strategies that have been proposed to prevent reflux after esophagectomy, such as creating an anastomotic fundoplication, intercostal muscle flap, or diaphragmatic slings. They are complex to create and their efficacy remains unproven, and therefore these operations have not been widely accepted.

## SUMMARY

Esophagectomy is a complex surgical procedure that routinely impacts quality of life. Improved results associated with early diagnosis in Barrett's screening programs and improved neoadjuvant protocols increase the potential for cure in patients with esophageal cancer who are treated surgically.

Surgeons must recognize that there are important technical issues associated with gastric conduit construction, anastomosis construction and location, and approaches to intraoperative pyloric management and postoperative nutritional management, and that these issues will impact the incidence and severity of postoperative functional problems.

Surgeons must also be able to identify the signs and symptoms of DGE, dumping, and anastomotic strictures, be prepared to advise patients regarding lifestyle and medical management and, when appropriate, initiate endoscopic and surgical intervention.

## REFERENCES

1. Siegel R, Ma J, Zou Z, et al. Cancer statistics, 2014. CA Cancer J Clin 2014;64:9–29.
2. O'Rourke I, Tait N, Bull C, et al. Oesophageal cancer: outcome of modern surgical management. Aust N Z J Surg 1995;65:11–6.
3. Lewis I. The surgical treatment of carcinoma of the oesophagus; with special reference to a new operation for growths of the middle third. Br J Surg 1946; 34:18–31.
4. McKeown KC. Total three-stage oesophagectomy for cancer of the oesophagus. Br J Surg 1976;63: 259–62.
5. Orringer MB, Sloan H. Esophagectomy without thoracotomy. J Thorac Cardiovasc Surg 1978;76: 643–54.
6. Ochsner A, DeBakey M. Surgical aspects of carcinoma of esophagus: review of literature and report of four cases. J Thorac Surg 1941;10:401–45.
7. Adelstein DJ, Rice TW, Becker M, et al. Use of concurrent chemotherapy, accelerated fractionation radiation, and surgery for patients with esophageal carcinoma. Cancer 1997;80:1011–20.
8. Keller SM, Ryan LM, Coia LR, et al. High dose chemoradiotherapy followed by esophagectomy for adenocarcinoma of the esophagus and gastroesophageal junction: results of a phase II study of the Eastern Cooperative Oncology Group. Cancer 1998;83:1908–16.
9. Kelsen DP, Ginsberg R, Pajak TF, et al. Chemotherapy followed by surgery compared with surgery alone for localized esophageal cancer. N Engl J Med 1998;339:1979–84.
10. Wright CD, Wain JC, Lynch TJ, et al. Induction therapy for esophageal cancer with paclitaxel and hyperfractionated radiotherapy: a phase I and II study. J Thorac Cardiovasc Surg 1997;114:811–5.
11. Ando N, Ozawa S, Kitagawa Y, et al. Improvement in the results of surgical treatment of advanced squamous esophageal carcinoma during 15 consecutive years. Ann Surg 2000;232:225–32.
12. Law S, Wong KH, Kwok KF, et al. Predictive factors for postoperative pulmonary complications and mortality after esophagectomy for cancer. Ann Surg 2004;240:791–800.
13. Siewert JR, Stein HJ, Feith M, et al. Histologic tumor type is an independent prognostic parameter in

esophageal cancer: lessons from more than 1,000 consecutive resections at a single center in the Western world. Ann Surg 2001;234:360–7.

14. American Cancer Society. Cancer facts and figures 2014. Atlanta (GA): American Cancer Society; 2014. Available at: http://www.cancer.org/research/cancerfactsstatistics/cancerfactsfigures2014/#. Accessed May 21, 2014.

15. Hiebert C, Bredenberg C. Selection and placement of conduits. In: Pearson F, Cooper J, Deslauriers R, et al, editors. Esophageal surgery. 2nd edition. New York: Churchill Livingstone; 2002. p. 794–801.

16. Muller JM, Erasmi H, Stelzner M, et al. Surgical therapy of oesophageal carcinoma. Br J Surg 1990;77:845–57.

17. Stelzner F, Kunath U. Results of esophago-intestinal anastomoses and studies of gastric perfusion in the stomach mobilized for that purpose. Chirurg 1977;48:651–6 [in German].

18. Beitler AL, Urschel JD. Comparison of stapled and hand-sewn esophagogastric anastomoses. Am J Surg 1998;175:337–40.

19. Kim RH, Takabe K. Methods of esophagogastric anastomoses following esophagectomy for cancer: a systematic review. J Surg Oncol 2010;101:527–33.

20. Gockel I, Gonner U, Domeyer M, et al. Long-term survivors of esophageal cancer: disease-specific quality of life, general health and complications. J Surg Oncol 2010;102:516–22.

21. Sutcliffe RP, Forshaw MJ, Tandon R, et al. Anastomotic strictures and delayed gastric emptying after esophagectomy: incidence, risk factors and management. Dis Esophagus 2008;21:712–7.

22. Fok M, Cheng SW, Wong J. Pyloroplasty versus no drainage in gastric replacement of the esophagus. Am J Surg 1991;162:447–52.

23. Mannell A, McKnight A, Esser JD. Role of pyloroplasty in the retrosternal stomach: results of a prospective, randomized, controlled trial. Br J Surg 1990;77:57–9.

24. Collard JM, Otte JB, Reynaert M, et al. Quality of life three years or more after esophagectomy for cancer. J Thorac Cardiovasc Surg 1992;104:391–4.

25. Hinder RA, Esser J, DeMeester TR. Management of gastric emptying disorders following the Roux-en-Y procedure. Surgery 1988;104:765–72.

26. Kraft R, Fry W, Deweese M. Postvagotomy gastric atony. Arch Surg 1964;88:865–74.

27. Miedema BW, Sarr MG, van Heerden JA, et al. Complications following pancreaticoduodenectomy. Current management. Arch Surg 1992;127:945–9.

28. Gawad KA, Hosch SB, Bumann D, et al. How important is the route of reconstruction after esophagectomy: a prospective randomized study. Am J Gastroenterol 1999;94:1490–6.

29. Imada T, Ozawa Y, Minamide J, et al. Gastric emptying after gastric interposition for esophageal carcinoma: comparison between the anterior and posterior mediastinal approaches. Hepatogastroenterology 1998;45:2224–7.

30. van Lanschot JJ, van BM, Oei HY, et al. Randomized comparison of prevertebral and retrosternal gastric tube reconstruction after resection of oesophageal carcinoma. Br J Surg 1999;86:102–8.

31. Cheung HC, Siu KF, Wong J. Is pyloroplasty necessary in esophageal replacement by stomach? A prospective, randomized controlled trial. Surgery 1987;102:19–24.

32. Urschel JD, Blewett CJ, Young JE, et al. Pyloric drainage (pyloroplasty) or no drainage in gastric reconstruction after esophagectomy: a meta-analysis of randomized controlled trials. Dig Surg 2002;19:160–4.

33. Burt M, Scott A, Williard WC, et al. Erythromycin stimulates gastric emptying after esophagectomy with gastric replacement: a randomized clinical trial. J Thorac Cardiovasc Surg 1996;111:649–54.

34. Bagheri R, Fattahi SH, Haghi SZ, et al. Botulinum toxin for prevention of delayed gastric emptying after esophagectomy. Asian Cardiovasc Thorac Ann 2013;21:689–92.

35. Cerfolio RJ, Bryant AS, Canon CL, et al. Is botulinum toxin injection of the pylorus during Ivor Lewis [corrected] esophagogastrectomy the optimal drainage strategy? J Thorac Cardiovasc Surg 2009;137:565–72.

36. Eldaif SM, Lee R, Adams KN, et al. Intrapyloric botulinum injection increases postoperative esophagectomy complications. Ann Thorac Surg 2014;97:1959–64.

37. Salameh JR, Aru GM, Bolton W, et al. Electrostimulation for intractable delayed emptying of intrathoracic stomach after esophagectomy. Ann Thorac Surg 2008;85:1417–9.

38. Wormuth JK, Heitmiller RF. Esophageal conduit necrosis. Thorac Surg Clin 2006;16:11–22.

39. Geer RJ, Richards WO, O'Dorisio TM, et al. Efficacy of octreotide acetate in treatment of severe postgastrectomy dumping syndrome. Ann Surg 1990;212:678–87.

40. McLarty AJ, Deschamps C, Trastek VF, et al. Esophageal resection for cancer of the esophagus: long-term function and quality of life. Ann Thorac Surg 1997;63:1568–72.

41. Orringer MB, Stirling MC. Esophageal resection for achalasia: indications and results. Ann Thorac Surg 1989;47:340–5.

42. Wang LS, Huang MH, Huang BS, et al. Gastric substitution for resectable carcinoma of the esophagus: an analysis of 368 cases. Ann Thorac Surg 1992;53:289–94.

43. Woodward ER, Bushkin FL. The early postprandial dumping syndrome: prevention and treatment. Major Probl Clin Surg 1976;20:14–27.

44. Woodward ER, Neustein CL. The late postprandial dumping syndrome. Major Probl Clin Surg 1976; 20:28–33.

45. Andreasen JJ, Orskov C, Holst JJ. Secretion of glucagon-like peptide-1 and reactive hypoglycemia after partial gastrectomy. Digestion 1994;55:221–8.

46. Shultz KT, Neelon FA, Nilsen LB, et al. Mechanism of postgastrectomy hypoglycemia. Arch Intern Med 1971;128:240–6.

47. Gitzelmann R, Hirsig J. Infant dumping syndrome: reversal of symptoms by feeding uncooked starch. Eur J Pediatr 1986;145:504–6.

48. Harju E, Larmi TK. Efficacy of guar gum in preventing the dumping syndrome. JPEN J Parenter Enteral Nutr 1983;7:470–2.

49. Kneepkens CM, Fernandes J, Vonk RJ. Dumping syndrome in children. Diagnosis and effect of glucomannan on glucose tolerance and absorption. Acta Paediatr Scand 1988;77:279–86.

50. Chandos B. Dumping syndrome and the regulation of peptide YY with verapamil. Am J Gastroenterol 1992;87:1530–1.

51. Christoffersson E, Wallensten S. Drug therapy in the dumping syndrome. Nord Med 1971;86:1589–90 [in Norwegian].

52. Shibata C, Funayama Y, Fukushima K, et al. Effect of steroid therapy for late dumping syndrome after total gastrectomy: report of a case. Dig Dis Sci 2004;49: 802–4.

53. Sigstad H. Effect of tolbutamide on the dumping syndrome. Scand J Gastroenterol 1969;4:227–31.

54. Dewar L, Gelfand G, Finley RJ, et al. Factors affecting cervical anastomotic leak and stricture formation following esophagogastrectomy and gastric tube interposition. Am J Surg 1992;163:484–9.

55. Law S, Fok M, Chu KM, et al. Comparison of hand-sewn and stapled esophagogastric anastomosis after esophageal resection for cancer: a prospective randomized controlled trial. Ann Surg 1997;226:169–73.

56. Orringer MB, Marshall B, Iannettoni MD. Eliminating the cervical esophagogastric anastomotic leak with a side-to-side stapled anastomosis. J Thorac Cardiovasc Surg 2000;119:277–88.

57. Bailey SH, Bull DA, Harpole DH, et al. Outcomes after esophagectomy: a ten-year prospective cohort. Ann Thorac Surg 2003;75:217–22.

58. Zieren HU, Muller JM, Pichlmaier H. Prospective randomized study of one- or two-layer anastomosis following oesophageal resection and cervical oesophagogastrostomy. Br J Surg 1993;80:608–11.

59. Trentino P, Pompeo E, Nofroni I, et al. Predictive value of early postoperative esophagoscopy for occurrence of benign stenosis after cervical esophagogastrostomy. Endoscopy 1997;29:840–4.

60. Kochhar R, Makharia GK. Usefulness of intralesional triamcinolone in treatment of benign esophageal strictures. Gastrointest Endosc 2002;56:829–34.

61. Ramage JI Jr, Rumalla A, Baron TH, et al. A prospective, randomized, double-blind, placebo-controlled trial of endoscopic steroid injection therapy for recalcitrant esophageal peptic strictures. Am J Gastroenterol 2005;100:2419–25.

62. Zein NN, Greseth JM, Perrault J. Endoscopic intralesional steroid injections in the management of refractory esophageal strictures. Gastrointest Endosc 1995;41:596–8.

63. Ramboer C, Verhamme M, Dhondt E, et al. Endoscopic treatment of stenosis in recurrent Crohn's disease with balloon dilation combined with local corticosteroid injection. Gastrointest Endosc 1995; 42:252–5.

64. Miyashita M, Onda M, Okawa K, et al. Endoscopic dexamethasone injection following balloon dilatation of anastomotic stricture after esophagogastrostomy. Am J Surg 1997;174:442–4.

65. Rupp T, Earle D, Ikenberry S, et al. Randomized trial of savary dilation with/without intralesional steroids for benign gastroesophageal reflux strictures. Gastrointest Endosc 1995;41:357.

66. Gandhi RP, Cooper A, Barlow BA. Successful management of esophageal strictures without resection or replacement. J Pediatr Surg 1989;24:745–9.

67. Simmons DT, Baron TH. Electroincision of refractory esophagogastric anastomotic strictures. Dis Esophagus 2006;19:410–4.

68. Park JY, Song HY, Kim JH, et al. Benign anastomotic strictures after esophagectomy: long-term effectiveness of balloon dilation and factors affecting recurrence in 155 patients. AJR Am J Roentgenol 2012; 198:1208–13.

69. Urschel JD, Urschel DM, Miller JD, et al. A meta-analysis of randomized controlled trials of route of reconstruction after esophagectomy for cancer. Am J Surg 2001;182:470–5.

70. Sharma P, Kozarek R. Role of esophageal stents in benign and malignant diseases. Am J Gastroenterol 2010;105:258–73.

71. Barthel JS, Kelley ST, Klapman JB. Management of persistent gastroesophageal anastomotic strictures with removable self-expandable polyester silicon-covered (Polyflex) stents: an alternative to serial dilation. Gastrointest Endosc 2008;67:546–52.

72. Evrard S, Le MO, Lazaraki G, et al. Self-expanding plastic stents for benign esophageal lesions. Gastrointest Endosc 2004;60:894–900.

73. Fukumoto R, Orlina J, McGinty J, et al. Use of Polyflex stents in treatment of acute esophageal and gastric leaks after bariatric surgery. Surg Obes Relat Dis 2007;3:68–71.

74. Garcia-Cano J. Dilation of benign strictures in the esophagus and colon with the polyflex stent: a case series study. Dig Dis Sci 2008;53:341–6.

75. Holm AN, de la Mora Levy JG, Gostout CJ, et al. Self-expanding plastic stents in treatment of benign

esophageal conditions. Gastrointest Endosc 2008; 67:20–5.

76. Papachristou GI, Baron TH. Use of stents in benign and malignant esophageal disease. Rev Gastroenterol Disord 2007;7:74–88.

77. Pennathur A, Chang AC, McGrath KM, et al. Polyflex expandable stents in the treatment of esophageal disease: initial experience. Ann Thorac Surg 2008; 85:1968–72.

78. Wong RF, Adler DG, Hilden K, et al. Retrievable esophageal stents for benign indications. Dig Dis Sci 2008;53:322–9.

79. Martin RC, Woodall C, Duvall R, et al. The use of self-expanding silicone stents in esophagectomy

strictures: less cost and more efficiency. Ann Thorac Surg 2008;86:436–40.

80. Aly A, Jamieson GG. Reflux after oesophagectomy. Br J Surg 2004;91:137–41.

81. Gutschow C, Collard JM, Romagnoli R, et al. Denervated stomach as an esophageal substitute recovers intraluminal acidity with time. Ann Surg 2001;233:509–14.

82. Borst HG, Dragojevic D, Stegmann T, et al. Anastomotic leakage, stenosis, and reflux after esophageal replacement. World J Surg 1978;2:861–4.

83. McKeown KC. Total oesophagectomy—three-staged resection. In: Jamieson G, editor. Surgery of the oesophagus. Edinburgh (United Kingdom): Churchill Livingstone; 1988. p. 677–85.

# Complications Following Surgery for Gastroesophageal Reflux Disease and Achalasia

Samad Hashimi, MD, Ross M. Bremner, MD, PhD*

## KEYWORDS

- Achalasia • Antireflux surgery • Complications • Nissen fundoplication • Toupet fundoplication
- Treatment of complications

## KEY POINTS

- A thorough preoperative workup is essential for good outcomes in surgery for achalasia or reflux disease.
- An understanding of the evolution and advances of laparoscopic surgery paired with careful surgical technique improve patient satisfaction and outcomes.
- Although unusual, complications do occur. The surgeon must be adept at managing these problems.
- Reoperations for functional esophageal disorders are far more complicated than first-time operations and should be performed in high-volume centers that have extensive experience performing reoperations.

## INTRODUCTION

Gastroesophageal reflux disease (GERD) and motility disorders of the esophagus, such as achalasia, are functional disorders with a broad spectrum of presenting symptoms. Good surgical outcomes are dependent on the physician's clear understanding of the pathophysiology of the disease and on the selection of an appropriate surgical procedure. To achieve good postoperative outcomes, a thorough diagnostic examination and individualized, carefully performed surgical techniques are critical.

Operative techniques for laparoscopic antireflux surgery and achalasia have evolved over the past 20 years, and are now relatively standardized.

The LOTUS trial reported use of certain standardized surgical maneuvers with impressive postoperative results, including an overall postoperative complication rate of only 3%.[1] Almost all operations for reflux or achalasia are now attempted laparoscopically, at least for first-time surgery. Compared with open surgery, the laparoscopic approach is associated with fewer complications and shorter hospital stays,[2] and conversion to open surgery is needed in fewer than 2.5% of cases.[3,4] Because the laparoscopic approach to antireflux surgery was adopted hastily in the early 1990s, undesirable results sometimes occurred in the early era. Proponents of laparoscopy are still trying to recover from the tarnished reputation of laparoscopic antireflux surgery; however, surgical

Disclosure Statement: Neither the authors nor their institution have any personal, financial, or institutional interest in any of the materials or devices described in this article.
Department of Thoracic Disease and Transplantation, Norton Thoracic Institute, St. Joseph's Hospital and Medical Center, 500 W. Thomas Road, Suite 500, Phoenix, AZ 85013, USA
* Corresponding author.
E-mail address: Ross.Bremner@dignityhealth.org

thoracic.theclinics.com

treatment of patients with achalasia, hiatal hernia, and GERD has evolved into what should now be recognized as highly successful, cost-effective management for these diseases. As reported by Stefanidis and colleagues,[5] the results of at least 7 randomized controlled trials (RCTs) have been published that show antireflux surgery to be superior to medical management for alleviating symptoms of GERD. As with any surgical intervention, complications do occur. Some are unpredictable; however, surgeons who pay close attention to a patient's initial symptoms, possess a clear understanding of the underlying pathophysiology of that particular patient, and apply modern laparoscopic techniques will reliably achieve good outcomes. Complications occur at least twice as frequently in reoperations.[6] Reoperations should therefore be performed at centers of excellence by experienced surgeons.[7]

Unfortunately, the esophagus is a relatively unforgiving organ and the best time to repair a functional disorder is at the time of the first surgery. Bearing this in mind, we cannot emphasize enough that great care must be exercised before functional surgery is offered to a patient who presents with foregut symptoms.

## ANTIREFLUX SURGERY
### Preoperative Examination

A considerable amount of research has been published regarding the necessary tests that should be performed before antireflux surgery is considered. At Norton Thoracic Institute in Phoenix, AZ, we routinely perform endoscopy, manometry, and barium esophagograms, gleaning complementary information from each study. This helps us to understand the whole picture, to better comprehend the patient's symptoms, and to select the best course of treatment. Impedance and pH studies should be carried out when significant diagnostic uncertainty exists or when a diagnosis of GERD cannot be made based on endoscopy. The pH studies are useful to rule out reflux as a potential source of the problem in patients with complex symptoms.

Proton pump inhibitors (PPIs) can alleviate symptoms for most patients with mild GERD or a minimal hiatal hernia. The widespread use of PPIs has resulted in a shift in the presenting symptoms of patients referred for surgery over the past 2 decades, as PPIs have been shown to control heartburn symptoms relatively well, even for extended periods of time. Patients are now more commonly referred for surgical correction of a large paraesophageal hernia or for an intrathoracic stomach. These patients frequently have symptoms related to the hernia itself, including anemia, chest pain or discomfort, early satiety, and bloating. Although surgery for these patients is often complicated, it can still usually be performed laparoscopically. Specific techniques that should be considered for these cases are discussed below.

## COMPLICATIONS OF ANTIREFLUX SURGERY

Major complications associated with antireflux surgery are uncommon, and perioperative mortality rates are very low. In 2006, Dominitz and colleagues[8] reported a perioperative mortality rate of 0.8% after antireflux surgery, but a more recent study using the Nationwide Inpatient Sample of more than 15,000 patients showed a much lower mortality rate of 0.08%.[9] Moreover, this report also demonstrated that, despite the progressive age increase in patients undergoing antireflux surgery and their larger number of comorbidities, the operative mortality of antireflux surgery has decreased by 50% over the past decade.[9]

### Intraoperative Complications

#### Aspiration during intubation
Patients undergoing antireflux surgery usually have a hiatal hernia and the lower esophageal sphincter (LES) is frequently defective. Great care should be exercised when these patients are intubated for an operation, as they are at very high risk of aspiration. Rapid-sequence induction with cricoid pressure and inclining the torso 45° are useful techniques to avoid aspiration. If aspiration is suspected, a bronchoscopy should be performed immediately to evaluate the extent of pulmonary soilage and to clear the airways. If gross soilage is suspected, it may be prudent to cancel the procedure and reschedule it for a later time, after the patient has had an opportunity to recover from the aspiration event.

#### Viscus injury from trocar insertion
Intestinal injuries usually can be repaired laparoscopically. Trocar injuries are now quite infrequent as a result of increased surgeon experience and blunt-tipped trocars, some of which offer camera visualization of the layers of the abdominal wall. Once the camera port is inserted, all other port insertions should be performed under camera visualization. Some surgeons still prefer the use of a traditional spring-loaded Veress needle. In all cases, it is critical that the surgeon pay close attention if the patient has had previous abdominal surgery, as intra-abdominal adhesions may exist.

#### Complications after retractor placement
Retractors are usually needed to retract the liver, but injury to the liver may result from their use.[10]

With modern increased rates of obesity, a large, fatty liver may impede access to the hiatus. To improve hiatal access, the diaphragmatic ligaments that hold the left lobe of the liver over the hiatus may need to be taken down. Small tears and injury to the liver caused by instrumentation can usually be controlled with electrocautery or hemostatic agents and the application of pressure. Cardiac tamponade after a retractor-caused injury also has been described.[11]

### Capnothorax
One or both pleural spaces are frequently entered during dissection in the mediastinum. This is more common with reoperations or with large hiatal hernias, and it occurs while the surgeon is resecting the sac of the hernia. The capnothorax may cause a mild hemodynamic effect intraoperatively, as intra-abdominal pressure is transmitted into the chest. Fluid administration by the anesthesiologist can improve venous return and stabilize hemodynamics. Occasionally, intraperitoneal pressure needs to be decreased. Once the pneumoperitoneum is released at the end of the procedure, the anesthesiologist should give several large positive pressure breaths to reexpand the lung before extubation. Although a significant capnothorax may be evident on the postoperative chest radiograph, it rarely requires any intervention other than oxygen administration if the patient is otherwise stable. Carbon dioxide dissolves very rapidly, and the capnothorax usually will resolve within hours.

### Esophageal perforation
Esophageal perforation occurs occasionally, but it is more commonly associated with dissection of giant hiatal hernias than with smaller, simple hernias. Traction injury to the esophagus also can occur when the esophagus is directly retracted or is retracted via a Penrose drain, which encircles the esophagus. We suggest always having a nasogastric tube or an endoscope in the esophagus during retraction. We routinely use an intraoperative endoscope, as this facilitates identification of the esophagus (especially in cases of reoperation). The endoscope allows visualization of the esophagogastric mucosal integrity when injury is suspected. Intraoperative repair of a small esophageal laceration usually is successful, but an overlooked perforation can lead to devastating mediastinitis and sepsis.[12] Sutures through the esophagus anchoring the Nissen also can be passed too deeply, resulting in a small mucosal tear that can leak later. The esophageal lumen is home to multiple bacteria, including oral flora and anaerobes, and mediastinitis and peritonitis can be severe.

Perforation of the esophagus by the bougie that is commonly used during fundoplication procedures also has been described; in one study, the bougie was associated with esophageal injury in 1.2% of cases.[13] Injury can occur anywhere along the length of the esophagus and should be repaired immediately, if possible. We use a bougie only in select cases, and it is usually unnecessary for Toupet or partial fundoplications. However, in the case of a Collis lengthening procedure, a bougie is necessary to prevent overnarrowing of the gastric tube. A Collis operation also has been associated with leaks from the staple line, but this is an unusual complication occurring up to 2.7% of the time in experienced hands.[14]

### Intra-abdominal catastrophe
A severe esophageal tear or a delayed diagnosis of an esophageal leak causing sepsis and a hostile inflammatory phlegmon are complex problems, and may be impossible to repair acutely. Adequate drainage and stents have been used successfully to treat these complications, but an esophageal diversion may be necessary. If the esophagus is to be stapled at the gastroesophageal (GE) junction or just above it, it is useful to have a drain in the lumen of the distal esophagus (the drain exits through an abdominal site), as this can help drain salivary secretions and can aid in later reoperation for esophageal reconstruction.

Gastric necrosis necessitating gastric resection has been described in cases of giant hiatal hernias.[15] Gastric necrosis is thought to result from devascularization of the proximal stomach from injury to the left gastric artery or from takedown of the short gastric vessels and excessive skeletonization of the greater curvature, especially if some of these vessels are taken down before a giant hernia is reduced. At Norton Thoracic Institute, we have treated several patients who were referred to us after gastric necrosis. Adequate debridement and drainage, maintenance of nutritional support, and a delayed reconstruction months later is the best approach. A Roux-en-Y esophagojejunostomy is a sound surgical option that reconstructs the alimentary tract while obviating any future GE reflux, but a more extensive operation using a colon interposition may be required.

### Splenic injury
In the former era of open surgery, between 1% and 20% of antireflux procedures were complicated by the need for splenectomy.[16,17] In the laparoscopic era, however, this number has fallen to less than 1%,[15] possibly as a result of the use of improved thermocoagulation devices such as the

Harmonic scalpel (Ethicon, Cincinnati, OH) and the decreased incidence of traction injury. Occasionally a portion of the spleen may infarct after takedown of the short gastric vessels, and this infarction may be noted intraoperatively or incidentally on a postoperative computed tomography (CT) scan, but it is usually of no clinical consequence. Bleeding from the short gastric vessels or from a minor tear of the capsule can still occur intraoperatively despite the use of thermocoagulation devices, but usually can be controlled by applying gentle pressure with an intra-abdominal sponge and the use of endoclips.

### Bleeding

Although it is uncommon, severe intraoperative bleeding does occur occasionally, and it is more likely to occur in reoperation than in initial surgery. Bleeding also can occur in the immediate postoperative period, and postoperative hypotension is a red flag, as a significant amount of blood can be hidden in the abdomen, especially in obese patients. Postoperative bleeding may necessitate a return to the operating suite, and an open operation may be required to control this bleeding. **Fig. 1** shows the anatomy of the hiatus and

potential sites of bleeding during an antireflux operation, as summarized in **Box 1**.

### Early Postoperative Complications

#### Dysphagia

Dysphagia in the early postoperative period is common and is usually due to edema of the fundoplication, but in some cases it indicates a narrow fundoplication or a tight crural closure. Patients can usually easily swallow liquids within a day of surgery and generally remain on a liquid diet for a week or 2 after surgery until the edema subsides. Mild dysphagia usually resolves a few weeks after surgery, so the patient and surgeon alike are urged to be patient. Mild dysphagia also may be related to poor perioperative motility. A patient with known poor peristalsis preoperatively is more likely to be patient with "expected" mild dysphagia postoperatively.

If the patient has significant difficulty swallowing liquids, barium studies may be warranted and the surgeon may consider endoscopy. If there has been a technical error, an early operation to remove a crural stitch or loosen the wrap is far easier than a delayed operation in a

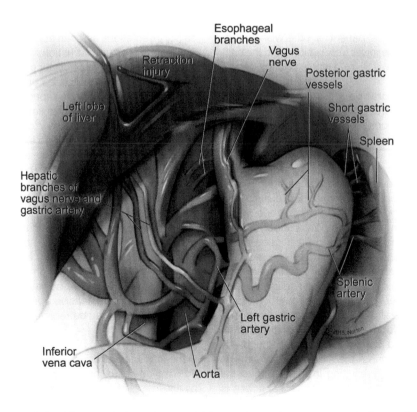

**Fig. 1.** Anatomy of the hiatus and sites of potential hemorrhage that can occur during antireflux surgery. (*Courtesy of* Norton Thoracic Institute, Phoenix, AZ.)

---

**Box 1**
**Common sources of bleeding**

Bleeding Sites

Spleen

Short gastric vessels

Posterior gastric vessels

Gastrohepatic ligament (along the hepatic branch of the vagus)

Vessels in the sac

Aortic perforators

Aorta

Vena cava

---

malnourished patient. These complications are unusual, especially if a bougie was used to help size the fundoplication.

### Early recurrence of hiatal hernia

Severe bucking or heaving after emergence from anesthesia has been reported to increase the risk of long-term reherniation, but they also can induce acute reherniation.[15,18] Extubation while the patient is still under deep anesthesia can help reduce the incidence of reherniation, as can perioperative administration of antiemetics, such as ondansetron. Hiatal hernia is usually diagnosed after a barium study or after a CT scan is performed for a patient with abdominal pain. Acute reherniation usually requires immediate surgical repair.

### Consequences of vagus nerve injury

Vagal injury can occur during operations on the lower esophagus, and this type of injury is more common in reoperations and procedures to repair very large hiatal hernias. Giant hiatal hernias and the so-called "intrathoracic stomach" are best repaired by takedown of the sac from the inner aspect of the crura and blunt dissection of the entire intrathoracic sac, in turn resulting in reduction of the hernia and its contents. The vagal fibers may be displaced and difficult to detect. The vagus nerve is often easier to identify high in the hiatus, and it can then be traced down toward the GE junction. Traction injury is likely more common than realized, and the redundant sac should be removed cautiously to avoid inadvertent transection of the nerve. Damage to only one nerve is usually tolerated over the course of time, but transection of both nerves can lead to a variety of both short-term and long-term gastrointestinal complaints, such as bloating, early satiety from delayed gastric emptying, and varying degrees of diarrhea, including classic dumping syndrome.[19] Lindeboom and colleagues[20] used both gastric emptying and vagal nerve function studies to study 41 patients before and after laparoscopic partial fundoplication. Some degree of vagal nerve injury was detected in 10% of patients, but the size of hiatal hernia was not reported, and this percentage likely represented patients with small hernias only. Gastric emptying was generally accelerated after fundoplication, consistent with previous reports.[21] Lindeboom and colleagues[20] did not report an association between mild injury and significant delay in gastric emptying.

Patients with GERD frequently suffer from irritable bowel syndrome, and this can cloud the picture of postoperative symptoms. Cholecystectomy performed concurrently with surgical treatment for GERD increases the risk of postoperative diarrhea.[22] Gastrointestinal side effects after Nissen fundoplication may not be directly related to the antireflux procedure. They are frequently mild and often abate with time.[23]

### Ileus

Although less common after laparoscopic procedures compared with open surgery, ileus can occur. If it is severe and if gastric distension is significant, it should be treated with nasogastric drainage. Ileus occurs more frequently after reoperation than first-time surgery.[15] A gastric ileus may occur for a few days after surgery in cases of repair of a larger hernia, the procedure for which may last several hours and include a fair amount of manipulation of the stomach. Injury to the vagus nerve during dissection may exacerbate the ileus. Our practice is to leave a nasogastric tube in overnight and to endoscopically inject botulinum toxin A into the pylorus (discussed later in this article) in patients with giant hernias or in whom some vagal injury is suspected. Prokinetic agents and methylnaltrexone also may be useful. Nasogastric drainage is occasionally needed for longer periods.

### Deep vein thrombosis and pulmonary embolism

Patients undergoing repair of a massive hiatal hernia are at significant risk for deep vein thrombosis (DVT) and subsequent pulmonary embolism (PE). One study from the early laparoscopic era reported these complications in up to 1% of patients.[24] Many factors can contribute to this risk: older age, obesity, duration of the procedure, and the reverse Trendelenburg position with resultant venous stasis. Use of subcutaneous heparin before anesthesia and postoperatively, along with sequential compression devices intraoperatively and postoperatively, can limit the incidence of DVT and PE. Ambulation on the day of surgery also is vital.

## Later Postoperative Complications

### Dysphagia

As seen in **Box 2**, there are many possible causes of persistent or delayed-onset dysphagia. Although it is uncommon, dysphagia can significantly inhibit a patient's lifestyle. It is important to note that antireflux surgery is usually associated with an improvement in preoperative dysphagia, but surgery also can trigger dysphagia as a new symptom for a patient who has undergone fundoplication. Reported incidences vary greatly in the literature, but larger studies have shown the incidence of mild dysphagia to be less than 20% 1 year postoperatively, with only 5% to 8% of patients suffering from long-term dysphagia.[25] Postoperative dysphagia is less common after a partial fundoplication than after a 360° complete fundoplication.[25] Some series report up to 6% of patients requiring esophageal dilation to treat dysphagia, and this is usually successful.[26] Reoperation may be necessary to modify a long or too-tight fundoplication. A recent article noted a trend toward greater dysphagia in patients with a longer Nissen (3 cm) than in patients with a shorter Nissen (1.5 cm).[26] Significant dysphagia associated with reherniation or with a low wrap or "slipped" Nissen may require revision surgery.

### Gas bloat

Patients with GERD are habitual swallowers, and some patients swallow twice as frequently as patients without reflux disorders.[27] Fundoplication limits belching, yet the patient's subconscious habit of swallowing sometimes continues, trapping small amounts of swallowed air in the stomach, exacerbating bloating. Carbonated beverages compound the problem and should be avoided. Patients may report an increase in flatulence; for these patients, simethicone is available over the counter and can be useful, but the symptom usually resolves over time. Gas bloat, especially troublesome for patients with concomitant irritable bowel syndrome, is generally less common after a partial fundoplication, because some belching may be possible.[25]

Vagal damage and delayed gastric emptying are possible complications of difficult surgical procedures, reoperations, or reduction of large paraesophageal hernias. A gastric emptying study can be useful, but a gastric bezoar or retained gastric food seen on endoscopy after an overnight fast usually indicates poor emptying. Prokinetic agents can be used, but metoclopramide should not be used for extended lengths of time, and erythromycin can have other intestinal side effects. Pyloric dilation or endoscopic injection of botulinum toxin A can help alleviate symptoms.[28] Patients with a history of major depression have been shown to have a higher incidence of this symptom postoperatively. Toupet fundoplication is advised in these cases.[29]

### Recurrence of hiatal hernia

Perhaps the most frustrating long-term complication for surgeons and patients alike is the recurrence of a hiatal hernia, reported in up to 40% of patients undergoing repair of large paraesophageal hernias.[30] Possible causes of recurrence are a fibrosed, shortened esophagus; weak diaphragmatic tissue; very large defects that require tension for closure; or postoperative stressors on the repair, such as trauma, vomiting, chronic cough, or obesity. Some investigators tout the liberal use of the Collis gastroplasty; however, even in some of the largest reported series, recurrence rates remain the same between Collis gastroplasty and standard fundoplication.[14,31] The use of a patch appears to help, but the investigators of one study of an absorbable biologic mesh showed that although early recurrence decreased,[32] long-term recurrence did not.[32,33] Permanent mesh placement has been associated with some catastrophic complications, such as erosion into the esophagus[34]; therefore, its use should be avoided. Our own practice has been to use an absorbable onlay patch of a biocompatible synthetic tissue scaffold (Gore Bio-A Tissue Reinforcement; W. L. Gore and Associates, Flagstaff, AZ) to encourage ingrowth of collagen I. The early results of our cohort of more than 800 patients are encouraging, but long-term follow-up results are not yet available.

---

**Box 2**
**Causes of persistent dysphagia**

Tight crural closure

Long or narrow/tight fundoplication

Problems with a Collis (if performed)

Fibrotic reaction or erosion of pledgets or mesh

Persistent or new-onset esophageal stricture (reflux- or pill-induced)

Underlying motility disorder (especially hypomotility)

Concomitant cricopharyngeal disorder (eg, Zenker diverticulum)

Recurrent hiatal hernia (especially paraesophageal component)

"Slipped" Nissen (a Nissen riding on the top of the stomach)

Recurrences are possible, and this is not surprising when one considers all of the forces on the diaphragm at the hiatus, especially when the hiatus has been weakened by a large hernia. Chronic coughing, heaving, or retching; abdominal trauma; and weight gain all contribute to increased long-term transdiaphragmatic pressure gradients and subsequent reherniation. Reoperation should be considered only for symptomatic patients: it is critical to be mindful of the difference between radiographic and symptomatic recurrence, as many of the former remain innocuous and asymptomatic. The overall reoperation rate for hiatal hernias ranges between 2% and 5%.[35,36] A small recurrence often can be managed conservatively, as these hernias rarely become large enough to warrant surgery, although scant data exist to show the progression of these small hernias with time. **Fig. 2** shows several examples of failure or loosening of fundoplications and recurrence of hernias, as seen on endoscopy.

### Recurrence of reflux and regurgitation

It is possible for a fundoplication to unravel and cause a recurrence of GERD and typical heartburn. Patients undergoing a partial fundoplication may experience a progressive worsening of heartburn, as the fundoplication may loosen over time (**Fig. 2**A). This loosening is more common after an anterior rather than a posterior fundoplication, and the anterior fundoplication should be avoided for patients with reflux disease.[37] In the absence of recurrent hiatal hernia, it is often sufficient to manage most of these patients with medication.

### Mesh or pledget erosion

Endoscopy for dysphagia or chest discomfort after a Nissen fundoplication occasionally reveals a foreign body in the distal esophagus or proximal stomach. This may be a remnant from a previous pledget or a previously placed permanent mesh (**Fig. 3**).[34] A suture or small piece of pledget can

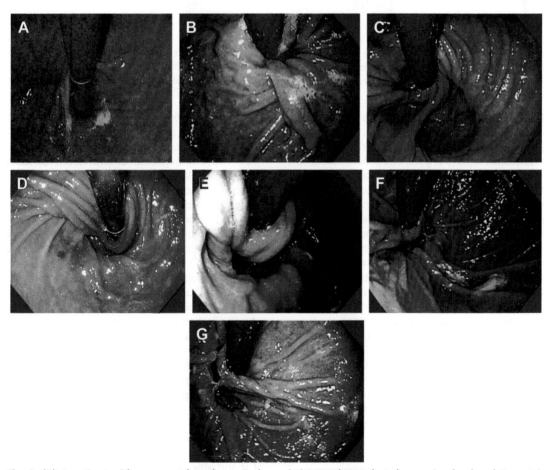

**Fig. 2.** (*A*) A patient with recurrent heartburn. Endoscopic image shows that the previously placed Toupet is intact but has loosened over time. Retroflex maneuver showing the opening of the fundoplication with easy eructation during insufflation. (*B*, *C*) A fundoplication that has herniated into the chest. (*D–G*) Endoscopic images depicting a paraesophageal recurrence of hiatal hernia with partial dehiscence of the diaphragmatic closure. (*Courtesy of* Norton Thoracic Institute, Phoenix, AZ.)

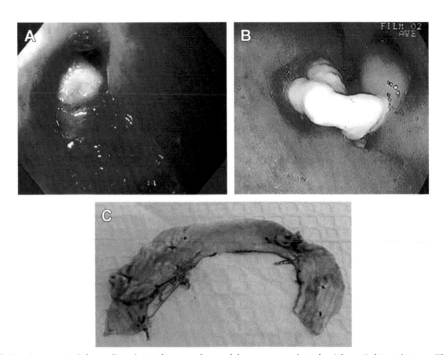

**Fig. 3.** (*A*) Foreign material eroding into the esophageal lumen associated with a tight stricture. This patient required resection of this area with a Roux-en-Y esophagojejunostomy. (*B*) Endoscopic view showing a permanent mesh that has eroded into the esophageal lumen. (*C*) The permanent mesh resected during reoperation. (*Courtesy of* Norton Thoracic Institute, Phoenix, AZ; and Sumeet Mittal, Omaha, NE; with permission.)

be removed endoscopically, but this finding generally necessitates reoperation (**Fig. 3**C). The GE junction often cannot be salvaged in this situation, and despite reports of gallant treatment modalities, such as stenting after removal, resection of either the esophagus or the proximal stomach is often required.[34] If the esophagus still has some peristalsis and if intestinal metaplasia is not present, a distal esophagectomy and proximal gastrectomy with a Roux-en-Y esophagojejunostomy is a good option, as it avoids removal of the entire esophagus while obviating any future reflux problems. If the patient has an aperistaltic esophagus, intestinal metaplasia (certainly with any degree of dysplasia), or the mesentery of the small bowel does not reach to the healthy intrathoracic esophagus, an esophagectomy may be needed. An intrathoracic anastomosis should be performed in this circumstance because the proximal stomach is usually somewhat devitalized and cervical anastomoses have been associated with a high rate of complications after a previous antireflux procedure.[38]

## Reoperation

Reoperation deserves special mention, as patients who undergo reoperation present a special series of challenges. Not only is their symptomatology complex; these patients are understandably

more anxious about surgery, and the outcomes for reoperation are less successful than first-time procedures.[39] Barium studies, pH testing, manometry, and gastric emptying are all tests that play a role in the workup of these patients. We prefer to do an endoscopy as a standalone procedure to better understand what procedures have been done previously and to visualize the anatomy. It can be difficult for the untrained eye to detect small paraesophageal recurrences, a low or slipped Nissen (especially in the presence of Barrett esophagus) (**Fig. 4**), or to evaluate the stability of a previously placed fundoplication. A clear antegrade view to look for rugal folds above a fundoplication and a retroflexed view with gastric air distention are critical, informative maneuvers. The surgeon should also note any foreign material or sutures in the gastric lumen. A transoral incisionless fundoplication has a typical appearance as shown in **Fig. 5**.

Reoperation involves takedown of the previous fundoplication (with extreme care to avoid vagal injury if possible), reduction of a hernia, rerepair of a diaphragmatic dehiscence or an onlay patch of absorbable mesh, and refundoplication. Reoperations have higher conversion rates to open surgery than first-time surgery, and the operations last longer.[40,41] As mentioned previously, if any vagal injury is perceived or if the vagus nerves

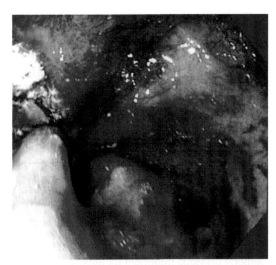

**Fig. 4.** A fundoplication placed below the gastro-esophageal junction, referred to as a "slipped Nissen." The rugal folds of the stomach are seen above the fundoplication. Foreign material and esophagitis are also evident. The fundoplication usually appears normal from below using a retroflexed maneuver. (*Courtesy of* Norton Thoracic Institute, Phoenix, AZ.)

cannot be well visualized secondary to scar tissue or previous injury, or if there is significant delayed gastric emptying on preoperative studies, the treating physician should consider opening the pylorus with either a formal pyloroplasty, or by injecting botulinum toxin A submucosally (100–200 IU in

1-mL aliquots in 4 quadrants). Dilation even up to a 20-mm-diameter balloon may be unsuccessful, especially in larger male patients. Placement of a gastrostomy tube and/or a perihiatal drain should be considered, depending on the level of difficulty of the procedure.

Although reoperations often can be performed laparoscopically, anything beyond a second operation usually requires an open approach. A surgeon may note at the third or fourth operation that the fundus or esophagus is too damaged from scarring, fibrosis, or foreign body migration, and is unusable for further fundoplication. Enterotomies are more common in reoperations and more commonly involve the stomach. Intraoperative endoscopy is advised for all of these cases, not only because it helps identify anatomy during dissection, but also because it can help identify any mucosal barrier breaches. It is imperative to repair these when they are appreciated intraoperatively. After multiple operations, there is a much higher likelihood of permanent vagal nerve damage and gastric dysfunction, and a Roux-en-Y procedure is a very useful surgical option.[42] If the anastomosis must be done above the LES, an esophagojejunostomy is performed, and a transoral circular stapler anvil (Orvil Device; Covidien, New Haven, CT) is a useful tool in this situation. If the GE junction can be preserved, it also may be possible to preserve the left gastric artery and a very small pouch of stomach, allowing a well-vascularized gastrojejunal anastomosis to be performed.

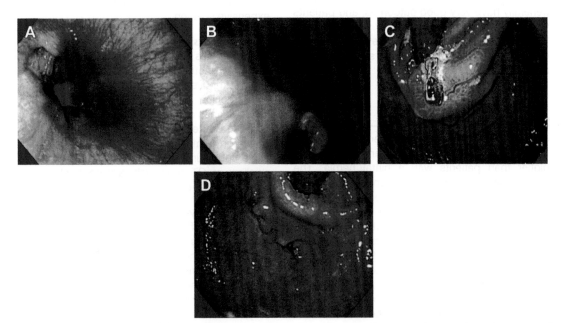

**Fig. 5.** (*A–D*) Foreign material that may be seen after endoscopic antireflux procedures such as the transoral incisionless fundoplication procedure. (*Courtesy of* Norton Thoracic Institute, Phoenix, AZ.)

## COMPLICATIONS OF SURGERY FOR ACHALASIA

Myotomy, a procedure originally described by Heller in 1913,[43] has been modified in the laparoscopic era to involve only one side of the esophageal wall and to extend for a short distance onto the stomach. The excellent outcomes associated with this modified approach make this the surgical treatment of choice for most patients. Overall, the procedure is very safe, with the hospital stay usually limited to less than 1 day, and perioperative complications in the low 4% range.[44] The modified Heller myotomy has been further fine-tuned over the past 15 years, and more recently the advent of the peroral endoscopic myotomy (POEM) shows promise as a myotomy that requires no incisions. Robotic surgery does not show a clear benefit over laparoscopic surgery for GERD, but may have a place in the treatment of achalasia.

### Preoperative Examination for Achalasia Surgery

Achalasia is a disease with 2 essential components: a nonrelaxing LES and an aperistaltic esophageal body. Surgery is designed only to relieve the functional outflow obstruction; peristalsis will not return. The Chicago classification, based on manometric features, clarifies which patients are likely to have good outcomes after Heller myotomy.[45,46] In brief, patients with manometric features of Type II achalasia (classic achalasia) generally have very good outcomes, and patients with Type III achalasia (formerly referred to as "vigorous achalasia") have a less predictable outcome, probably related to the spastic involvement of the esophageal body.

### Anesthesia

A patient with achalasia is at extreme risk of aspiration at the time of induction of anesthesia, even higher than patients with a hiatal hernia. The dilated esophagus, especially a megaesophagus, will likely contain some fluid even if the patient has consumed nothing the night before surgery. Rapid-sequence induction with the head of the bed elevated and the use of cricoid pressure during induction are helpful ways to prevent aspiration. A liquid-only diet for at least 3 days preoperatively is recommended, but this should be extended for a patient with a megaesophagus. An esophagus filled with fluid at the time of procedure usually can be drained with an endoscope or a nasoesophageal tube.

### Trocar and Retractor Injuries

These complications, generally uncommon, are similar to those described previously for antireflux surgery. Similarly, wound infections and port-site herniation are rare, and rates of these complications are certainly lower than they are for open surgery.

### Complications of Myotomy

#### Mucosal injury

Mucosal injuries are reported in up to 10% of laparoscopic cases[47]; however, Nau and Rattner[48] reported only one perforation in their recent study of 206 consecutive patients. Mucosal injuries during myotomy are more likely in patients who have undergone previous treatment for achalasia, such as dilation or botulinum toxin A injection.[49] Previous therapy, especially multiple treatments, is thought to result in a scarred submucosa, which causes difficulty when muscle layers are dissected away from the mucosa. Mucosal injury is more common on the gastric side, and should be repaired with fine absorbable monofilament suture, such as 4–0 PDS sutures (Ethicon, Cincinnati, OH). Intraoperative endoscopy can help identify these injuries and test the effectiveness of the repair.

Some studies have reported a mucosal injury rate of 0% with the use of the robotic approach.[50,51] Magnification, stereoscopic vision, and the fine movements of the instruments likely facilitate dissection of the muscle fibers. No RCT exists as of yet, however, and the robotic approach is an expensive solution.

#### Subcutaneous neck and facial emphysema

Subcutaneous neck and facial emphysema after myotomy should alert the surgeon to a possible leak.[52] Emphysema is most commonly associated with tracking of the pneumoperitoneum along fascial planes through the mediastinum and also can occur after repair of a large hiatal hernia. If the emphysema is accompanied by a fever, high white cell count, or chest discomfort, a contrast swallow or CT scan with oral contrast may be needed to rule out a leak.

#### Incomplete myotomy

Persistence of early postoperative dysphagia suggests an incomplete myotomy or a tight fundoplication,[53] whereas late recurrence indicates fibrosis at the myotomy site or progressive dilation and redundancy of the esophagus.[54] Early dysphagia may be secondary to incomplete myotomy, and there is ongoing debate regarding the appropriate length of the optimal myotomy. Most surgeons extend the myotomy 4 to 6 cm onto the esophagus and 2 to 3 cm onto the stomach.[55,56] Failed myotomy is commonly associated with inadequate extension onto the stomach. An intraoperative endoscope can ensure adequacy of the myotomy and the postoperative mucosal integrity.[47] Inadequate myotomy with persistent dysphagia can be managed with postoperative pneumatic dilation, but reoperation may be warranted.

### Reflux esophagitis

Surgical treatment of achalasia balances relief of outflow obstruction of the esophagus at the expense of an increased risk of GE reflux. In the era before PPIs, there was much debate about how long to extend the myotomy to palliate the patient without causing severe reflux and perhaps even peptic stricture.[11,54] The laparoscopic approach used now generally includes extension onto the stomach, and the most common long-term complication after an effective modified Heller myotomy is GE reflux. Esophageal exposure to refluxed gastric juice is worsened by a depressed clearance mechanism of the aperistaltic esophageal body.

It is now generally accepted that some form of fundoplication is a necessary part of most surgical procedures. In a large meta-analysis, Campos and colleagues[57] showed that adding an antireflux procedure to myotomy decreased reflux symptoms from 31% to 9%, and objective abnormal pH testing dropped from 42% to 15%. A recent review of 2 meta-analyses, 3 RCTs, and 3 prospective trials has shown that some form of antireflux procedure is necessary to decrease reflux.[58] The optimal fundoplication type, however, is still being debated. A complete Nissen fundoplication has been associated with an increased incidence of dysphagia, and it is generally agreed that a partial fundoplication is preferable.[58] One advantage of an anterior Dor fundoplication is that it does not require posterior esophageal dissection or takedown of the short gastric vessels, and it can cover the exposed myotomy, sealing any potential delayed leaks. A Toupet fundoplication holds the myotomized muscle edges apart and may provide better long-term reflux control. However, a Toupet fundoplication does require posterior esophageal dissection and takedown of the short gastric vessels. Although Mayo and colleagues' review[58] showed no difference between the Toupet and the Dor procedures in terms of symptom management, Wei and colleagues[59] noted that the Dor fundoplication may be associated with higher rates of postoperative GERD. At the very least, a partial fundoplication is necessary after an effective cardiomyotomy, and some reflux should be expected in some patients. Fortunately, PPIs are usually very effective and we advise our patients that they may be needed long-term after myotomy.

### The peroral endoscopic myotomy

Discussed briefly earlier in this article, the POEM is a new, evolving myotomy technique that accesses natural orifices to treat achalasia. This technique involves opening the mucosa endoscopically in the mid esophagus and using the endoscope and a small electrocautery device (microknife) to develop a submucosal tunnel to access the thickened circular fibers of the spastic LES. These muscle fibers are then cut endoscopically with the microknife. After the scope is withdrawn, the mucosal entry point is closed with endoclips. A steep learning curve has been associated with the POEM.[60]

First described by Inoue and colleagues[61] in 2009, centers in Japan appear to have the greatest experience with the POEM.[62] There are now several centers in the United States that are increasing the experience with the procedure, and although the early results seem promising, long-term results are unavailable. A potentially high incidence of postoperative GERD is a concern, as no antireflux measure is performed as part of the procedure. Proponents of the procedure indicate that preservation of the longitudinal muscle fibers may provide some form of antireflux barrier.

Familiari and colleagues[63] recently published a review of 100 Italian patients who underwent the POEM with a mean follow-up of 11 months. Clinical success was documented in 94.5% of patients, and 24-hour pH monitoring documented GERD in 53.4% of patients. However, only a minority of patients had heartburn (24.3%) or esophagitis (27.4%), and these complications were successfully treated with PPIs. Wang and colleagues[64] noted that a modified POEM with shorter myotomy under endotracheal anesthesia and $CO_2$ insufflations resulted in a safe procedure with excellent short-term efficacy in a series of 46 patients treated for achalasia. A drawback of the procedure is that many patients develop a pneumoperitoneum, and $CO_2$ used to insufflate the tunnel appears to be absorbed more rapidly than air. A decompression needle in the abdomen may be required during the procedure.

Although their study was not prospectively randomized, Bhayani and colleagues[65] compared POEM to laparoscopic myotomy with partial fundoplication with similar early results. The POEM also has been successful in treating patients with previous failed Heller myotomy.[66]

As noted, POEM is still an emerging technique, and few centers in the United States have significant experience. Little is known about long-term complications associated with the procedure, but short-term results are positive and the procedure seems to be safe when performed by experienced practitioners. Long-term GERD may be an ongoing problem for some patients.

## SUMMARY

Surgery for GERD and achalasia, usually performed laparoscopically, has excellent outcomes. Complications are unusual, but the surgeon should be prepared to manage them when they occur. Reoperations are sometimes needed, but these difficult procedures should be performed at centers with sufficient experience.

## REFERENCES

1. Attwood SE, Lundell L, Ell C, et al. Standardization of surgical technique in antireflux surgery: the LOTUS Trial experience. World J Surg 2008;32(6):995–8.
2. Peters MJ, Mukhtar A, Yunus RM, et al. Meta-analysis of randomized clinical trials comparing open and laparoscopic anti-reflux surgery. Am J Gastroenterol 2009;104(6):1548–61 [quiz: 1547, 1562].
3. Mahon D, Rhodes M, Decadt B, et al. Randomized clinical trial of laparoscopic Nissen fundoplication compared with proton-pump inhibitors for treatment of chronic gastro-oesophageal reflux. Br J Surg 2005;92(6):695–9.
4. Mehta S, Bennett J, Mahon D, et al. Prospective trial of laparoscopic Nissen fundoplication versus proton pump inhibitor therapy for gastroesophageal reflux disease: seven-year follow-up. J Gastrointest Surg 2006;10(9):1312–6 [discussion: 1316–7].
5. Stefanidis D, Hope WW, Kohn GP, et al. Guidelines for surgical treatment of gastroesophageal reflux disease. Surg Endosc 2010;24(11):2647–69.
6. Wang YR, Dempsey DT, Richter JE. Trends and perioperative outcomes of inpatient antireflux surgery in the United States, 1993-2006. Dis Esophagus 2011; 24(4):215–23.
7. Funch-Jensen P, Bendixen A, Iversen MG, et al. Complications and frequency of redo antireflux surgery in Denmark: a nationwide study, 1997-2005. Surg Endosc 2008;22(3):627–30.
8. Dominitz JA, Dire CA, Billingsley KG, et al. Complications and antireflux medication use after antireflux surgery. Clin Gastroenterol Hepatol 2006;4(3): 299–305.
9. Funk LM, Kanji A, Scott Melvin W, et al. Elective antireflux surgery in the US: an analysis of national trends in utilization and inpatient outcomes from 2005 to 2010. Surg Endosc 2014;28(5):1712–9.
10. Pasenau J, Mamazza J, Schlachta CM, et al. Liver hematoma after laparoscopic Nissen fundoplication: a case report and review of retraction injuries. Surg Laparosc Endosc Percutan Tech 2000;10(3): 178–81.
11. Firoozmand E, Ritter M, Cohen R, et al. Ventricular laceration and cardiac tamponade during laparoscopic Nissen fundoplication. Surg Laparosc Endosc 1996;6(5):394–7.
12. Rantanen TK, Salo JA, Sipponen JT. Fatal and life-threatening complications in antireflux surgery: analysis of 5,502 operations. Br J Surg 1999;86(12): 1573–7.
13. Patterson EJ, Herron DM, Hansen PD, et al. Effect of an esophageal bougie on the incidence of dysphagia following Nissen fundoplication: a prospective, blinded, randomized clinical trial. Arch Surg 2000;135(9):1055–61 [discussion: 1061–2].
14. Nason KS, Luketich JD, Awais O, et al. Quality of life after Collis gastroplasty for short esophagus in patients with paraesophageal hernia. Ann Thorac Surg 2011;92(5):1854–60 [discussion: 1860–1].
15. Pohl D, Eubanks TR, Omelanczuk PE, et al. Management and outcome of complications after laparoscopic antireflux operations. Arch Surg 2001; 136(4):399–404.
16. DeMeester TR, Bonavina L, Albertucci M. Nissen fundoplication for gastroesophageal reflux disease. Evaluation of primary repair in 100 consecutive patients. Ann Surg 1986;204(1):9–20.
17. Rogers DM, Herrington JL Jr, Morton C. Incidental splenectomy associated with Nissen fundoplication. Ann Surg 1980;191(2):153–6.
18. Iqbal A, Kakarlapudi GV, Awad ZT, et al. Assessment of diaphragmatic stressors as risk factors for symptomatic failure of laparoscopic Nissen fundoplication. J Gastrointest Surg 2006;10(1):12–21.
19. Oelschlager BK, Yamamoto K, Woltman T, et al. Vagotomy during hiatal hernia repair: a benign esophageal lengthening procedure. J Gastrointest Surg 2008;12(7):1155–62.
20. Lindeboom MY, Ringers J, van Rijn PJ, et al. Gastric emptying and vagus nerve function after laparoscopic partial fundoplication. Ann Surg 2004; 240(5):785–90.
21. Hinder RA, Stein HJ, Bremner CG, et al. Relationship of a satisfactory outcome to normalization of delayed gastric emptying after Nissen fundoplication. Ann Surg 1989;210(4):458–64 [discussion: 464–5].
22. Klaus A, Hinder RA, DeVault KR, et al. Bowel dysfunction after laparoscopic antireflux surgery: incidence, severity, and clinical course. Am J Med 2003;114(1):6–9.
23. Hazan TB, Gamarra FN, Stawick L, et al. Nissen fundoplication and gastrointestinal-related complications: a guide for the primary care physician. Southampt Med J 2009;102(10):1041–5.

24. Jamieson GG, Watson DI, Britten-Jones R, et al. Laparoscopic Nissen fundoplication. Ann Surg 1994;220(2):137–45.

25. Varin O, Velstra B, De Sutter S, et al. Total vs partial fundoplication in the treatment of gastroesophageal reflux disease: a meta-analysis. Arch Surg 2009; 144(3):273–8.

26. Mickevicius A, Endzinas Z, Kiudelis M, et al. Influence of wrap length on the effectiveness of Nissen and Toupet fundoplication: a prospective randomized study. Surg Endosc 2008;22(10):2269–76.

27. Bremner RM, Hoeft SF, Costantini M, et al. Pharyngeal swallowing. The major factor in clearance of esophageal reflux episodes. Ann Surg 1993;218(3): 364–9 [discussion: 369–70].

28. Hooft N, Smith M, Huang J, et al. Gastroparesis is common after lung transplantation and may be ameliorated by botulinum toxin-A injection of the pylorus. J Heart Lung Transplant 2014;33(12): 1314–6.

29. Kamolz T, Granderath FA, Pointner R. Does major depression in patients with gastroesophageal reflux disease affect the outcome of laparoscopic antireflux surgery? Surg Endosc 2003;17(1):55–60.

30. Hashemi M, Peters JH, DeMeester TR, et al. Laparoscopic repair of large type III hiatal hernia: objective followup reveals high recurrence rate. J Am Coll Surg 2000;190(5):553–60 [discussion: 560–1].

31. Luketich JD, Nason KS, Christie NA, et al. Outcomes after a decade of laparoscopic giant paraesophageal hernia repair. J Thorac Cardiovasc Surg 2010; 139(2):395–404, 404.e1.

32. Oelschlager BK, Pellegrini CA, Hunter J, et al. Biologic prosthesis reduces recurrence after laparoscopic paraesophageal hernia repair: a multicenter, prospective, randomized trial. Ann Surg 2006; 244(4):481–90.

33. Oelschlager BK, Pellegrini CA, Hunter JG, et al. Biologic prosthesis to prevent recurrence after laparoscopic paraesophageal hernia repair: long-term follow-up from a multicenter, prospective, randomized trial. J Am Coll Surg 2011;213(4):461–8.

34. Stadlhuber RJ, Sherif AE, Mittal SK, et al. Mesh complications after prosthetic reinforcement of hiatal closure: a 28-case series. Surg Endosc 2009;23(6): 1219–26.

35. Luketich JD, Raja S, Fernando HC, et al. Laparoscopic repair of giant paraesophageal hernia: 100 consecutive cases. Ann Surg 2000;232(4):608–18.

36. Pierre AF, Luketich JD, Fernando HC, et al. Results of laparoscopic repair of giant paraesophageal hernias: 200 consecutive patients. Ann Thorac Surg 2002;74(6):1909–15 [discussion: 1915–6].

37. Engstrom C, Lonroth H, Mardani J, et al. An anterior or posterior approach to partial fundoplication? Long-term results of a randomized trial. World J Surg 2007;31(6):1221–5 [discussion: 1226–7].

38. Shen KR, Harrison-Phipps KM, Cassivi SD, et al. Esophagectomy after anti-reflux surgery. J Thorac Cardiovasc Surg 2010;139(4):969–75.

39. Furnee EJ, Draaisma WA, Broeders IA, et al. Surgical reintervention after failed antireflux surgery: a systematic review of the literature. J Gastrointest Surg 2009;13(8):1539–49.

40. Iqbal A, Awad Z, Simkins J, et al. Repair of 104 failed anti-reflux operations. Ann Surg 2006;244(1): 42–51.

41. Oelschlager BK, Lal DR, Jensen E, et al. Medium- and long-term outcome of laparoscopic redo fundoplication. Surg Endosc 2006;20(12):1817–23.

42. Awais O, Luketich JD, Reddy N, et al. Roux-en-Y near esophagojejunostomy for failed antireflux operations: outcomes in more than 100 patients. Ann Thorac Surg 2014;98(6):1905–11 [discussion 1911–3].

43. Heller E. Extramukose cardioplastik beim chronischen cardiospasmus mit dilatation des oesophagus. Mitt Grenzeg Med Chir 1913;27:141.

44. Parise P, Santi S, Solito B, et al. Laparoscopic Heller myotomy plus Dor fundoplication in 137 achalasic patients: results on symptoms relief and successful outcome predictors. Updates Surg 2011;63(1):11–5.

45. Bredenoord AJ, Fox M, Kahrilas PJ, et al. Chicago classification criteria of esophageal motility disorders defined in high resolution esophageal pressure topography. Neurogastroenterol Motil 2012;24(Suppl 1): 57–65.

46. Muller M. Impact of high-resolution manometry on achalasia diagnosis and treatment. Ann Gastroenterol 2015;28(1):3–9.

47. Chuah SK, Chiu CH, Tai WC, et al. Current status in the treatment options for esophageal achalasia. World J Gastroenterol 2013;19(33):5421–9.

48. Nau P, Rattner D. Laparoscopic Heller myotomy as the gold standard for treatment of achalasia. J Gastrointest Surg 2014;18(12):2201–7.

49. Smith CD, Stival A, Howell DL, et al. Endoscopic therapy for achalasia before Heller myotomy results in worse outcomes than Heller myotomy alone. Ann Surg 2006;243(5):579–84 [discussion: 584–6].

50. Galvani C, Gorodner MV, Moser F, et al. Laparoscopic Heller myotomy for achalasia facilitated by robotic assistance. Surg Endosc 2006;20(7): 1105–12.

51. Shaligram A, Unnirevi J, Simorov A, et al. How does the robot affect outcomes? A retrospective review of open, laparoscopic, and robotic Heller myotomy for achalasia. Surg Endosc 2012;26(4):1047–50.

52. Tanaka E, Murata H, Minami H, et al. Anesthetic management of peroral endoscopic myotomy for esophageal achalasia: a retrospective case series. J Anesth 2014;28(3):456–9.

53. Luckey AE 3rd, DeMeester SR. Complications of achalasia surgery. Thorac Surg Clin 2006;16(1):95–8.

54. Frobese AS, Hawthorne HR, Nemir P Jr. The surgical management of achalasia of the esophagus. Ann Surg 1956;144(4):653–69.

55. Chen Z, Bessell JR, Chew A, et al. Laparoscopic cardiomyotomy for achalasia: clinical outcomes beyond 5 years. J Gastrointest Surg 2010;14(4): 594–600.

56. Oelschlager BK, Chang L, Pellegrini CA. Improved outcome after extended gastric myotomy for achalasia. Arch Surg 2003;138(5):490–5 [discussion: 495–7].

57. Campos GM, Vittinghoff E, Rabl C, et al. Endoscopic and surgical treatments for achalasia: a systematic review and meta-analysis. Ann Surg 2009;249(1): 45–57.

58. Mayo D, Griffiths EA, Khan OA, et al. Does the addition of a fundoplication improve outcomes for patients undergoing laparoscopic Heller's cardiomyotomy? Int J Surg 2012;10(6):301–4.

59. Wei MT, He YZ, Deng XB, et al. Is Dor fundoplication optimum after laparoscopic Heller myotomy for achalasia? A meta-analysis. World J Gastroenterol 2013;19(43):7804–12.

60. Kurian AA, Dunst CM, Sharata A, et al. Peroral endoscopic esophageal myotomy: defining the learning curve. Gastrointest Endosc 2013;77(5):719–25.

61. Inoue H, Minami H, Satodate H, et al. First clinical experience of submucosal endoscopic esophageal myotomy for esophageal achalasia with no skin incision. Gastrointest Endosc 2009;69(5):AB122.

62. Minami H, Inoue H, Haji A, et al. Per-oral endoscopic myotomy: emerging indications and evolving techniques. Dig Endosc 2015;27(2):175–81.

63. Familiari P, Gigante G, Marchese M, et al. Peroral endoscopic myotomy for esophageal achalasia: outcomes of the first 100 patients with short-term follow-up. Ann Surg 2014. [Epub ahead of print].

64. Wang J, Tan N, Xiao Y, et al. Safety and efficacy of the modified peroral endoscopic myotomy with shorter myotomy for achalasia patients: a prospective study. Dis Esophagus 2014. [Epub ahead of print].

65. Bhayani NH, Kurian AA, Dunst CM, et al. A comparative study on comprehensive, objective outcomes of laparoscopic Heller myotomy with per-oral endoscopic myotomy (POEM) for achalasia. Ann Surg 2014;259(6):1098–103.

66. Onimaru M, Inoue H, Ikeda H, et al. Peroral endoscopic myotomy is a viable option for failed surgical esophagocardiomyotomy instead of redo surgical Heller myotomy: a single center prospective study. J Am Coll Surg 2013;217(4):598–605.

# Prevention and Management of Complications Following Tracheal Resection

Smita Sihag, MD, Cameron D. Wright, MD*

## KEYWORDS

- Outcomes • Complications • Tracheal resection

## KEY POINTS

- Tracheal resections are generally performed at specialized centers with experienced teams of thoracic surgeons, anesthesiologists, otolaryngologists, and intensivists.
- Serious complications following tracheal surgery may be avoided by using intraoperative techniques that preserve adequate blood supply and eliminate tension on the tracheal end-to-end anastomosis.
- Careful preoperative evaluation for selecting appropriate surgical candidates and determining optimal timing of surgery is critical to avoiding complications.
- Primary preoperative factors that increase the risk of anastomotic complications after tracheal surgery are reoperation, increased length of resection (with need for release maneuvers), and need for preoperative tracheostomy.
- Strategies to avoid or detect postoperative complications early center on slow diet advancement to prevent aspiration, aggressive clearance of secretions, voice rest (for laryngotracheal resections), guardian chin stitch, and surveillance bronchoscopy.

## INTRODUCTION

Techniques of tracheal surgery have advanced significantly over the past 65 years since the initial tracheobronchial resections and reconstructions that were performed in the 1950s. In particular, airway management during tracheal resection and surgical maneuvers to release tension on the end-to-end tracheal anastomosis are the areas of greatest development that have led to improved safety and outcomes. At present, tracheal surgery is typically performed at specialized, high-volume centers where teams of experienced thoracic surgeons, anesthesiologists, otolaryngologists, and intensivists work together to manage the care of these patients.

The most common indications for tracheal resection and reconstruction are as follows:

- Postintubation or posttracheostomy circumferential tracheal stenosis, which is the result of high-pressure endotracheal or tracheostomy cuffs, inflammation, infection, and necrosis of the trachea.[1,2]
- Tracheal tumors, both primary and secondary. Squamous cell carcinoma and adenoid cystic carcinoma are the most common primary tracheal malignancies. Secondary

Disclosures: The authors have no relevant financial disclosures to report.
Department of Thoracic Surgery, Harvard Medical School, Massachusetts General Hospital, 55 Fruit Street, Blake 1570, Boston, MA 02114, USA
* Corresponding author.
E-mail address: cdwright@partners.org

1547-4127/15/$ – see front matter © 2015 Elsevier Inc. All rights reserved.

thoracic.theclinics.com

malignancies invading the trachea usually arise from bronchogenic or thyroid neoplasms.[3,4]

- Idiopathic laryngotracheal stenosis (ILTS) (laryngotracheal resection) is relatively rare but is seen with increasing frequency. This disease almost entirely affects younger women and primarily involves the cricoid.[5]
- Tracheoesophageal and tracheoinnominate fistulas, also a consequence of long-term high-pressure endotracheal tube and tracheostomy cuffs, which cause areas of granulation, malacia, and eventual erosion into surrounding structures. Fistulas may also occur due to penetrating trauma to the airway.[6]
- Congenital and postinfectious lesions are relatively rare and can represent a wide spectrum of disease from short- or long-segment stenosis, cartilaginous fibrosis, or calcified nodules.

Although many of these indications are serious and if left untreated can progress to detrimental airway compromise, almost none of them signify true emergencies. It is important to emphasize this point because careful and extensive preoperative evaluation and determining the appropriate timing of surgery are key measures to avoiding complications downstream.[7] The exception is tracheoinnominate fistula, for which immediate and definitive intervention may be necessary to control hemorrhage. Otherwise, the following temporizing measures can be used until the optimal time for elective tracheal resection and reconstruction:

- Rigid bronchoscopy with dilation or tumor coring for airway obstruction
- Flexible bronchoscopy with balloon dilation of airway stenosis
- Therapeutic flexible bronchoscopy for clearance of secretions or hemoptysis
- Tracheostomy, particularly in the situation of tracheoesophageal fistula (TEF) such that the cuff is inflated and occlusive distal to the fistula to protect the airway

Of note, placement of a covered expandable stent in the trachea is not a preferred option for bridging a patient to surgery because of the increase in inflammation and granulation and should be mainly used in palliative circumstances when resection and reconstruction are not possible.[8]

Preoperative evaluation and selection of patients centers on computed tomographic (CT) imaging and flexible and rigid bronchoscopy to assess the length of diseased trachea, laryngeal involvement, and vocal cord function, as well as presence of secretions, infection, inflammation, granulation, or obstruction. Biopsy is indicated for any endobronchial lesions. Nebulizers and intravenous antibiotics may be used to treat signs of purulent secretions and active infection, and any airway surgery should be postponed in this scenario. Patients should not be ventilator dependent, so as to prevent exposure of a fresh anastomosis to positive pressure ventilation, foreign body, and airway colonization postoperatively. Active airway inflammation may be treated with a course of corticosteroid therapy, but if possible, steroids should be discontinued well before tracheal surgery. Tracheostomy stomas should be mature or well healed before surgery. Radiation therapy in the surgical field should likewise be avoided preoperatively, because it greatly increases the risk of anastomotic separation.[9] No trials demonstrate any role for neoadjuvant radiation in the treatment of tracheal malignancies, although there is evidence of benefit in the palliative or adjuvant setting, especially in the case of a positive margin or incomplete resection.[10] Any plans for reoperative tracheal surgery should be delayed at least several months after the initial operation, if possible, while the airway may be stabilized with a T-tube.[11]

## SURGICAL TECHNIQUE

The first attempt at tracheal resection and reconstruction is often the best chance at achieving a positive outcome for the patient. The operation can divided into 4 phases[12]:

### Induction

The procedure begins with flexible/rigid bronchoscopy to inspect the airway and clear secretions. The patient is positioned supine with the neck extended if the approach is via a low collar incision or median sternotomy, although lesions near the carina require a right-sided posterolateral thoracotomy in the left lateral decubitus position. Usually, the airway is intubated under direct visualization distal to the lesion if possible with a flexible, armored single-lumen endotracheal tube. A total intravenous anesthetic is preferable throughout the operation, as opposed to inhaled agents.

### Resection

The region of interest of the trachea is exposed and dissected carefully so as not to cause injury to the recurrent laryngeal nerves or innominate artery or devascularize the trachea. The oral endotracheal tube is then withdrawn, and once the airway is transected, cross-table ventilation involving a flexible, armored single-lumen endotracheal tube or jet catheter is initiated via the distal airway. The appropriate length of trachea is then resected by trimming each end to healthy mucosa and cartilage. Approximately 4.5 cm of the cervical trachea can be resected safely with neck flexion and pretracheal mobilization alone in ideal patients. Up to 50% of the total tracheal length may be resected at maximum with the use of more complex release maneuvers, although the risk of anastomotic separation increases markedly with increasing length resected because of excess tension.

## Reconstruction

Once the resection is complete, 2-0 vicryl full-thickness traction sutures are placed in the midline laterally on both sides of the trachea. These sutures are brought together to assess tension. Release maneuvers such as (1) neck flexion, (2) blunt finger dissection in the pretracheal plane down to the carina (as is done for a mediastinoscopy) for pretracheal mobilization, (3) suprahyoid laryngeal release,[13] (4) takedown of the inferior pulmonary ligament, (5) division of the left mainstem bronchus, or (6) intrapericardial hilar release may be used to bring the ends of the trachea together without tension. The anastomosis is then performed using lubricated 4-0 vicryl sutures placed in an interrupted manner 3 mm apart, and 3 mm from the cut edge of the trachea. Once the sutures are placed, the oral endotracheal tube is then advanced distal to the anastomosis, and the sutures are tied down sequentially (traction sutures first) with the knots on the exterior of the airway. A pedicled tissue flap, most often one of the strap muscles, may be used to buttress the anastomosis and seal it from surrounding structures such as the esophagus and innominate artery. A closed suction drain is left in the wound before closure.

## Extubation

The goal is to extubate the patient at the end of the procedure. If there are concerns regarding the airway or postoperative edema and swelling, a small tracheostomy may be placed proximal or distal to the anastomosis as necessary. A guardian stitch is placed between the chin and chest to keep the neck in a slightly flexed to neutral position to prevent neck hyperextension as additional anastomotic protection. Patients are typically monitored in the intensive care unit for 24 to 48 hours postoperatively.

In summary, during tracheal surgery, it is crucial to abide by 3 main principles:

- Preservation of blood supply to the trachea (by limiting dissection to just beyond the area of resection)
- Elimination of tension (by judicious airway length resection and use of release maneuvers)
- Construction of an air-/water-tight anastomosis (by meticulous attention to detail)

Postoperative management entails slow diet advancement to prevent aspiration, aggressive pulmonary toilet to clear secretions, and voice rest (if a laryngotracheal resection was performed). Laryngeal manipulation or release can affect swallowing function, and these patients should undergo formal evaluation before starting oral intake. Antibiotics and steroids are used selectively. Surveillance bronchoscopy at 1 week or sooner is the key to recognizing anastomotic complications early because ischemia can be detected by endoscopy earlier than when it presents with a wound infection.

## CLINICAL OUTCOMES AND COMPLICATIONS

By far, the largest experience in a review of anastomotic complications of tracheal surgery comes from the Massachusetts General Hospital (MGH), published in 2004 by Wright and colleagues.[14] This experience includes 901 patients from 1975 to 2003 who underwent tracheal resection and reconstruction for indications of postintubation stenosis (PITS), tumor, TEF, and idiopathic ILTS. Overall morbidity and mortality were reported at 18.2% and 1.2%, respectively. The highest rates of morbidity and mortality were observed in patients with TEF followed by those with tracheal tumors, whereas the lowest rates were seen in patients with ILTS. This result is likely attributable to the difference in patient populations, as well as the length and complexity of repairs. Patients with ILTS tend to be young healthy women requiring short resections for focal disease, whereas those with TEF are generally sicker with a tracheostomy in place, have poor tissue quality, and require a more lengthy resection and repair. Patients with tracheal malignancies likewise tend to be older and also may require longer resections to achieve negative margins.

Overall, anastomotic complications were seen in 9% of patients, and the trend was similar with the highest rates of anastomotic complications in patients with TEF and PITS. A complication with the anastomosis results in significant morbidity and prolonged hospitalization, and it is the single greatest predictor of death following tracheal surgery. Thus, unsurprisingly, patients with TEF also had the highest mortality rate. Anastomotic complications can be defined along a spectrum ranging from granulation tissue formation at the suture line, scarring and stenosis, to separation and dehiscence. Granulation tissue formation presumably is a consequence of an inflammatory reaction from the suture material (although mitigated by the use of absorbable polyglactin), low-grade stretch or separation of the anastomosis that leads to tissue ingrowth, or the patient's own individual wound healing capability. Stenosis may also be due to low-grade tension and ischemia to the anastomosis that ultimately causes scar formation and contracture of the tissues. Last, disruption of the anastomotic suture line can be either focal or more catastrophic resulting in anastomotic failure and, although ischemia may play a role, excess tension is the primary culprit. Based on multivariate analysis, notable risk factors for anastomotic complications following tracheal surgery included young age (less than 17 years), diabetes, preoperative tracheostomy, length of resection greater than 4 cm, need for intraoperative release maneuver, laryngotracheal resection (as opposed to simple tracheal resection), and reoperation. Length of resection greater than 4 cm should prompt consideration for need for a release maneuver, although the approach used to mitigate tension is at the discretion of the surgeon. The correlation between length of resection and anastomotic failure is demonstrated in **Fig. 1**. While obesity and steroid use were not significant risk factors in this analysis, a history of diabetes, which is known to affect the microcirculation and wound healing, did increase the risk of postoperative anastomotic complications with an odds ratio of 2.72 (confidence interval, 1.53–4.82; $P = .0004$). Need for tracheostomy preoperatively suggests a marginal airway at baseline with greater potential for bacterial colonization, inflammation, scarring, and malacic segments. Reoperation, even though usually successful when carefully planned and executed at least 4 to 6 months after the initial reconstruction, poses additional challenges to tracheal mobilization because of adhesions and fibrosis that may contribute to increased tension and compromised blood supply aside from merely adding to the length of resection. Laryngeal anastomoses tend to be more technically demanding and complex than simple tracheal end-to-end anastomoses, and the end product is more fragile and susceptible to breakdown. Based on clinical observation, the maximum length of trachea that may be safely resected in children and adolescents is

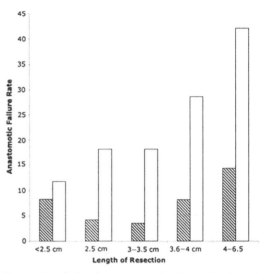

**Fig. 1.** Correlation between tracheal resection length and anastomotic failure rate. The open bars represent reoperative tracheal resections. The bars with diagonal lines represent first-time tracheal resections. As expected, reoperative tracheal surgery has a higher failure rate. (*From* Wright CD, Grillo HC, Wain JC, et al. Anastomotic complications after tracheal resection: prognostic factors and management. J Thorac Cardiovasc Surg 2004;128(5):734; with permission.)

considerably less and approximates 30%.[15] For reasons that are not entirely well understood, pediatric patients have a lower threshold for tension than adults.

In all, most patients who experienced anastomotic complications were successfully managed without a temporary artificial airway or reintervention. In this series, 6 of the 81 patients with evidence of anastomotic separation did eventually die of loss of airway, and anastomotic failure increased the risk of mortality by an odds ratio of 13.0 ($P = .001$). Causes of death in patients who did not have an anastomotic failure were myocardial infarction, pulmonary embolism, and aspiration pneumonia.

Another series of 94 patients reported by Bibas and colleagues[16] from Brazil shows a 21% rate of anastomotic complications, recurrent stenosis being most common in their experience. The investigators used similar operative techniques as those described by Grillo[17] and Pearson and colleagues.[18] All patients underwent tracheal resection and reconstruction for a diagnosis of benign tracheal or laryngotracheal stenosis. Risk factors for anastomotic complications were essentially the same: previous tracheal resection and length of resection greater than 4 cm. Rates of major complications largely related to the anastomosis from other single-institution series reported in the literature are summarized in **Table 1**.

Nonanastomotic, airway-related complications such as glottic edema and/or vocal cord edema and need for temporary tracheostomy occur at an exceedingly low rate, but all are more prevalent following laryngotracheal resection by an order of twofold or more compared with straightforward tracheal resection. Laryngeal reconstruction can predictably generate some degree of glottic edema and laryngeal dysfunction. Both of these adversely impact the normal swallowing mechanism and pose a greater risk of aspiration. Severe upper airway swelling with stridor and airway compromise necessitates temporary tracheostomy placement. Injury to the recurrent laryngeal nerve with vocal cord paralysis was observed in less than 2% of patients.

## MANAGEMENT OF POSTOPERATIVE COMPLICATIONS
### Anastomotic Complications

Granulation tissue formation at the site of the anastomosis is relatively rare as reported in the MGH experience (7 of 901 patients, or .007%). However, other series report the incidence to be as high as 33%, despite using a similar technique to that described by Grillo and colleagues[25] at MGH for construction of the anastomosis. However, the number of patients analyzed in this series is considerably smaller at only 12. Some degree of granulation tissue is to be expected postoperatively, but in the worst-case scenario, granulation tissue can cause obstruction of the airway. The time course of developing symptomatic granulation tissue is generally days to weeks, and patients present with stridor. As in the case of any airway symptoms following tracheal surgery, prompt evaluation with flexible bronchoscopy is indicated to assess the problem (**Figs. 2** and **3**). Management options include rigid bronchoscopy with direct debridement of granulation tissue if the proliferation is focal. Injection with corticosteroids has also been described with some effect. Laser ablation and brachytherapy are reasonable treatment strategies for benign granulation tissue of the airway from tracheal stents and tracheostomies in nonsurgical candidates; however, safety and efficacy following airway reconstruction has not been extensively studied. Silicone Montgomery T-tubes (Hood Laboratories, Pembroke, MA) can be used if the proliferation is severe and recurrent and the threat of reobstruction is high.

Restenosis of the airway following reconstruction is more common than granulation tissue formation but still occurs at a rate of less than 1%. As with granulation tissue formation, patients with a history of PITS are at highest risk. Residual stenosis is possible due to inadequate resection of initial tracheal stenosis, especially if presentation is earlier than expected. However, low-grade ischemia to the anastomosis is the more likely cause. The time course of restenosis is more insidious, and symptoms may develop over several months. The diagnosis is confirmed using flexible bronchoscopy, and the mainstay of management is dilation (**Fig. 4**). Either graduated rigid bronchoscopes or a pneumatic balloon dilator may be used to dilate the anastomosis because both techniques are effective. If dilations are required more often than every 3 to 6 months, reoperation should be considered. Results of initial operative intervention for tracheal stenosis (idiopathic or postintubation) are quite good with success rates reported as high as greater than 95%. If there is adequate amount of residual trachea, reoperation for postoperative recurrent tracheal stenosis also carries a remarkably high success rate of 92% despite the increased risk of anastomotic complications if deferred for 6 months to 1 year allowing for complete resolution of postoperative healing.[26] Use of silicone stents or a Montgomery T-tube may be necessary for long-term management of restenosis that is not amenable to reresection.

**Table 1**
**Rates of major complications following tracheal reconstruction**

| Author | No. of Patients | Major Complications (%) | Mortality (%) |
| --- | --- | --- | --- |
| Couraud et al,[19] 1994 | 217 | 4.6 | 3.2 |
| Rea et al,[20] 2002 | 65 | 12.3 | 1.5 |
| Amoros et al,[21] 2006 | 54 | 9.2 | 1.85 |
| D'Andrilli et al,[22] 2008 | 35 | 14.3 | 0 |
| Cordos et al,[23] 2009 | 60 | 13.3 | 5 |
| Marulli et al,[24] 2008 | 37 | 8.1 | 0 |

*Data from Refs.[19–24]*

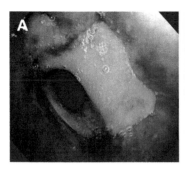
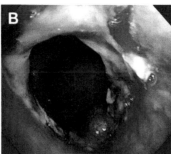

Fig. 2. (A) Obstructing fibrinous debris on a tracheal anastomosis 7 days after resection. The patient had mild stridor. (B). The same anastomosis immediately after bronchoscopic debridement of the fibrinous debris demonstrating a markedly improved airway.

Anastomotic dehiscence is usually the most serious of all complications following tracheal surgery. Separation of the suture line to some degree was detected in less than 1% of patients (37 of 901 patients) in the MGH experience. Presentation is early within days or 1 to 2 weeks of surgery, and clinical manifestations may be stridor, cough, increased secretions, hemoptysis, subcutaneous emphysema, or a wound infection. Total loss of airway is exceedingly rare, but it carries a very high mortality rate. CT imaging can assist in initial evaluation of dehiscence and may demonstrate air or fluid collections in the neck or mediastinum, as well as pneumonia (**Fig. 5**). Urgent bronchoscopy is necessary to evaluate the integrity of the anastomosis (**Fig. 6**). The anterior wall of the anastomosis is usually the site of initial separation because of increased effect of tension. Small separations in the suture line can be watched, especially if the anastomosis is buttressed with a vascularized tissue flap. A dehiscence larger than several millimeters is typically managed with a Montgomery T-tube at the authors' institution to avoid loss of airway. The T-tube can be inserted directly through the defect and surrounding muscle, and tissue can be used to seal off the area. Any air or fluid collections should be drained, and broad-spectrum antibiotic therapy should be initiated. In some patients, this dehiscence may eventually heal over a long period with the T-tube being subsequently removed. After 6 months, reoperation may be considered if there is no improvement, but this should be delayed as long as reasonably possible. Immediate reoperation can be considered in certain select situations where an episode of violent coughing or neck hyperextension causes the anastomosis to come apart in the very early postoperative period.

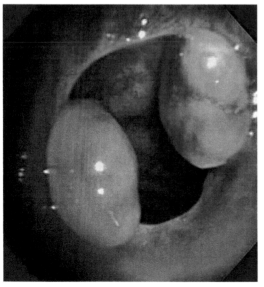

Fig. 3. Polypoid granulations 2 months after tracheal resection due to exposed lateral stay sutures; these were easily removed by rigid bronchoscopy.

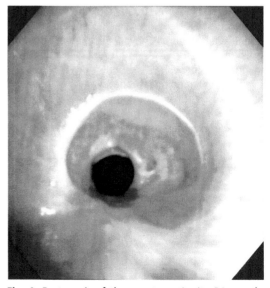

Fig. 4. Restenosis of the anastomotic site 34 months after resection of 3.5 cm of trachea in a young woman with postintubation tracheal stenosis. She had mild dyspnea on exertion.

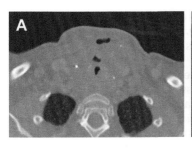
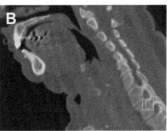

**Fig. 5.** (*A*) Axial CT image 6 days after laryngotracheal resection with some necrosis of the anterior aspect of the anastomosis with a small air leak. (*B*) Sagittal CT image. This patient went on to drainage of the anterior aspect of the incision, hyperbaric oxygen therapy, and subsequent healing without further sequelae.

Impaired wound healing of the anastomosis is a complication that is often recognized early on, at the initial surveillance bronchoscopy at 1 week or less from surgery (**Fig. 7**). Presumably, wound healing problems such as focal areas of ischemic or necrotic cartilage or even partial separation eventually lead to the more severe long-term anastomotic complications of restenosis and dehiscence, and possibly even granulation tissue formation. At the authors' institution, hyperbaric oxygen therapy administered at 2 atm; 100% oxygen for at least 90 minutes daily over 5 to 14 days has led to a substantial improvement in healing as monitored by frequent bronchoscopy.[27] An initial series of 5 patients was reported in 2014, and hyperbaric oxygen therapy continues to be an ongoing area of study. While short-term findings seem promising, long-term outcomes still need to be examined.

## Fistulas

Tracheoinnominate fistula is the most feared and catastrophic complication following tracheal surgery but happens with extraordinarily low frequency. In the MGH experience, only 3 patients developed this complication, although 2 of them died. A small-scale, so-called sentinel bleed may present before signs of significant hemorrhage into the airway are apparent. The main tenet in dealing with this issue is avoiding it in the first place, because this complication is usually the result of technical missteps. The surgical principles that must be adhered to in order to prevent this problem are (1) not dissecting out the artery completely so as to leave the adventitia exposed, (2) covering any anastomosis in proximity to the artery with a vascularized muscle flap, and (3) not overresecting the airway so as to leave the reconstruction at greater tension and threat of dehiscence. If a sentinel bleed is perceived,

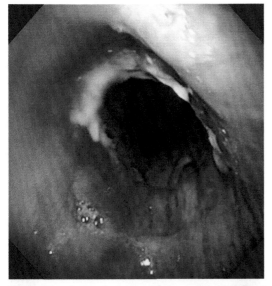

**Fig. 6.** Bronchoscopic image of the patient in **Fig. 5** with small amount of necrotic anterior cartilage from 9- to 3-o'clock position. Although the anastomosis was intact, it did leak air into the neck and caused a neck wound infection that required drainage and packing.

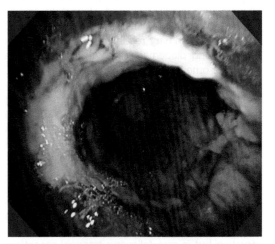

**Fig. 7.** Bronchoscopic image of a patient with a right main to trachea anastomosis demonstrating ischemic anterior cartilages; this healed uneventfully with the help of hyperbaric oxygen therapy.

bronchoscopy and CT scan can be pursued to rule out communication with the innominate artery if the patient remains hemodynamically stable. Usually, some degree of anastomotic separation will be evident on bronchoscopy. In the setting of catastrophic hemorrhage into the airway, the wound may need to be reopened at the bedside and digital pressure applied while the patient is emergently transported to the operating room for reexploration. Securing the airway in this scenario is always challenging. Once in the operating room, the prior incision is reopened and a partial (or complete) sternotomy is needed to obtain adequate exposure. The innominate artery should be clamped and divided proximal to the carotid-subclavian bifurcation. Each end should be oversewn and reinforced with a vascularized tissue flap. The risk of cerebral ischemia is very low, although a bypass graft should be considered if changes in the electroencephalogram are observed. In addition, repairing and buttressing of the tracheal anastomosis should also be performed at the same time.

TEF, on the other hand, is a consequence of breakdown of the membranous wall of the anastomosis. This breakdown creates an infected field posteriorly and allows for fistula formation to the esophagus. Unrecognized injury to the esophagus during the index operation or resection of part of the wall of the esophagus to obtain a negative margin during tumor resection may also be possible causes. Cough, dysphagia, and aspiration pneumonia are the hallmark clinical signs. Both bronchoscopy and barium swallow can confirm the diagnosis. This complication is similarly quite uncommon and was detected again in only 3 of 901 patients in the MGH series, although all were successfully salvaged. Ultimately, operative exploration with tracheal reresection and anastomosis, primary repair of the esophagus in 2 layers, and placement of a vascularized strap muscle or omental flap between suture lines represents definitive treatment of this problem. However, in the short term, tracheostomy placement with an occlusive cuff distal to the fistula, enteral feeding, drainage, and broad-spectrum antibiotics are indicated to clear any infection before an attempt at repair.

### Laryngeal Complications

The incidence of glottic edema is relatively high following laryngotracheal resection and reconstruction but is rare following tracheal resection. Rates of glottic edema are reported at 5% in patients who underwent laryngotracheal reconstruction. Symptoms of hoarseness and stridor should

prompt bronchoscopic evaluation to make the diagnosis (**Fig. 8**). Mild-to-moderate edema of the vocal cords can be easily managed with voice rest, steroids, aspiration precautions, diuretics, epinephrine nebulizers, and most importantly, patience. An assessment of whether or not the patient has an adequate airway must be made, because significant glottic edema can occasionally lead to obstruction. In this instance, tracheostomy placement above or below the anastomosis is indicated. Recurrent laryngeal nerve injury only occurs at a rate of less than 2% in most reported series, even in laryngotracheal resection despite the proximity of the nerve to the field of dissection. The approach among surgeons at the authors' institution is to dissect in the peritracheal planes immediately adjacent to the airway and to deliberately avoid violating the tracheoesophageal groove or trying to identify the path of the nerve. Hoarseness of the voice and weak cough are usually fairly easy to discern postoperatively. A laryngologist may be consulted to assist with diagnosis and management. Awake bedside flexible laryngoscopy is performed to inspect the vocal cords. Minor cord dysfunction is likely to improve over time and may be a consequence of traction injury to the nerve. However, if there is complete cord paralysis either in the abducted or adducted position, a temporizing laryngoplasty procedure (vocal cord injection with collagen) should be undertaken during the early postoperative course to prevent aspiration. Bilateral recurrent laryngeal nerve injury

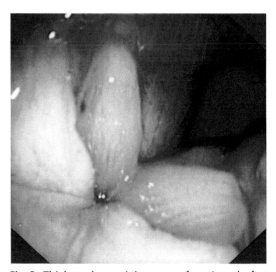

**Fig. 8.** This bronchoscopic image was from 1 week after a high laryngotracheal resection in a patient who had severe vocal cord edema. She was aphonic and had mild stridor. She improved with intravenous dexamethasone and with time without further intervention.

is an indication for tracheostomy due to glottic obstruction.

Swallowing dysfunction is not common after tracheal surgery, but needs to be appropriately assessed if suspected. The assessment should begin preoperatively with a thorough evaluation of glottic function before laryngotracheal or tracheal resection. Several patients with PITS, for example, may have glottic injury from traumatic endotracheal intubation. Elderly patients, patients who have been intubated for a prolonged period, and those who have undergone a suprahyoid laryngeal release procedure are most at risk. Eliciting the help of a speech and swallow pathology specialist is recommended. A modified barium swallow study can reveal the extent of swallowing dysfunction. The swallowing mechanism should improve with time and exercises, but enteral feeding may be required via a gastrostomy tube; any suspected significant aspiration event should be investigated further with bronchoscopy. In the MGH series, 24 of 901 patients exhibited swallowing dysfunction with evidence of an aspiration event postoperatively. Severe aspiration pneumonia with progression to acute respiratory distress syndrome is obviously rare, but the occasional patient has required prolonged ventilatory support, and even venovenous extracorporeal membrane oxygenation.

## SUMMARY

Strict adherence to the principles of tracheal surgery by preserving adequate blood supply, eliminating tension, and using meticulous anastomotic technique represents the best strategy to avoid complications of tracheal surgery. Furthermore, careful preoperative evaluation and appropriate selection of patients also play important roles in achieving a positive outcome. In experienced centers, rates of significant morbidity and mortality approximate 10% and 2%, respectively. The range of postoperative complications after tracheal reconstruction includes edema, granulation, fistula, separation, and restenosis. Anastomotic complications, in particular, lead to an increased risk of mortality and must be treated aggressively to secure the airway. Early detection via bronchoscopy and effective airway management with dilation, T-tube stenting, or tracheostomy often yields successful results.

## REFERENCES

1. Cooper JD, Grillo HC. Analysis of problems related to cuffs on intratracheal tubes. Chest 1972;62(2 Suppl):21S–7S.

2. Grillo HC, Donahue DM. Postintubation tracheal stenosis. Chest Surg Clin N Am 1996;6(4):725–31.

3. Grillo HC, Mathisen DJ. Primary tracheal tumors: treatment and results. Ann Thorac Surg 1990; 49(1):69–77.

4. Gaissert HA, Honings J, Grillo HC, et al. Segmental laryngotracheal and tracheal resection for invasive thyroid carcinoma. Ann Thorac Surg 2007;83(6): 1952–9.

5. Grillo HC. Management of idiopathic tracheal stenosis. Chest Surg Clin N Am 1996;6(4):811–8.

6. Muniappan A, Wain JC, Wright CD, et al. Surgical treatment of nonmalignant tracheoesophageal fistula: a thirty-five year experience. Ann Thorac Surg 2013;95(4):1141–6.

7. Mathisen DJ. Complications of tracheal surgery. Chest Surg Clin N Am 1996;6(4):853–64.

8. Gaissert HA, Grillo HC, Wright CD, et al. Complication of benign tracheobronchial strictures by self-expanding metal stents. J Thorac Cardiovasc Surg 2003;126(3):744–7.

9. Muehrcke DD, Grillo HC, Mathisen DJ. Reconstructive airway operation after irradiation. Ann Thorac Surg 1995;59(1):14–8.

10. Chow DC, Komaki R, Libshitz HI, et al. Treatment of primary neoplasms of the trachea. The role of radiation therapy. Cancer 1993;71(10):2946–52.

11. Gaissert HA, Grillo HC, Mathisen DJ, et al. Temporary and permanent restoration of airway continuity with the tracheal T-tube. J Thorac Cardiovasc Surg 1994;107(2):600–6.

12. Grillo HC. Surgery of the trachea and bronchi. Hamilton (Ontario): BC Decker Inc; 2004.

13. Montgomery WW. Suprahyoid release for tracheal anastomosis. Arch Otolaryngol 1974;99(4):255–60.

14. Wright CD, Grillo HC, Wain JC, et al. Anastomotic complications after tracheal resection: prognostic factors and management. J Thorac Cardiovasc Surg 2004;128(5):731–9.

15. Wright CD, Graham BB, Grillo HC, et al. Pediatric tracheal surgery. Ann Thorac Surg 2002;74(2):308–13 [discussion: 314].

16. Bibas BJ, Terra RM, Oliveira Junior AL, et al. Predictors for postoperative complications after tracheal resection. Ann Thorac Surg 2014;98(1):277–82.

17. Grillo HC. Primary reconstruction of airway after resection of subglottic laryngeal and upper tracheal stenosis. Ann Thorac Surg 1982;33(1):3–18.

18. Pearson FG, Cooper JD, Nelems JM, et al. Primary tracheal anastomosis after resection of the cricoid cartilage with preservation of recurrent laryngeal nerves. J Thorac Cardiovasc Surg 1975;70(5): 806–16.

19. Couraud L, Jougon J, Velly JF, et al. Iatrogenic stenoses of the respiratory tract. Evolution of therapeutic indications. Based on 217 surgical cases. Ann Chir 1994;48(3):277–83 [in French].

20. Rea F, Callegaro D, Loy M, et al. Benign tracheal and laryngotracheal stenosis: surgical treatment and results. Eur J Cardiothorac Surg 2002;22(3): 352–6.

21. Amoros JM, Ramos R, Villalonga R, et al. Tracheal and cricotracheal resection for laryngotracheal stenosis: experience in 54 consecutive cases. Eur J Cardiothorac Surg 2006;29(1):35–9.

22. D'Andrilli A, Ciccone AM, Venuta F, et al. Long-term results of laryngotracheal resection for benign stenosis. Eur J Cardiothorac Surg 2008;33(3):440–3.

23. Cordos I, Bolca C, Paleru C, et al. Sixty tracheal resections–single center experience. Interact Cardiovasc Thorac Surg 2009;8(1):62–5 [discussion: 65].

24. Marulli G, Rizzardi G, Bortolotti L, et al. Single-staged laryngotracheal resection and reconstruction for benign strictures in adults. Interact Cardiovasc Thorac Surg 2008;7(2):227–30 [discussion: 230].

25. Marques P, Leal L, Spratley J, et al. Tracheal resection with primary anastomosis: 10 years experience. Am J Otolaryngol 2009;30(6):415–8.

26. Donahue DM, Grillo HC, Wain JC, et al. Reoperative tracheal resection and reconstruction for unsuccessful repair of postintubation stenosis. J Thorac Cardiovasc Surg 1997;114(6):934–8 [discussion: 938–9].

27. Stock C, Gukasyan N, Muniappan A, et al. Hyperbaric oxygen therapy for the treatment of anastomotic complications after tracheal resection and reconstruction. J Thorac Cardiovasc Surg 2014; 147(3):1030–5.

# Prevention and Management of Nerve Injuries in Thoracic Surgery

Hugh G. Auchincloss, MD, MPH[a], Dean M. Donahue, MD[b],*

## KEYWORDS

- Peripheral nerves • Anatomy • Physiology • Thoracic surgery • Complications
- Peripheral nerve injury

## KEY POINTS

- Understanding of the basic anatomy and physiology of the peripheral nerves of the chest is important for thoracic surgeons.
- Peripheral nerves may be injured during an operation by partial or complete transection, thermal insult, crush, stretch, or exposure to a toxic environment.
- Progress has been made in the field of nerve repair and regeneration, but there is no treatment that is as reliable as avoiding these injuries.

## INTRODUCTION

Nerve injuries have the potential to cause substantial morbidity after thoracic surgical procedures. For the most part, these injuries are preventable, provided that the surgeon has a thorough understanding of the relevant anatomy and follows important surgical principles. When nerve injuries do occur, it is important for the surgeon to recognize the options available in the immediate and postoperative settings, including expectant management, immediate nerve reconstruction, or auxiliary procedures to mitigate the consequences of loss of the damaged nerve's function. This article covers the basic anatomy and physiology of nerves and nerve injuries, an overview of techniques in nerve reconstruction, and a guide to the nerves most commonly involved in thoracic operative procedures.

## ANATOMY AND PHYSIOLOGY OF NERVES AND NERVE INJURY

Extensive knowledge of the complex peripheral nervous system is unnecessary for the practice of safe thoracic surgery. However, surgeons should have an understanding of the basic anatomy and physiology of peripheral nerves. This understanding helps to eliminate surgical techniques that put nerves at risk for injury, and fosters an appreciation for the natural history of nerve injuries and nerve repair.

### Anatomy and Physiology of Peripheral Nerves

The peripheral nervous system is composed of 2 cell types: neurons and neuroglia. An individual neuron consists of a cell body and an axon. Multiple dendrites are associated with the cell body and transmit synaptic information inward, whereas a single axon conveys information away from the cell body. Neuroglia exist to provide the scaffolding and nutrient milieu for neurons. In some cases neuroglia produce myelin, a substance that insulates the long axonal processes of most neurons and improves the speed of conduction. Myelinated and unmyelinated axons are invested in several layers of connective tissue called endoneurium, perineurium, and epineurium. The epineurium contains the vascular and lymphatic

[a] Department of Thoracic Surgery, Massachusetts General Hospital, Blake 1570, Boston, MA 02114, USA;
[b] Department of Thoracic Surgery, Harvard Medical School, Massachusetts General Hospital, Blake 1570, 55 Fruit Street, Boston, MA 02114, USA
* Corresponding author.
E-mail address: ddonahue@partners.org

Thorac Surg Clin 25 (2015) 509–515
http://dx.doi.org/10.1016/j.thorsurg.2015.07.012

network that supplies individual neurons. The viability of the epineurial layer is a key determinant to how well a nerve may recover after injury, with or without repair.

Neurons can be classified in multiple ways. Neurons belonging to the somatic nervous system provide voluntary skeletal motor control and precise sensory information, whereas neurons belonging to the autonomic nervous system provide involuntary motor and sensory information to and from the viscera and smooth muscle. Within the autonomic nervous system, a further subdivision exists between sympathetic ("fight or flight") and parasympathetic ("rest and digest") neurons. These distinctions are of little importance to surgeons with respect to the handling of individual peripheral nerves, because most peripheral nerves contain neurons of all different types enclosed within a single epineurial sheath. Injury to a nerve is likely to affect all neurons equally.

### Classification of Peripheral Nerve Injury

A peripheral nerve may be damaged in several ways during the course of an operation, including by partial or complete transection, thermal insult, crush, stretch, or exposure to a toxic environment. The pattern of injury that results from these injuries exists along a spectrum with important implications for immediate management and prognosis for recovery. The severity of peripheral nerve injury is determined first by whether or not there is axonal damage, and then by the degree to which there is connective tissue damage. A classification of peripheral nerve injuries was originally proposed by Seddon in 1943, expanded by Sunderland in the 1950s, and is still widely in use today.

- Neurapraxia (Sunderland class I injury) refers to temporary interruption of normal nerve conduction without axonal or connective tissue damage. Neuropraxial injuries are the mildest form of peripheral nerve trauma. Usually the cause is mild crush, stretch, or thermal injury to the nerve that in turn causes demyelination. The mechanism by which demyelination is triggered is not understood fully, but may be related to transient ischemia or local inflammatory response. However, because the axon itself remains intact, full recovery of nerve function is expected in days or weeks.
- Axonotmesis (Sunderland class II injury) is defined as axonal injury without damage to the connective tissue scaffolding of the nerve. Typically, this injury is caused by prolonged stretch, crush, or ischemia with resultant axonal damage. An axon that is damaged

cannot repair itself and undergoes a process of Wallerian degeneration, whereby the distal part of the axon degenerates and the resultant products are scavenged by macrophages. Renervation of the target organ can be achieved by collateralization or axonal regeneration. Collaterization occurs if only some of the axons leading to a target organ are damaged, allowing the tissue innervated by the remaining axons to hypertrophy and preserve the function of the organ. If the majority of axons have been destroyed, then regeneration must take place for function to be maintained. This is possible because the connective tissue scaffolding of the nerve remains intact. After a period of Wallerian degeneration, axons begin to regrow at rate of 1 to 3 mm per day along their endoneurial tubes, nourished by the surrounding epineurium. If they reach the target organ within 12 to 18 months, renervation can occur, albeit with somewhat abnormal conduction. Beyond that window, a process of denervation-related fibrosis makes muscle recovery unlikely; however, some sympathetic and sensory nerve targets have been shown to maintain renervation potential as far out as 3 years.
- Neurotmesis (Sunderland class III/V injury) is axonal damage along with some degree of connective tissue damage. If the endoneurium alone is disrupted, then axonal regeneration may be possible. However, if damage extends to the epineurium (ie, complete transection of the nerve), surgical repair is required.

Special consideration exists for nerve injuries caused by thermal insult, local anesthetic toxicity, or exposure to damaging environmental factors. Thermal injuries are unique in that the degree of destruction to both the axons and the connective tissue scaffolding of the nerve may be more severe than is perceived by the surgeon. Total disruption of the epineurial layer with subsequent fibrosis may occur in the absence of obvious physical signs of damage. For this reason, thermal nerve injuries are often not identified at the time of surgery. If they are, however, the safest course is to resect the affected nerve along with proximal and distal margin and reconstruct the remaining tissue. The severity of local anesthetic toxicity may also be difficult to judge in the immediate period. Infiltration of local anesthetic agent directly into the epineurial layer typically results in neuropraxial injury. However, if high enough concentrations are achieved axonal death and even connective tissue damage are possible. Last, experimental models suggest that certain environments, particularly extreme acidity, can result in severe nerve injury. This theoretic risk has led the manufacturers of certain topical hemostatic agents whose mechanism of action produces local acidity to caution against the use of their products in the area of important peripheral nerves. However, there are no data to suggest that this concern is justified, and in practice topical hemostatic agents are often used as a way to avoid the need for electrocautery around peripheral nerves.

### Repair of Peripheral Nerves

Peripheral nerves may be repaired in several ways. If a nerve is transected and the bridging distance is short, a primary repair is used. For longer defects and situations in which tension limits primary repair, an interposition graft using either native nerve (eg, sural nerve) or synthetic material may be used. Peripheral nerve repair is beyond the scope of practice for thoracic surgeons and should be done by plastic surgeons trained in microsurgery. Repair is typically done using fine nonabsorbable monofilament suture under an operating microscope.

## NERVE INJURIES IN THORACIC SURGERY

Despite the progress made in the field of peripheral nerve repair and reconstruction, the results remain modest and avoidance of nerve injuries remains paramount for the thoracic surgeon.

Consideration begins with careful positioning of the patient. In the supine position, attention should be paid to padding of the elbows and gentle supination of the forearms and wrists. Upper extremities should not be extended, abducted, or externally rotated beyond 90°. In the lateral decubitus position, care is taken to avoid overextension of the upper shoulder and unevenly distributed pressure on the dependent shoulder.

Sophisticated knowledge of the anatomy of the peripheral nerves of the thorax along with their common anatomic variants is essential to the safe practice of surgery. Extra care must be taken when the patient's pathology distorts normal anatomy. Important structures should be identified during dissection and this identification should be explicit, particularly when operating with trainees whose perception of the situation may differ from that of an experienced surgeon. When operating in the vicinity of an important peripheral nerve or when the relevant anatomy is ambiguous, sharp dissection or bipolar cautery is favored over standard cautery. Care is taken to avoid excessive retraction or handling of nerves. These points

assume particular importance when the operation becomes challenging or stressful; hemostasis achieved at the expense of damage to an important peripheral nerve may proved to be a pyrrhic victory.

### Phrenic Nerve

The phrenic nerve provides motor, sensory, and sympathetic input to and from the diaphragm. It also provides some of the innervation to the mediastinal pleura. The phrenic nerve arises from the ventral rami of the third, fourth, and fifth cervical nerves. It follows a similar course on the right and left sides. In the neck, the phrenic nerve is found on the anterior aspect of the anterior scalene muscle. It then course inferiorly and passes medial to the insertion of the anterior scalene onto the first rib. As the nerve exits the thoracic inlet and enters the superior mediastinum, it is found anterior to the subclavian artery and posterior to the confluence of the subclavian and internal jugular veins. It then travels on the lateral aspect of the superior vena cava (on the right) and the proximal aortic arch anterior to the first intercostal vein (on the left) before continuing along the mediastinal pleura anterior to the pulmonary hilum. It is accompanied at this level by the pericardiophrenic artery and vein, which are branches of the internal mammary artery and vein, respectively. The nerve then inserts on the central portion the diaphragm. Occasionally, an accessory phrenic nerve arises from the cervical nerve roots and follow a similar course.

Injury to the phrenic nerve is of considerable concern to the thoracic surgeon for 2 reasons. First, the location of the nerve in the neck and the anterior hilum put it at risk during the majority of thoracic operative procedures in the neck, hemithorax, or mediastinum. Second, the phrenic nerve provides the only source of motor control to the diaphragm, meaning that neuropraxial injury to the nerve places the patient at high risk for postoperative respiratory complications, and significant injury results in unilateral diaphragmatic paralysis. Protection of the phrenic nerve depends on careful identification and sharp dissection (as with anterior scalenectomy during supraclavicular first rib resection), extreme caution (as with thymectomy, where the nerve frequently appears around the superior pole of the thymus in a deceptively anterior location), or outright avoidance (as with decortication for empyema, during which stripping of the mediastinal pleura should be undertaken judiciously). The phrenic nerve can also be injured during cryoablation or pulmonary vein isolation for the treatment of atrial arrhythmias, radiofrequency ablation of lung tumors, or by excessive cooling of the heart during cardiopulmonary bypass.

A full-thickness injury to the phrenic nerve recognized at the time of surgery should be treated with repair or interposition graft. For an injury too extensive to permit reconstruction, some surgeons consider performing plication of the diaphragm at the same operation. More often, however, phrenic nerve injury is unrecognized until the postoperative period when a chest radiograph demonstrates an elevated hemidiaphragm. In this case, there are few immediate surgical options. The best course is to wait a period of months to observe whether diaphragmatic function returns. After 12 to 18 months, if there has been no change in function and the patient is symptomatic, diaphragmatic plication should be considered.

## Vagus Nerve

The vagus nerve (cranial nerve X) constitutes the parasympathetic innervation of the cervical, thoracic, and abdominal viscera. Importantly, it also carries motor and sensory fibers that innervate the larynx via the superior and recurrent laryngeal nerves (RLNs). The vagus nerve arises in the brainstem, exits the skull through the jugular foramen, and enters the neck in the posterior of the carotid sheath along with the internal jugular vein. It enters the chest anterior to the subclavian artery and posterior to the innominate vein, in a more medial position than the phrenic nerve. On the right the RLN branches off the vagus nerve at the level of the subclavian, whereas on the left it arises at level of the aortic arch. In the superior mediastinum, the vagus nerve runs posteroinferiorly along the trachea, lateral to the vena cava (on the right) and the aortic arch (on the left) before passing posterior to the pulmonary hilum. In the upper and middle thorax, the vagus nerve gives rise to extensive cardiac, pulmonary, and esophageal plexuses. Caudally, the left and right vagi pass through the esophageal hiatus anterior and posterior to the esophagus, respectively, although the communication between the 2 nerves is extensive.

The vagus nerve may be at risk for injury during extensive posterior hilar dissection or sampling of subcarinal or paratracheal lymph nodes. The left vagus is also in the immediate vicinity during left upper lobectomy or sampling of aortopulmonary lymph nodes. The latter is significant because injury to the vagus nerve at this level also compromises the left RLN. Distal to this, however, injury to the vagus nerve (particularly unilateral injury) is probably of little consequence. Indeed, both vagi are routinely sacrificed during esophageal surgery with marginal effect on patient outcomes. Injury to both vagi proximal to the cardiac plexus would theoretically result in unopposed sympathetic innervation to the heart, as seen after cardiac transplantation; however, this scenario is exceedingly unlikely. In practice, most surgeons would not repair an injured vagus nerve.

## Recurrent Laryngeal Nerve

The RLN is a branch of the vagus nerve and provides innervation to all the muscles of the ipsilateral larynx with the exception of the cricothyroid. Additionally, the nerve carries sensory information from the larynx and cervical esophagus. On the right side, the RLN arises at the level of the subclavian artery, hooks around the artery posteriorly, and then courses superiorly in the tracheoesophageal groove. On the left, the RLN arises at the level of the aortic arch, hooks around the arch posteriorly lateral to the ligamentum arteriosum, and runs superiorly in the tracheoesophageal groove. Both nerves insert on the inferior lateral larynx at the approximate level of the inferior parathyroid gland. However, considerable variability exists. The course of the RLN is said to be more consistent on the left than on the right. An infrequent anatomic variant is the nonrecurrent laryngeal nerve. This occurs predominantly on the right in association with vascular anomalies (ie, right subclavian arising directly from the aortic arch). In this case, the nerve travels along either the superior or inferior thyroid artery.

Injury to the RLN can occur in the chest during vascular procedures on the right subclavian artery or aortic arch, during sampling of aortopulmonary lymph nodes, or by aggressive biopsy technique or use of cautery on the left side of the trachea during mediastinoscopy. However, injury to the RLN is more common in the neck during procedures involving the thyroid or parathyroid glands, trachea, or cervical esophagus. Considerable debate exists among endocrine surgeons regarding the best way to avoid RLN injury during thyroidectomy or parathyroidectomy, with some favoring continuous nerve monitoring to facilitate identification of the nerve and others arguing that the RLN should be avoided altogether. During tracheal resection and reconstruction, the RLN is avoided by keeping the dissection as close to the trachea as possible. For procedures on the cervical esophagus such as cricopharyngeal myotomy for Zenker's diverticulum, the esophagus is approached posterolaterally to reflect the RLN anteriorly and avoid injury.

Unilateral injury to the RLN results in paralysis of the ipsilateral vocal cord and hoarseness. Bilateral

RLN injury results in potentially catastrophic airway compromise if unrecognized, and should prompt immediate tracheostomy if the injury is felt to be significant. If injury to the RLN is suspected during the course of surgery and circumstances permit (eg, total thyroidectomy for small papillary thyroid cancer), surgery on the contralateral thyroid lobe should be abandoned.

The routine use of continuous nerve monitoring during thyroid surgery has led to increased intraoperative detection of RLN injuries. The majority of these injuries are neuropraxial and do not require further intervention. For more severe injuries, including those that involve complete transection of the nerve, there is controversy regarding the most appropriate management. Classic teaching held that repair of the nerve was contraindicated because of the potential for laryngeal synkinesis. Synkinesis is the process of misdirected renervation of the complex musculature of the larynx, leading to paradoxic motion and in rare cases airway compromise. In contrast, spontaneous nerve regeneration (which can occur for distal injuries even if the connective tissue layers of the nerve are damaged) was thought to lead to better functional outcome. Newer data suggest that this is probably not the case, and the current practice of most surgeons is to perform nerve repair if significant injury is recognized. Alternatively, the ansa cervicalis may be located on the lateral aspect of the carotid sheath and anastomosed to the distal end of the transected nerve. This does not restore function to the larynx, but does seem to provide tone to the associated muscles and improve the functional outcome of spontaneous regeneration.

Management of a unilateral RLN nerve injury detected postoperatively is an extensive topic. There are multiple techniques for restoring maximal airway patency and phonation, including gelfoam injection, cord medicalization, and laryngoplasty. None of these techniques should be used in the immediate postoperative period because the potential for delayed nerve recovery is substantial. Current recommendations are that for a stable patient with no significant aspiration risk, no irreversible procedures should be performed in the first 12 to 18 months.

### Stellate Ganglion/Sympathetic Trunk

The stellate (or cervicothoracic) ganglion is formed by the fusion of the inferior cervical ganglion and superior thoracic ganglion. It is the most superior ganglion in the thoracic sympathetic trunk. The sympathetic trunk contains the postsynaptic cell bodies of the sympathetic autonomic nervous system. After receiving input from presynaptic nerves with bodies located in the spinal cord, these postsynaptic nerve fibers form splanchnic nerves that terminate in the cardiac, pulmonary, or esophageal plexus, or rejoin spinal nerves and provide motor innervation to the blood vessels, hair follicles, and sweat glands of the body wall and upper extremity. The stellate ganglion is located on the anterior surface of the transverse process of the C7 vertebral body immediately superior to the posterior insertion of the first rib. Extending caudally, each successive vertebral body is associated with a ganglion of the sympathetic chain with connections to the ganglia located above and below. The sympathetic ganglion immediately inferior to the stellate ganglion may also communicate directly with the intercostal nerve above via the nerve of Kuntz. In the posterior thorax, the sympathetic trunk is found deep to the parietal pleura with each ganglion located anterior and superior to the costovertebral junction of its associated rib.

Temporary or permanent interruption of the stellate ganglion or sympathetic trunk may be desirable in certain circumstances. Regional block of the stellate ganglion has been used with limited success for temporary palliation of upper extremity Raynaud syndrome, complex regional pain disorders, and refractory angina. Permanent division of the sympathetic trunk at the level of T3 or T4 is a well-described treatment for palmar hyperhidrosis. In these instances, the negative effects of sympathectomy are weighed carefully against potential benefit; the same cannot be said in the case of inadvertent injury. The stellate ganglion in particular can be damaged during resection of the first rib for thoracic outlet syndrome if division of the posterior rib occurs too medially. It may also be involved directly by a superior sulcus (Pancoast) tumor or be damaged during tumor resection. The sympathetic chain is more protected in its posterior location in the thorax. However, injury is possible during pleurectomy for benign or malignant disease, or during anterior exposure of the thoracic spine. Reconstruction of the sympathetic chain with sural nerve graft has been described, but is probably not indicated in most cases. Once injured, no reconstruction options exist for the stellate ganglion because it contains the neuronal cell and innumerable synaptic connections.

Disruption of the stellate ganglion results in ipsilateral Horner syndrome (a triad of ptosis, meiosis, and facial anhydrosis caused by a lack of sympathetic input to the face). Injury to the inferior sympathetic trunk produces variable results depending on the level at which the injury occurs. Sympathectomy performed at the level of T2 or higher seems to result in some changes in cardiac physiology, namely depression in resting heart rate, shortening of QTc interval, and possibly blunting of exercise response. Cases of life-threatening bradycardia have been reported, but for the most part these changes are mild and clinically unimportant. Compensatory truncal or gustatory sweating (caused by disruption of excessive sudomotor function in the ipsilateral upper extremity) is more apparent and probably occurs in more than one-half of patients after sympathectomy for hyperhidrosis. It is not clear whether these results can be applied to patients with normal preoperative sudomotor function.

### Brachial Plexus

The brachial plexus is the most anatomically complex nerve structure routinely encountered by thoracic surgeons. Typically, the plexus is formed by the ventral rami the spinal nerves originating from C5, C6, C7, C8, and T1. Occasionally it is formed from the spinal nerves of C4 through C8 or C6 through T2, leading to a prefixed or postfixed brachial plexus, respectively. The 5 nerve roots of the plexus join to form upper, middle, and lower trunks, followed by divisions, cords, and ultimately terminal branches (the musculocutaneous, axillary, radial, median, and ulnar nerve). At its origin, the brachial plexus emerges between the anterior and middle scalene muscles and follows a course along with the subclavian artery that leads superior to the first rib, through the axilla, and into the medial aspect of the upper extremity. Proximal branches such as the long thoracic nerve (C5, C6, and C7), dorsal scapular nerve (C5), median pectoral nerve (C8 and T1), and thoracodorsal nerve (C6, C7, and C8) exit the plexus superior to the first rib and run along the lateral chest wall.

The brachial plexus provides essentially the entire motor and sensory innervation to the upper extremity as well as some of the muscles of the chest wall. Traumatic or iatrogenic injury to the main plexus or any of its branches results in deficits that range from minor sensory loss to moderate functional difficulty (eg, scapula alata or "winged scapula" from long thoracic nerve injury) to extreme disability (eg, "Erb's palsy" from avulsion of the upper brachial plexus).

The brachial plexus may be damaged during any procedure by poor patient positioning. Abduction, external rotation, or overextension of the shoulder, particularly when coupled with contralateral head flexion, can cause traction injury to the superior nerve roots. An unsupported and dependent shoulder in the lateral decubitus position is at particularly high risk. The resulting palsy is usually temporary;

however, the deficit is occasionally permanent. Intraoperatively, the brachial plexus is encountered during procedures involving the thoracic outlet. This includes first rib resection and scalenectomy and resection of superior sulcus tumors. First rib resection involves careful identification and dissection of the 3 trunks of the brachial plexus with judicious use of bipolar cautery; monopolar cautery should never be used. Paralytic agents are not used during the procedure so that inadvertent stimulation of the plexus (or the adjacent phrenic nerve) is immediately apparent. Special care is taken to avoid excessive retraction on the nerve trunks during exposure of the first rib. As a general rule, if exposure is excellent, retraction is too vigorous. Superior sulcus tumors represent another challenge for the surgeon because the patient's tumor may invade the plexus directly and the surrounding anatomy may be fibrotic from neoadjuvant chemoradiation. The surgeon may choose to sacrifice a portion of the brachial plexus as part of a thorough oncologic operation. This possibility should be discussed with the patient preoperatively.

## SUMMARY

A nerve injury after thoracic surgery often feels like a technical failure to surgeon and patient alike. For the surgeon, there is the knowledge that the relevant anatomy was misidentified or poor surgical technique was used and a preventable error resulted; for the patient, there is temporary or lasting functional deficit that may result in substantial morbidity and decrease quality of life. Progress has been made in the field of nerve repair and regeneration; prompt identification and appropriate management can significantly mitigate the morbidity of nerve injuries. However, the surgeon should be mindful that there is no current remedy for these injuries that is as reliable as avoidance.

## FURTHER READINGS

Arcasoy SM, Jett JR. Superior pulmonary sulcus tumors and Pancoast's syndrome. N Engl J Med 1997; 337(19):1370–6.

Illig K, Thompson R, Frieschlag J, et al. Thoracic outlet syndrome. 1st edition. New York: Springer-Verlag; 2013.

Kwong KF, Cooper LB, Bennett LA, et al. Clinical experience in 397 consecutive thoracoscopic sympathectomies. Ann Thorac Surg 2005;80(3):1063–6 [discussion: 1066].

Macchiarini P, Dartevelle P, Chapelier A, et al. Technique for resecting primary and metastatic nonbronchogenic tumors of the thoracic outlet. Ann Thorac Surg 1993;55(3):611–8.

Menorca RM, Fussell TS, Elfar JC. Nerve physiology: mechanisms of injury and recovery. Hand Clin 2013;29(3):317–30.

Randolph G. Surgery of the thyroid and parathyroid glands. 2nd edition. Philadelphia: Elsevier/Saunders; 2013.

Seddon HJ, Medawar PB, Smith H. Rate of regeneration of peripheral nerves in man. J Physiol 1943;102(2): 191–215.

Selke F, del Nido P, Swanson S. Sabiston and Spencer surgery of the chest. 8th edition. Philadelphia: Elsevier/Saunders; 2010.

Shields T, Locicero J III, Reed C, et al. General thoracic surgery. 7th edition. Philadelphia: Lippincott Williams and Wilkins; 2009.

Sunderland S. A classification of peripheral nerve injuries producing loss of function. Brain 1951;74(4): 491–516.

# Chest Wall Resection and Reconstruction
## Management of Complications

Kweku Hazel, MD, Michael J. Weyant, MD*

## KEYWORDS

- Chest wall resection • Prosthetic reconstruction • Complications of chest wall resection

## KEY POINTS

- The main complications after chest wall resection and reconstruction include respiratory complications and wound/prosthetic complications.
- The main risk factors for complications after chest wall resection include age, size of defect, and concomitant lung resection.
- It is critical to provide adequate tissue coverage over the prosthesis to minimize wound complications.
- A rigid prosthesis should be considered to reconstruct the largest of anterolateral chest wall defects.

## BACKGROUND

Chest wall resections are most commonly performed for tumors, infection, radiation necrosis, and trauma.[1] Chest wall resections are defined as the removal of a full-thickness portion of the chest wall, including muscle, bone, and possibly skin. The decision to perform a reconstruction of the chest wall after resection depends on the propensity of the defect to cause paradoxic chest wall motion and possibly respiratory failure as well as the cosmetic result of the defect. Defects in the anterior chest less than 5 cm and posterior defects less than 10 cm generally do not need to be reconstructed with prosthetic material. Modern prosthetic materials available for the replacement of the bony chest wall are far superior to the autogenous or cadaveric biological materials used in early reconstructive attempts.[2,3] The combination of these prosthetic materials as well as advances in the knowledge and use of myocutaneous and pedicled tissue flaps allow even the largest of defects to be reconstructed.[4]

Despite the advances in surgical reconstructive techniques and prosthetic materials, complications after chest wall resection are common and are reported to occur in 24% to 46% of patients (**Table 1**).[1–7] In general, the complications associated with chest wall resection can be thought of in 3 general areas:

1. Complications arising from being subjected to a large invasive procedure (deep venous thrombosis, urinary tract infection, anesthetic complications, renal failure)
2. Respiratory complications arising from either poor pulmonary toilet or potentially a remaining flail segment produced by the chest wall defect or
3. Surgical complications directly related to the reconstructive efforts (hemorrhage, flap hematoma, flap necrosis, wound infections, erosion of prosthesis, prosthetic infections, and so forth)

Section of General Thoracic Surgery, Division of Cardiothoracic Surgery, University of Colorado Denver School of Medicine, 12631 East 17th Avenue, MS C310, Aurora, CO 80045, USA
* Corresponding author.
*E-mail address:* Michael.weyant@ucdenver.edu

Thorac Surg Clin 25 (2015) 517–521
http://dx.doi.org/10.1016/j.thorsurg.2015.07.013
1547-4127/15/$ – see front matter © 2015 Elsevier Inc. All rights reserved.

**Table 1**
**Morbidity and mortality rates of chest wall resection and reconstruction**

| Author, Year | N | Respiratory Complications | Morbidity (%) | Mortality (%) |
|---|---|---|---|---|
| Lans et al,[5] 2009 | 220 | NR | 34.0 | 2.3 |
| Weyant et al,[6] 2006 | 262 | 11.0 | 33.2 | 3.8 |
| Mansour et al,[1] 2002 | 200 | 20.0 | 24.0 | 7.0 |
| Deschamps et al,[4] 1999 | 197 | 24.4 | 46.0 | 4.1 |
| Pairolero, 1995 | 500 | NR | NR | 3.0 |
| McKenna et al,[7] 1988 | 112 | NR | NR | 3.6 |

The most frequent complications described are respiratory in nature and are reported to occur in up to 24% of patients.[1,6]

## RESPIRATORY COMPLICATIONS

Given the high incidence and level of morbidity associated with respiratory complications after chest wall resection, a great deal of attention has been paid to postulating the mechanism behind these risks. Much debate exists as to whether there are superior reconstructive techniques that may lead to a decreased incidence of pulmonary complications. Randomized trials do not exist comparing types of prosthetic materials; populations of patients undergoing chest wall resection are quite heterogeneous, making level 1 evidence nearly impossible to obtain. The large retrospective series available suggest that over time morbidity from respiratory complications seems to be diminishing, with one of the most recent series demonstrating a respiratory complication rate of 11%[6] (see **Table 1**). These findings raise the question as to whether reconstructing the chest wall with a truly rigid prosthesis, such as a methyl methacrylate marlex mesh composite (MMMM), is more beneficial than a prosthetic mesh alone, such as polytetrafluoroethylene (PTFE) or polypropylene mesh (PPM). It is important to note that even though a lower rate of respiratory complications was reported in that study, 7 of the 10 deaths in the series were caused by respiratory complications indicating a need for continued study to reduce these events.

The available data that suggest that prosthetic reconstruction of the chest wall is beneficial is inferred from historical literature. In 1978, Thomas and colleagues[8] reported on the possible benefit of surgical stabilization of the chest wall in patients with severe flail chest. Lardinois and colleagues[9] also reported results in 55 patients with severe anterolateral flail chest who had improved respiratory mechanics after surgical chest wall stabilization. Niwa and colleagues[10] reported data in a canine model of controlled chest wall resection comparing a group who had reconstruction with prosthetic mesh and a group who had only skin closure. In this study, the size of the chest wall resection could be tightly controlled. The group of animals who did not undergo any chest wall reconstruction had significantly poorer respiratory mechanics after the procedure.

Other investigators have attempted to directly compare the type of prosthesis used and assess outcomes. Kilic and colleagues[11] reported a series of patients comparing a rigid prosthesis (MMMM) versus PTFE. The investigators reported reduced paradoxic respiratory motion, lower operative morbidity, and shorter length of stay in patients having the rigid prosthesis in this nonrandomized study. In a series of patients having MMMM reconstruction, Lardinois and colleagues[12] report no difference in preoperative and postoperative forced expiratory volume in the first second of expiration even after concomitant lung resection.[12] The finding that respiratory function can be unaltered with the use of a rigid prosthesis is enticing, but without an adequate comparison with nonrigid reconstruction the question remains open.

Given the lack of prospective randomized trials it is unclear whether the surgical technique or type of prosthesis clearly influences the incidence of respiratory complications. Advances in anesthetic techniques or critical care may also be playing a role. Overall it is reasonable to consider the use of a rigid prosthesis in carefully selected patients with large anterolateral chest wall defects.

## WOUND AND PROSTHETIC COMPLICATIONS

Wound complications and complications related to the prosthesis are second in incidence to respiratory complications after chest wall resection and reconstruction. These complications are reported to occur in 7% to 20% of patients.[6,7] The main complications related to the wound and prosthesis are wound infection, wound dehiscence, and dislodgement or fracture of the prosthesis

(**Figs. 1** and **2**). Complications that are directly related to the plastic surgical reconstructive efforts include flap hematoma and flap loss/necrosis.

Any wound infection after reconstruction of the chest wall with prosthetic material should raise the suspicion of an underlying infection or compromise of the prosthesis. Wound complications after prosthetic chest wall reconstruction often do not present with signs of overt sepsis but with more indolent findings, such as drainage of the wound without cellulitis. These complications most often present weeks to months after surgery. The presence of a wound infection, however, should not trigger an immediate return to the operating room to remove the prosthesis. The combination of the use of imaging studies and clinical impression should be used to determine the need for prosthesis removal. Computed tomography is the main imaging tool used to evaluate a possibly compromised prosthesis. This imaging modality can illustrate whether there is fluid and air surrounding the prosthesis indicating a deeper wound infection (see **Fig. 1**).

Wound infections are reported to occur in approximately 5% of chest wall resections reconstructed with a prosthesis.[4,6] Weyant and colleagues[6] report that only 8 of 14 (57%) patients who developed a wound infection required removal of the prosthesis. Deschamps and colleagues[4] reported similarly that only 5 of 9 patients who developed wound infections required prosthesis removal.[4] Given the possibility of retaining the prosthesis even in the event of a wound

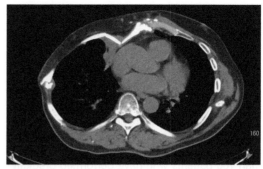

**Fig. 2.** Computed tomographic image of a patient 2 years after resection of a large anterior chest wall tumor. The patient suffered a traumatic fracture of the prosthesis. The fracture's end is adjacent to the right atrium. The prosthesis was removed without complication.

infection, a through inspection of the wound and imaging modalities should be used to make the decision to remove the prosthesis. These reports also suggest that the type of prosthesis and prosthetic material may influence the need for prosthesis removal in the event of a deep wound infection. Deschamps and colleagues[4] report that only patients who had PPM implants required prosthesis removal, whereas none of the patients who had PTFE and a wound infection needed to have the prosthesis removed. Weyant and colleagues[6] report that the rate of prosthesis removal was similar in rigid and nonrigid (PTFE, PPM) groups; however, the patients who had a rigid MMMM prosthesis used had a significantly higher overall wound complication rate. These results are tempered by the finding that patients who had a rigid prosthesis had significantly larger chest wall defects compared with the nonrigid group. Although it is unclear whether it is the material used for reconstruction or the size of the lesion that is responsible for more prosthetic complications, these data suggest that adequate soft tissue coverage over a rigid or polypropylene prosthesis is critical to the success of the operation.

It is reported that autologous tissue transfer is used in 19% to 57% of patients, and advances in these techniques have significantly improved our ability to perform chest wall reconstruction.[1,6] The most commonly used autografts are latissimus flaps, pectoralis flaps, transverse rectus abdominis musculocutaneous flaps, pedicled omentum flaps, and skin grafts. These procedures can lead to complications both at the donor site as well as the location of transposition. Flap hematomas are reported to occur in 3% to 5% of patients and usually require nothing more than a procedure to evacuate the hematoma in the

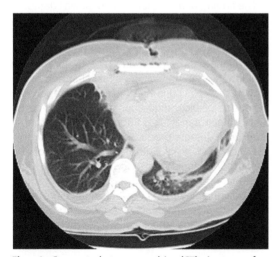

**Fig. 1.** Computed tomographic (CT) image of a patient 3 weeks after sternal resection and reconstruction with an MMMM prosthesis. CT image demonstrates both fluid and air around the prosthesis as well as a draining sinus tract to the skin. The prosthesis was removed with no difficulty.

operating room. Flap loss from ischemia occurs in up to 5% of patients and can be a difficult problem to treat, requiring alternative methods of soft tissue coverage.[5] Donor site complications are rare but include donor site hernias and infection.

## PREDICTORS OF COMPLICATIONS

Very few studies have provided analysis if predictors of complications after chest wall resection and reconstruction. The two series with greater than 100 patients who have performed predictive analysis are summarized in **Box 1**. Many univariate predictors have been evaluated, but relatively few turn out to be significant predictors of postoperative complications. The most significant predictors of complications seem to be the size of the lesion, patient age, concomitant lung resection, ulceration of the chest wall lesion before resection, and the use of omentum in the reconstruction.

Regarding the size of the lesion, most historical studies have quantified the size of the lesions resected by stating the number of ribs resected in the specimen. Weyant and colleagues[6] used the area (square centimeters) measurements from pathology reports to more accurately describe the size of the lesions. For example, the mean number of ribs removed in all of the prosthesis groups was 3, yet there were significant differences in the size based on area measurements. Using more precise size measurements should allow for more accurate description of complications.

The report by Weyant and colleagues[6] reports that concomitant lung resection is a significant predictor of postoperative complications. This finding is not entirely surprising given the additional respiratory compromise produced by the added lung resection. In their series, concomitant lung resection was performed in 141 (54%) of patients. The increased risk of postoperative complications seemed to be specific to anatomic lung resections (segmentectomy, lobectomy, bilobectomy, pneumonectomy), whereas the addition of a wedge resection did not increase the risk of respiratory complications. Importantly, although mortality predictors cannot be reliably analyzed because of the small sample size, it seems that there is significant risk of death when combining chest wall resection with pneumonectomy. The report from Weyant and colleagues[6] contained 9 patients who had combined pneumonectomy with chest wall resection. These patients had a postoperative mortality rate of 44% (4 of 9), indicating the need for caution in deciding on operative therapy for these patients.

The finding of ulceration of a chest wall defect to be a predictor of postoperative wound complications is not surprising, but it helps to illustrate possible ways of preventing these complications. Ulcerations can be produced by a tumor eroding through the skin or necrosis of skin harmed by radiation therapy. Lans and colleagues[5] report the incidence of ulcerating chest wall wounds to be 14% in their series. It is important to note that in chest wall defects produced by radiation therapy, the ulcerated area is the proverbial tip of the iceberg; in planning for these resections, a wider area than is visible usually needs to be resected. An additional anecdotal preventive measure in patients with ulcerating chest wounds is to consider antibiotic therapy and local wound debridement before the definitive resection.

## RECENT ADVANCES

The high incidence of complications after chest wall resection has led to a continued interest in improving materials and surgical techniques to

---

**Box 1**
**Multivariate predictors of complications after chest wall resection**

*Factors Analyzed in Univariate Analysis*

Type of prosthesis

Anatomic location

Sternal resection

Concomitant lung resection

Medical comorbidity

Prior radiotherapy

Prior chemotherapy

Reoperation

Soft tissue transfer

Drains

Age

Size (cm$^2$)

Tumor type

Ulceration

Use of omentum

*Significant Multivariate Predictors of Complications*

Age

Size of defect

Concomitant lung resection

Ulceration of chest wall lesion

Use of omentum

reduce morbidity after these operations. Recent development of titanium rib plating systems has led to the extrapolation of these techniques to chest wall resection. Fabre and colleagues[13] reported one of the largest series of chest wall reconstructions using a combination of titanium plates coupled with prosthetic materials. In this series of 24 patients, the investigators found no increase in complication rates compared with previous series and also demonstrate little change in spirometry values when comparing preoperative and postoperative values. It is unclear whether this technique represents any significant advantage over previously described techniques, but clearly it is a viable option to consider when reconstructing the chest wall.

Over the last 20 years, thoracic surgeons have been dedicated to using and applying minimally invasive surgical techniques to minimize the trauma of surgery for their patients. Recently, video-assisted thoracoscopic surgery (VATS) has been implemented in the arsenal of techniques used in chest wall resection. Hennon and colleagues[14] described their experience using VATS as an alternative to open chest wall resection during resection of lung tumors invading the chest wall where full-thickness resection of the bony chest wall is required. They reported on a series of 17 patients who had en bloc lung and chest wall resections using a VATS approach. Overall the complication and morbidity rates were not improved over previous reports; however, the mean age in this series was 76 years, indicating the investigators were attempting these procedures in the most frail of patients. Cleary, more study is warranted to establish these newer techniques in mainstream clinical practice.

## SUMMARY

Clear improvements have been made over time in our ability to technically perform chest wall resection and reconstructions. There continues to be a high morbidity rate after these procedures, the most significant of which are respiratory in nature. Caution should be used when considering the combination of a pneumonectomy and chest wall resection, as there is a significant mortality rate. Providing adequate soft tissue coverage over an inserted prosthesis can minimize wound and prosthetic complications, and working with an experienced plastic surgical team is extremely useful. There is no clear superior prosthetic material, although large anterolateral chest wall defects may be better served using a rigid prosthesis.

## REFERENCES

1. Mansour KA, Thourani VH, Losken A, et al. Chest wall resections and reconstruction: a 25-year experience. Ann Thorac Surg 2002;73:1720–6.
2. Carbone M, Pastorino U. Surgical treatment of chest wall tumors. World J Surg 2001;25:218–30.
3. Arnold PG, Pairolero PC. Chest wall reconstruction: an account of 500 consecutive patients. Plast Reconstr Surg 1996;98:804–10.
4. Deschamps C, Tirnaksiz BM, Darbandi R, et al. Early and long-term results of prosthetic chest wall reconstruction. J Thorac Cardiovasc Surg 1999;117: 588–92.
5. Lans TE, van der Pol C, Wouters MW, et al. Complications in wound healing after chest wall resection in cancer patients; a multivariate analysis of 220 patients. J Thorac Oncol 2009;4:639–43.
6. Weyant MJ, Bains MS, Venkatraman E, et al. Results of chest wall resection and reconstruction with and without rigid prosthesis. Ann Thorac Surg 2006;81: 279–85.
7. McKenna RJ Jr, Mountain CF, McMurtrey MJ, et al. Current techniques for chest wall reconstruction: expanded possibilities for treatment. Ann Thorac Surg 1988;46:508–12.
8. Thomas AN, Blaisdell FW, Lewis FR Jr, et al. Operative stabilization for flail chest after blunt trauma. J Thorac Cardiovasc Surg 1978;75(6):793–801.
9. Lardinois D, Krueger T, Dusmet M, et al. Pulmonary function testing after operative stabilisation of the chest wall for flail chest. Eur J Cardiothorac Surg 2001;20(3):496–501.
10. Niwa H, Yamakawa Y, Kobayashi S, et al. Preservation of pulmonary function by chest wall reconstruction. Nihon Geka Gakkai Zasshi 1991;92(9): 1359–62.
11. Kilic D, Gungor A, Kavukcu S, et al. Comparison of mersilene mesh-methyl metacrylate sandwich and polytetrafluoroethylene grafts for chest wall reconstruction. J Invest Surg 2006;19:353–60.
12. Lardinois D, Müller M, Furrer M, et al. Functional assessment of chest wall integrity after methylmethacrylate reconstruction. Ann Thorac Surg 2000; 69:919–23.
13. Fabre D, El Batti S, Singhal S, et al. A paradigm shift for sternal reconstruction using a novel titanium rib bridge system following oncological resections. Eur J Cardiothorac Surg 2012;42:965–70.
14. Hennon MW, Dexter EU, Huang M, et al. Does thoracoscopic surgery decrease the morbidity of combined lung and chest wall resection? Ann Thorac Surg 2015;99:1929–35.

# Postoperative Chylothorax

Nicola Martucci, MD, Maura Tracey, RN, Gaetano Rocco, MD, FRCSEd*

## KEYWORDS

- Chylothorax • Thoracic duct • Chylous effusion • Postoperative complication

## KEY POINTS

- Chylothorax is an unusual but serious complication of thoracic surgical procedures, and is associated with considerable morbidity if not addressed in a timely fashion.
- Thoracic surgeons should be familiar with the anatomy of the thoracic duct, the causes of chylothorax, and the implications of a prolonged chyle leak.
- Postoperative chylothorax is typically treated conservatively with reasonable success rates. The timing of direct intervention with percutaneous embolization of the cisterna chyli or thoracoscopic ligation of the thoracic duct is controversial, and direct intervention is often reserved for refractory cases.

## INTRODUCTION

Chylothorax is a potentially serious complication of thoracic surgical procedures, especially surgery of the esophagus, with an incidence ranging from 0.5% to 2%.[1–3] It is a pathologic condition characterized by the accumulation of chyle, a fluid rich in fats, in the pleural space, and is generally secondary to injury of the thoracic duct. Approximately 2.4 L of chyle are transported through the lymphatic system every day and damage to or rupture of the thoracic duct may cause a large and rapid accumulation of fluid in the pleural space, which is a severe complication with high mortality (up to 30% if untreated)[2,4] caused by nutritional deficiency, respiratory disorders, dehydration, and immunosuppression. The ideal treatment of this complication is still not completely defined; over the years various methods of treatment have been proposed, including simple chest drainage, total parenteral nutrition alone, and different surgical options.

## ELEMENTS OF ANATOMY

The thoracic duct arises from the cisterna chyli, or receptaculum chyli, described in 1651 by J. Pecquet.[5] The cisterna chyli is in the abdomen, located anterior to the second lumbar vertebra, posterior to and on the right of the abdominal aorta. The thoracic duct originates from the upper portion of the cisterna and vertically enters the chest through the aortic orifice of the diaphragm, passing between the azygos vein and the aorta. In the lower part of the posterior mediastinum, the thoracic duct runs to the right of the spine, in the space between the aorta and esophagus. Then, at the level of the fourth thoracic vertebra, the duct becomes oblique to the left, crosses the midline, and moves to the left of the spine along the back to the aortic arch and anterior to the subclavian vein until it reaches the apex of the chest. At this point, the thoracic duct forms an arch before the scalene muscle and then terminates at the junction between the left subclavian vein and the jugular vein. In total, the thoracic duct measures 36 to 45 cm in length and 2 to 3 mm in diameter. This anatomy of the thoracic duct is found in 65% of the population.[6] However, the thoracic duct presents different anatomic variants, because it is a double structure during embryogenesis and it can triple in up to 40% of individuals. The presence of anatomic variations

Division of Thoracic Surgery, Department of Thoracic Surgery and Oncology, Istituto Nazionale Tumori, Fondazione Pascale, IRCCS, Via Semmola 81, Naples 80131, Italy
* Corresponding author.
*E-mail address:* Gaetano.Rocco@btopenworld.com

Thorac Surg Clin 25 (2015) 523–528
http://dx.doi.org/10.1016/j.thorsurg.2015.07.014
1547-4127/15/$ – see front matter © 2015 Elsevier Inc. All rights reserved.

together with the presence of multiple small lymphatic vessel tributaries, shown by several anatomic studies, is probably responsible of the incidence of postoperative chylothorax, irrespective of the surgeon's meticulous attention and skill.

The primary role of the thoracic duct is to drain the lymph and the chyle that originate from the gastrointestinal tract: the chyle contains large amounts of cholesterol, triglycerides, chylomicrons, fat-soluble vitamins, and albumin, whereas the lymph consists of immunoglobulins, enzymes, digestive products, and white blood cells, most of which are lymphocytes.[7] In adults, the thoracic duct transports up to 4 L of a chyle per day and its flow depends on several factors, such as diet, medications, and gastrointestinal absorption. The flow is maintained by the combined effect of intra-abdominal and intrathoracic pressures, arterial compression of the neighboring vessels, and the contraction of the muscles of the duct.[8]

Rupture of the thoracic duct leads to a significant loss of fat, protein, and T lymphocytes with consequent disorders of the immunologic and nutritional profiles together with disorders related to the accumulation of large quantities of fluid in the pleural space.[9,10] In general, after an acute phase related to mechanical compression of the intrathoracic organs caused by accumulation of fluid, complications related to chylothorax depend on the consequences of the chronic loss of chyle, whereas immunosuppression occurs because of the loss of lymphocytes and immunoglobulins, making these patients vulnerable to infection. The loss of electrolytes can result in hypovolemia, hyponatremia, hypocalcemia, and metabolic acidosis, whereas malnutrition is the result of chronic loss of fatty acids and proteins. All these events result in the high mortality in untreated patients with chylothorax.[2,11]

## CAUSES

The causes of chylothorax can be divided into 3 main categories: congenital, neoplastic, and traumatic. The traumatic cause is the most common, and can be blunt trauma or vertebral fractures, as well as injuries during certain diagnostic procedures, such as catheterization of the subclavian vein, central venous catheterization, or surgery. Iatrogenic injuries may involve the entire thoracic duct; lesions of the abdominal tract can occur during sympathectomy or lymph node dissection, whereas lesions of the thoracic tract may result from lung and esophageal procedures. In addition, lesions of the cervical portion of the duct may develop during lymph node dissection or neck surgery.[10] Esophageal surgery is the most common cause of iatrogenic chylothorax, with an incidence ranging from 0.2% to 10.5%,[2] and seems to be more frequent with a transhiatal or thoracoscopic approach to the esophagus. Most of the lesions occur near the arch of the aorta and azygos, where the esophagus and the thoracic duct are the closest.[12] In lung surgery, chylothorax has been reported in 2.1% of the resections.[13] Reportedly, chylothorax after lung surgery is more common on the right side and after pneumonectomy and it is probably related to mediastinal lymphadenectomy after pulmonary resection for malignancy.[13,14] Recently, the incidence of postoperative chylothorax after video-assisted thoracic surgery (VATS) lung resection and mediastinal nodal dissection for primary lung cancer was estimated to be 2.6%.[15]

## CLINICAL FEATURES

In the postoperative period the presence of chylothorax should be suspected when an abundant pleural collection of more than 500 mL/d with milky features occurs between the second and tenth postoperative days. Usually, the effusion is evident when the patient resumes oral intake.[10] The different clinical aspects of chylothorax depend on the amount of chyle lost, as well as its cause. A rapid and abundant loss is generally associated with hypovolemia and respiratory distress from the accumulation of chyle in the pleural space. Malnutrition is caused by the loss of proteins, fat, and vitamins, whereas loss of electrolytes can cause hyponatremia and hypocalcemia.[9] The significant loss of immunoglobulins, T cells, and proteins can cause immunosuppression, which predisposes the patient to systemic opportunistic infections, whereas infection of the pleural effusion is rare because chyle is bacteriostatic.[16] Digoxin and amiodarone may be ineffective when administered to patients with chylothorax because they are expelled through the chyle in the pleural space.[1] Pleural effusion may be 1-sided, either right (50%), left (33%), or bilateral (16.66%), and its location depends on the point of duct injury. Lesions above the fifth thoracic vertebra determine left pleural effusion, whereas lesions below this level lead to right pleural effusion.[9,17]

## DIAGNOSIS

Diagnostic tests for suspected chylothorax begin with the confirmation of the diagnosis by chemical analysis of pleural fluid: a high content of lymphocytes and chylomicrons can confirm the diagnosis.[18] Radiological studies, such as traditional chest radiograph and computed tomography scan, do not allow diagnosis of chylothorax; they only indicate the presence of persistent postoperative pleural effusion. The definitive diagnosis is obtained by means of thoracentesis and subsequent laboratory analysis of collected pleural fluid. Laboratory analysis is necessary since the macroscopic features of the pleural collection may be misleading since the classic milky white color is found in only 50% of cases, because it is often serous fluid or bloody serum, or blood.[19] Therefore, chemical examination is necessary to make a diagnosis based on the presence of chylomicrons in the pleural fluid. Chylomicrons are molecular complexes of proteins and lipids synthesized in the jejunum and transported through the thoracic duct into the circulation. Pedal lymphography (PL) is considered the gold standard for the diagnosis of chylothorax and is a technique that allows the precise localization of the leak in the thoracic duct.[10,20,21] This diagnostic method also has some therapeutic effects, probably caused by tissue sclerosis induced by iodinated contrast material.[20] It is still debated whether to perform pedal lymphography only in those patients undergoing surgical repair of the leak or in all patients with postoperative chylothorax for diagnostic purposes.[14,22] The alternative to PL is intranodal lymphography (IL), which uses ultrasonography-guided detection of accessible nodes (ie, inguinal) and subsequent injection of these nodes with lipiodol. The advantages of the intranodal injection include bypassing of the lower extremities, thus yielding reduced duration of the procedure, as well as decreased radiation doses and volumes of contrast medium.[21] As a consequence, IL is preferentially used in children because of the small size of their lymphatic vessels and the commonly enlarged inguinal nodes.[21]

## TREATMENT

Treatment of postoperative chylothorax can be either conservative or surgical. Conservative therapy consists of reducing the flow of chyle by means of complete elimination of fat intake by establishing enteral or, preferably, parenteral feeding, which is considered the nutrition of choice in many studies.[10,23] Use of somatostatin or octreotide has been shown to be useful in the conservative treatment of chylothorax because these hormones reduce the production of intestinal chyle, decreasing the flow through the thoracic duct.[24–26]

Drainage of the pleural cavity is an indispensable procedure in conservative management and a chest tube without suction is always placed because suction does not allow the closure of the fistula.[10] Conservative treatment may also include talc pleurodesis, which can be performed by either talc slurry or by means of uniportal VATS in patients who are nonintubated and only sedated,[27] yielding a success rate of 73%, especially if full pulmonary reexpansion is obtained.[28] In addition, pleurodesis with OK-432, a lyophilized preparation of *Streptococcus pyogenes*, has shown an efficacy of up to 87%.[29,30] Conservative treatment including pleurodesis has been advocated as the first line of treatment of chylothorax resulting after lung surgery.[13]

Lymphangiography per se has been suggested to have a therapeutic effect in refractory postoperative chylothorax.[31] PL with subsequent catheterization of cisterna chyli or thoracic duct is another treatment option that allows percutaneous embolization and direct injection of sclerosing agents.[21,32] Reportedly, the success rate in identifying the leak with PL ranges between 64% and 86%.[21]

Percutaneous embolization of the cisterna chyli or the thoracic duct is usually performed with microcoils delivered through microcatheters and positioned both proximal and distal to the leak. In addition, cyanoacrylate glue is added to ensure complete occlusion of the duct.[21] According to the literature, the thoracic duct is successfully cannulated in only two-thirds of the patients with postoperative chylothorax. However, in these patients, successful occlusion of the thoracic duct is obtained in 90% of cases.[21] Main procedure-related complications include parenchymal bleeding, lipiodol embolization in the pulmonary system, and infection of the injection site.[21]

The timing of surgical ligation is still debated, with some surgeons suggesting that loss of more than 1 L of chyle per day for a week is evidence of failure of conservative treatment,[33] others resorting to surgery after 5 day of an output greater than 1 L per day,[34] and a few surgeons waiting for more than 2 weeks and intervening only if there are severe metabolic and nutritional imbalances.[1,35] According to some investigators,[29] early surgical treatment may be indicated if the drainage through the chest tube is greater than 500 mL during the first 24 hours after initiation of complete fasting and total parenteral nutrition.

Surgical treatment of postoperative chylothorax includes multiple options, among which the first is the direct ligation of the duct by means of a transthoracic access, proposed by Lampson[36] in 1948. The surgical ligation of the thoracic duct requires the location of the leak by means of a preoperative test, such as PL, which should help to plan the surgical procedure. Some investigators use preoperative or intraoperative administration of fats, through a nasogastric tube, which can facilitate the visualization of the leak in the thoracic duct by increasing the flow of lymph.[37] Besides the need to locate the leak, other challenges may be caused by the postoperative inflammation, with pleural thickening, which makes surgical dissection as well as suturing the inflamed tissue difficult.[10] Once the leak is identified it can be sutured or clipped, even if good results have been reported with the use of biological glues.[38] Surgery can be performed by means of thoracotomy, or more recently by VATS or a robotic approach. VATS has become the treatment of choice to reduce the invasiveness of the surgical repair of the defect in the thoracic duct.[39,40] In cases in which the loss of chyle is not identified either in thoracoscopy or thoracotomy a mass ligation of the duct may be indicated above the esophageal hiatus between the aorta, vertebral bodies, and the pericardium. This ensures duct ligation at its entry in the chest, sealing all the accessory ducts that could be the source of the chylothorax. The mass ligation of the thoracic duct is usually performed by means of thoracoscopy, especially if performed early.[41] Some investigators suggest that the ligation of the thoracic duct should be performed immediately behind the cisterna chyli using an abdominal approach.[42]

Chylothorax after esophagectomy can be an ominous event.[43] A literature and institutional review of the incidence of chylothorax in these patients was published in 2013 by Kranzfelder and colleagues.[44] Overall, there was a 2% incidence of postoperative chylothorax at their institution and 2.6% from the systematic review of the literature.[44] Early reoperation was the institutional preferred method to treat postoperative chylothorax, whereas the literature was split between studies favoring conservative treatment and those supporting a surgical approach.[44] No statistically significant difference was noted in terms of mortality and between transhiatal and transthoracic techniques.[44]

Cerfolio[4] reported a mortality of approximately 16% for patients undergoing surgical treatment of chylothorax after esophagectomy, compared with an 80% mortality after conservative treatment: these data alone seem to argue in favor of early surgical repair of leaks of the thoracic duct.[4,39]

One controversial issue is the concept of prophylactic ligation of the duct commonly performed during esophagectomy.[45,46] According to an analysis of the literature performed in 2012, enough evidence supporting prophylactic ligation during esophagectomy could be gathered.[47] However, recent evidence on 989 patients who underwent prophylactic ligation of the thoracic duct clearly showed no difference in the incidence of chylothorax in the event of prophylactic ligation, which also had an adverse effect on overall survival on multivariate analysis.[45]

In refractory cases and in cases of malignancy with patients unsuitable for surgical treatment, some investigators have described the use of a pleuroperitoneal shunt, which was first used in pediatric cases[48] and then in adults.[49] This device ensures a 1-way communication between the pleura and the peritoneum, through a pump system that is activated by a simple pressure by the patient. The shunt minimizes immunologic and nutritional deficiency and when the loss of chyle ends it can easily be removed.[8,23,50]

An alternative therapy for the treatment of postoperative chylothorax is radiotherapy, proposed because of the positive experience in the treatment of inguinal lymphatic fistulas[51] and in the management of malignant chylothorax.[52] Radiation therapy, in combination with a fat-free diet, may be an effective alternative to traditional surgical treatments but it still lacks reliable supportive data.[53]

## SUMMARY

Postoperative chylothorax is a challenging complication of major lung surgery and esophagectomy. Although it is still not certain whether it is best to proceed to concurrent thoracic duct ligation during esophagectomy or whether and when to begin conservative management, the treatment options are many and potentially effective in more than 1 clinical scenario. The association of diet and pleurodesis, the use of lymphangiography and percutaneous microcatheters to deliver microcoils and glue to achieve thoracic duct occlusion, and thoracoscopic/robotic ligation all represent minimally invasive alternatives to highly morbid repeat thoracotomies.

## REFERENCES

1. Nair SK, Petko M, Hayward MP. Aetiology and management of chylothorax in adults. Eur J Cardiothorac Surg 2007;32:362–9.
2. Wemyss-Holden SA, Launois B, Maddern GJ. Management of thoracic duct injuries after oesophagectomy. Br J Surg 2001;88:1442–8.
3. Sieczka EM, Harvey JC. Early thoracic duct ligation for postoperative chylothorax. J Surg Oncol 1996; 61:56–60.
4. Cerfolio RJ. Chylothorax after esophagogastrectomy. Thorac Surg Clin 2006;16:49–52.
5. Régnier C. Jean Pecquet (1622-1674) and his cistern. Rev Prat 1999;49:125–8.

6. Van Pernis PA. Variations of the thoracic duct. Surgery 1949;26:806–9.

7. Schlierf C, Falor WH, Wood PD, et al. Composition of human chyle chylomicrons following single fat feedings. Am J Clin Nutr 1969;22:79–86.

8. Paes ML, Powell H. Chylothorax: an update. Br J Hosp Med 1994;51:482–90.

9. McGrath EE, Blades Z, Anderson PB. Chylothorax: aetiology, diagnosis and therapeutic options. Respir Med 2010;104:1–8.

10. Chalret du Rieu M, Baulieux J, Rode A, et al. Management of postoperative chylothorax. J Visc Surg 2011;148:e346–52.

11. Wasmuth-Pietzuch A, Hansmann M, Bartmann P, et al. Congenital chylothorax: lymphopenia and high risk of neonatal infections. Acta Paediatr 2004;93:220–4.

12. Guo W, Zhao YP, Jiang YG, et al. Prevention of postoperative chylothorax with thoracic duct ligation during video-assisted thoracoscopic esophagectomy for cancer. Surg Endosc 2012;26:1332–6.

13. Cho HJ, Kim DK, Lee GD, et al. Chylothorax complicating pulmonary resection for lung cancer: effective management and pleurodesis. Ann Thorac Surg 2014;97:408–13.

14. Le Pimpec-Barthes F, D'Attellis N, Dujon A, et al. Chylothorax complicating pulmonary resection. Ann Thorac Surg 2002;73:1714–9.

15. Liu CY, Hsu PK, Huang CS, et al. Chylothorax complicating video-assisted thoracoscopic surgery for non-small cell lung cancer. World J Surg 2014;38:2875–81.

16. Dumont AE, Mayer DJ, Mulholland JH. The suppression of immunologic activity by diversion of thoracic lymph. Ann Surg 1964;160:373–83.

17. Bessone LN, Ferguson TB, Burford TH. Chylothorax. Ann Thorac Surg 1971;12:527–50.

18. Agrawal V, Doelken P, Sahn SA. Pleural fluid analysis in chylous pleural effusion. Chest 2008;133:1436–41.

19. Rahman NM, Chapman SJ, Davies RJ. Pleural effusion: a structured approach to care. Br Med Bull 2005;72:31–47.

20. Boffa DJ, Sands MJ, Rice TW, et al. A critical evaluation of a percutaneous diagnostic and treatment strategy for chylothorax after thoracic surgery. Eur J Cardiothorac Surg 2008;33:435–9.

21. Lee EW, Shin JH, Ko HK, et al. Lymphangiography to treat postoperative lymphatic leakage: a technical review. Korean J Radiol 2014;15:724–32.

22. Vallieres E, Shamji FM, Todd TR. Postpneumonectomy chylothorax. Ann Thorac Surg 1993;55(4):1006–8.

23. Riquet M, Assouad J, Le Pimpec Barthes F. Traitment du chylothorax. EMC-Chirurgie 2004;6:662–81.

24. Al-Zubairy SA, Al-Jazairi AS. Octreotide as a therapeutic option for management of chylothorax. Ann Pharmacother 2003;37:679–82.

25. Kalomenidis I. Octreotide and chylothorax. Curr Opin Pulm Med 2006;12:264–7.

26. Kelly RF, Shumway SJ. Conservative management of postoperative chylothorax using somatostatin. Ann Thorac Surg 2000;69:1944–5.

27. Rocco G, Martucci N, La Manna C, et al. Ten-year experience on 644 patients undergoing single-port (uniportal) video-assisted thoracoscopic surgery. Ann Thorac Surg 2013;96:434–8.

28. Akin H, Olcmen A, Isgorucu O, et al. Approach to patients with chylothorax complicating pulmonary resection. Thorac Cardiovasc Surg 2012;60:135–9.

29. Shimizu K, Yoshida J, Nishimura M, et al. Treatment strategy for chylothorax after pulmonary resection and lymph node dissection for lung cancer. J Thorac Cardiovasc Surg 2002;124:499–502.

30. Takuwa T, Yoshida J, Ono S, et al. Low-fat diet management strategy for chylothorax after pulmonary resection and lymph node dissection for primary lung cancer. J Thorac Cardiovasc Surg 2013;146:571–4.

31. Kawasaki R, Sugimoto K, Fujii M, et al. Therapeutic effectiveness of diagnostic lymphangiography for refractory postoperative chylothorax and chylous ascites: correlation with radiologic findings and preceding medical treatment. AJR Am J Roentgenol 2013;201:659–66.

32. Itkin M, Kucharczuk JC, Kwak A, et al. Non operative thoracic duct embolization for traumatic thoracic duct leak: experience in 109 patients. J Thorac Cardiovasc Surg 2010;139:584–9.

33. Patterson GA, Todd TR, Delarue NC, et al. Supradiaphragmatic ligation of the thoracic duct in intractable chylous fistula. Ann Thorac Surg 1981;32:44–9.

34. Platis IE, Nwogu CE. Chylothorax. Thorac Surg Clin 2006;16:209–14.

35. Selle JG, Snyder WH 3rd, Schreiber JT. Chylothorax: indications for surgery. Ann Surg 1973;177:245–9.

36. Lampson RS. Traumatic chylothorax; a review of the literature and report of a case treated by mediastinal ligation of the thoracic duct. J Thorac Surg 1948;17:778–91.

37. Shackcloth MJ, Poullis M, Lu J, et al. Preventing of chylothorax after oesophagectomy by routine preoperative administration of oral cream. Eur J Cardiothorac Surg 2001;20:1035–6.

38. Inderbitzi RG, Krebs T, Stirneman T, et al. Treatment of postoperative chylothorax by fibrin glue application under thoracoscopic view with use of local anesthesia. J Thorac Cardiovasc Surg 1992;104:209–10.

39. Rocco G. Chylothorax. In: Sabiston DC, Spencer EC, editors. Surgery of the chest. 8th edition. Philadelphia: WB Saunders; 2010. p. 427–30.

40. Thompson KJ, Kernstine KH, Grannis FW Jr, et al. Treatment of chylothorax by robotic thoracic duct ligation. Ann Thorac Surg 2008;85:334–6.

41. Kent RB 3rd, Pinson TW. Thoracoscopic ligation of the thoracic duct. Surg Endosc 1993;7:52–3.

42. Mason PF, Ragoowansi RH, Thorpe JA. Post-thoracotomy chylothorax - a cure in the abdomen? Eur J Cardiothorac Surg 1997;11:567–70.

43. Shah RD, Luketich JD, Schuchert MJ, et al. Postesophagectomy chylothorax: incidence, risk factors, and outcomes. Ann Thorac Surg 2012;93:897–903.

44. Kranzfelder M, Gertler R, Hapfelmeier A, et al. Chylothorax after esophagectomy for cancer: impact of the surgical approach and neoadjuvant treatment: systematic review and institutional analysis. Surg Endosc 2013;27:3530–8.

45. Hou X, Fu JH, Wang X, et al. Prophylactic thoracic duct ligation has unfavorable impact on overall survival in patients with resectable esophageal cancer. Eur J Surg Oncol 2014;40:1756–62.

46. Lai FC, Chen L, Tu YR, et al. Prevention of chylothorax complicating extensive esophageal resection by mass ligation of thoracic duct: a random control study. Ann Thorac Surg 2011;91:1770–4.

47. Choh CT, Khan OA, Rychlik IJ, et al. Does ligation of the thoracic duct during oesophagectomy reduce the incidence of post-operative chylothorax? Int J Surg 2012;10:203–5.

48. Azizkhan RG, Canfield J, Alford BA, et al. Pleuroperitoneal shunts in the management of neonatal chylothorax. J Pediatr Surg 1983;18:842–50.

49. Milsom JW, Kron IL, Rheuban KS, et al. Chylothorax: an assessment of current surgical management. J Thorac Cardiovasc Surg 1985;89:221–7.

50. Gupta D, Ross K, Piacentino V 3rd, et al. Use of LeVeen pleuroperitoneal shunt for refractory high-volume chylothorax. Ann Thorac Surg 2004;78: e9–12.

51. Dietl B, Pfister K, Aufschläger C, et al. Radiotherapy of inguinal lymphorrhea after vascular surgery. A retrospective analysis. Strahlenther Onkol 2005; 181:396–400 [in German].

52. Gerstein J, Kofahl-Krause D, Frühauf J, et al. Complete remission of a lymphoma-associated chylothorax by radiotherapy of the celiac trunk and thoracic duct. Strahlenther Onkologie 2008;184: 484–7.

53. Sziklavari Z, Allgäuer M, Hübner G, et al. Radiotherapy in the treatment of postoperative chylothorax. J Cardiothorac Surg 2013;8:72.

# Index

Note: Page numbers of article titles are in **boldface** type.

## A

AATS. See *American Association of Thoracic Surgeons.*

ACA/AHA. See *American College of Cardiology/American Heart Association.*

ACCP. See *American College of Chest Physicians.*

Acetaminophen
   for pain management, 397, 398

Achalasia surgery
   anesthesia for, 494
   complications of, 494–496
   and complications of myotomy, 494–496
   and fundoplication, 494, 495
   and peroral endoscopic myotomy, 495, 496
   preoperative examination for, 484
   and retractor injuries, 494
   and trocar injuries, 494

Acute respiratory distress syndrome
   and respiratory failure, 430–432

Aerodigestive fistulas
   and esophagogastric anastomotic leaks, 456, 457

Air leaks
   after pulmonary resection, 411–417
   and autologous blood patch, 416, 417
   and chest tube management, 414, 415
   and chest tube removal, 416
   and endobronchial valves, 417
   and Heimlich valve, 416
   intraoperative prevention of, 412–414
   invasive management of, 417
   and lung mobilization, 312
   noninvasive management of, 416, 417
   and pleural drainage systems, 415, 416
   and pleural tent, 412, 413
   and pleurodesis, 416, 417
   and pneumoperitoneum, 413
   postoperative management of, 414–416
   and staple-line buttressing, 413
   surgical intervention for, 417
   and surgical sealants, 413
   and tissue transposition, 413

Airway anastomosis
   and carinal resection and sleeve resection, 436–440, 443, 444

Airway dissection
   and carinal resection and sleeve resection, 437

American Association of Thoracic Surgeons
   guidelines for atrial fibrillation, 382, 383, 385, 387

American College of Cardiology/American Heart Association
   guidelines for myocardial infarction, 372, 374, 376

American College of Chest Physicians
   guidelines for myocardial infarction, 374
   guidelines for venous thromboembolic events, 377, 379

Amiodarone prophylaxis
   for atrial fibrillation, 383

Analgesia
   systemic vs. regional, 395

Anastomotic leakage following esophagectomy, **449–459**

Anastomotic stenosis
   and carinal resection and sleeve resection, 444

Anastomotic stricture
   and carinal resection and sleeve resection, 444
   and delayed gastric emptying, 476–478

Anesthesia
   for achalasia surgery, 494

Anticoagulation
   for atrial fibrillation, 385–387

Antiplatelet medications
   for coronary stents, 374–376

Antiplatelet therapy
   characteristics of, 375
   holding, 375
   and myocardial infarction, 374–376
   and performing surgery, 376

Antireflux surgery
   and aspiration during intubation, 486
   bleeding during, 488
   and capnothorax, 487
   and complications after retractor placement, 486, 487
   complications of, 486–494
   and deep vein thrombosis, 489, 490
   and dysphagia, 488–490
   early postoperative complications of, 488–490
   and esophageal perforation, 487
   and fundoplication, 487–494
   and gas bloat, 490
   and gastroesophageal reflux disease, 486–494
   and hiatal hernia recurrence, 489–491
   and ileus, 489
   and intra-abdominal catastrophe, 487
   intraoperative complications of, 486–488
   laster postoperative complications of, 490–494
   and mesh or pledget erosion, 491

Thorac Surg Clin 25 (2015) 529–535
http://dx.doi.org/10.1016/S1547-4127(15)00089-4
1547-4127/15/$ – see front matter © 2015 Elsevier Inc. All rights reserved.

# United States Postal Service

## Statement of Ownership, Management, and Circulation
### (All Periodicals Publications Except Requestor Publications)

**1. Publication Title**
Thoracic Surgery Clinics

**2. Publication Number**
0 1 3 - 1 2 6

**3. Filing Date**
9/18/15

**4. Issue Frequency**
Feb, May, Aug, Nov

**5. Number of Issues Published Annually**
4

**6. Annual Subscription Price**
$350.00

**7. Complete Mailing Address of Known Office of Publication** (Not printer) (Street, city, county, state, and ZIP+4®)

Elsevier Inc.
360 Park Avenue South
New York, NY 10010-1710

Contact Person
Stephen R. Bushing

Telephone (Include area code)
215-239-3688

**8. Complete Mailing Address of Headquarters or General Business Office of Publisher** (Not printer)

Elsevier Inc., 360 Park Avenue South, New York, NY 10010-1710

**9. Full Names and Complete Mailing Addresses of Publisher, Editor, and Managing Editor** (Do not leave blank)

**Publisher** (Name and complete mailing address)

Linda Belfus, Elsevier Inc., 1600 John F. Kennedy Blvd., Suite 1800, Philadelphia, PA 19103

**Editor** (Name and complete mailing address)

John Vassallo, Elsevier Inc., 1600 John F. Kennedy Blvd., Suite 1800, Philadelphia, PA 19103-2899

**Managing Editor** (Name and complete mailing address)

Adrianne Brigido, Elsevier Inc., 1600 John F. Kennedy Blvd., Suite 1800, Philadelphia, PA 19103-2899

**10. Owner** (Do not leave blank. If the publication is owned by a corporation, give the name and address of the corporation immediately followed by the names and addresses of all stockholders owning or holding 1 percent or more of the total amount of stock. If not owned by a corporation, give the names and addresses of the individual owners. If owned by a partnership or other unincorporated firm, give its name and address as well as those of each individual owner. If the publication is published by a nonprofit organization, give its name and address.)

| Full Name | Complete Mailing Address |
|---|---|
| Wholly owned subsidiary of | 1600 John F. Kennedy Blvd. Ste. 1800 |
| Reed/Elsevier, US holdings | Philadelphia, PA 19103-2899 |

**11. Known Bondholders, Mortgagees, and Other Security Holders Owning or Holding 1 Percent or More of Total Amount of Bonds, Mortgages, or Other Securities.** If none, check box ☐ None

| Full Name | Complete Mailing Address |
|---|---|
| N/A | |

**12. Tax Status** (For completion by nonprofit organizations authorized to mail at nonprofit rates) (Check one)
The purpose, function, and nonprofit status of this organization and the exempt status for federal income tax purposes:
☐ Has Not Changed During Preceding 12 Months
☐ Has Changed During Preceding 12 Months (Publisher must submit explanation of change with this statement)

**13. Publication Title**
Thoracic Surgery Clinics

**14. Issue Date for Circulation Data Below**
August 2015

| 15. Extent and Nature of Circulation | | | Average No. Copies Each Issue During Preceding 12 Months | No. Copies of Single Issue Published Nearest to Filing Date |
|---|---|---|---|---|
| **a. Total Number of Copies** (Net press run) | | | 644 | 504 |
| **b. Legitimate Paid and Or Requested Distribution (By Mail and Outside the Mail)** | (1) | Mailed Outside County Paid/Requested Mail Subscriptions stated on PS Form 3541. (Include paid distribution above nominal rate, advertiser's proof copies and exchange copies) | 281 | 199 |
| | (2) | Mailed In-County Paid/Requested Mail Subscriptions stated on PS Form 3541. (Include paid distribution above nominal rate, advertiser's proof copies and exchange copies) | | |
| | (3) | Paid Distribution Outside the Mails Including Sales Through Dealers And Carriers, Street Vendors, Counter Sales, and Other Paid Distribution Outside USPS® | 143 | 154 |
| | (4) | Paid Distribution by Other Classes of Mail Through the USPS (e.g. First-Class Mail®) | | |
| **c. Total Paid and or Requested Circulation** (Sum of 15b (1), (2), (3), and (4)) | | | 424 | 353 |
| **d. Free or Nominal Rate Distribution (By Mail and Outside the Mail)** | (1) | Free or Nominal Rate Outside-County Copies included on PS Form 3541 | 59 | 57 |
| | (2) | Free or Nominal Rate In-County Copies included on PS Form 3541 | | |
| | (3) | Free or Nominal Rate Copies mailed at Other classes Through the USPS (e.g. First-Class Mail®) | | |
| | (4) | Free or Nominal Rate Distribution Outside the Mail (Carriers or Other means) | | |
| **e. Total Nonrequested Distribution** (Sum of 15d (1), (2), (3) and (4)) | | | 59 | 57 |
| **f. Total Distribution** (Sum of 15c and 15e) | | | 483 | 410 |
| **g. Copies not Distributed** (See instructions to publishers #4 (page #3)) | | | 161 | 94 |
| **h. Total** (Sum of 15f and g) | | | 644 | 504 |
| **i. Percent Paid and/or Requested Circulation** (15c divided by 15f times 100) | | | 87.78% | 86.10% |

* If you are claiming electronic copies go to line 16 on page 3. If you are not claiming Electronic copies, skip to line 17 on page 3.

| 16. Electronic Copy Circulation | Average No. Copies Each Issue During Preceding 12 Months | No. Copies of Single Issue Published Nearest to Filing Date |
|---|---|---|
| a. Paid Electronic Copies | | |
| b. Total paid Print Copies (Line 15c) + Paid Electronic copies (Line 16a) | | |
| c. Total Print Distribution (Line 15f) + Paid Electronic Copies (Line 16a) | | |
| d. Percent Paid (Both Print & Electronic copies) (16b divided by 16c X 100) | | |

☐ I certify that 50% of all my distributed copies (electronic and print) are paid above a nominal price

**17. Publication of Statement of Ownership**
If the publication is a general publication, publication of this statement is required. Will be printed in the **November 2015** issue of this publication.

**18. Signature and Title of Editor, Publisher, Business Manager, or Owner**

*Stephen R. Bushing*
Stephen R. Bushing – Inventory Distribution Coordinator

**Date**
September 18, 2015

I certify that all information furnished on this form is true and complete. I understand that anyone who furnishes false or misleading information on this form or who omits material or information requested on the form may be subject to criminal sanctions (including fines and imprisonment) and/or civil sanctions (including civil penalties).

PS Form 3526, July 2014 (Page 3 of 3)

PS Form 3526, July 2014 (Page 1 of 3 (Instructions Page 3)) PSN 7530-01-000-9931 **PRIVACY NOTICE:** See our Privacy policy in www.usps.com

# Moving?

## Make sure your subscription moves with you!

To notify us of your new address, find your **Clinics Account Number** (located on your mailing label above your name), and contact customer service at:

**Email: journalscustomerservice-usa@elsevier.com**

**800-654-2452** (subscribers in the U.S. & Canada)
**314-447-8871** (subscribers outside of the U.S. & Canada)

**Fax number: 314-447-8029**

**Elsevier Health Sciences Division**
**Subscription Customer Service**
**3251 Riverport Lane**
**Maryland Heights, MO 63043**

*To ensure uninterrupted delivery of your subscription, please notify us at least 4 weeks in advance of move.

Printed and bound by CPI Group (UK) Ltd, Croydon, CR0 4YY

03/10/2024

01040379-0018